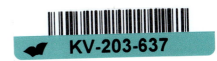

Relief of
Intractable Pain

Monographs in Anaesthesiology

VOLUME 18

Editors-in-Chief
A.R. HUNTER
and
T.E.J. HEALY

Elsevier · Amsterdam · New York · Oxford

Relief of
Intractable Pain

Edited by
MARK SWERDLOW
and
J. EDMOND CHARLTON

Fourth edition
Completely revised

1989
Elsevier · Amsterdam · New York · Oxford

1st edition © *1974, Excerpta Medica*
2nd, revised edition © *1978, Elsevier/North-Holland Biomedical Press*
3rd, revised edition © *1983, Elsevier Science Publishers B.V.*
4th, revised edition © *1989, Elsevier Science Publishers B.V. (Biomedical Division)*

The 1st and 2nd editions were originally published as Volume 1 in the series, the 3rd edition as Volume 13.

ISBN 0-444-81094-3 (volume)
ISBN 0-444-80023-9 (series)

This book is printed on acid-free paper.

Published by:

Elsevier Science Publishers B.V.
(Biomedical Division)
P.O. Box 211
1000 AE Amsterdam
The Netherlands

Sole distributors for the USA and Canada:

Elsevier Science Publishing Company, Inc.
655 Avenue of the Americas
New York, NY 10010
USA

Library of Congress Cataloging-in-Publication Data

Relief of intractable pain / edited by Mark Swerdlow and J. E. Charlton. − − 4th ed., completely rev.
    p. cm. − − (Monographs in anaesthesiology ; v. 18)
  Includes bibliographies and index.
  ISBN 0-444-81094-3 (alk. paper)
  1. Intractable pain − − Treatment. 2. Analgesia. I. Swerdlow, Mark. II. Charlton, J. E. (J. Edmond) III. Series.
RB127.R44 1989
616'.0472 − − dc20   89-7862
                                                              CIP

Printed in The Netherlands

To our wives Elizabeth and Laura

"But Pain
is perfect miserie
the
Worst of Evils..."

John Milton (1608–1674), Paradise Lost, Bk. VI

Contents

List of contributors   ix

Foreword   xi

Preface to the first edition   xiii

Preface to the fourth edition   xv

1. *Pain pathways and mechanisms*
   D. Bowsher   1

2. *The psychological treatment of pain*
   H. Merskey   23

3. *The structure and functions of a pain relief clinic*
   S.H. Butler and T.M. Murphy   67

4. *Assessment of the patient with chronic pain*
   S. Lipton   79

5. *Drug treatment of chronic pain*
   J.E. Charlton   93

6. *Non-invasive and other simple physical methods*
   G.M. Wyant   169

viii

7. *Peripheral nerve blocks in relief of intractable pain*
    M. Churcher   195

8. *Intrathecal and extradural block in pain relief*
    M. Swerdlow   223

9. *The sympathetic nervous system and pain relief*
    R.A. Boas   259

10. *Electrical stimulation for pain relief: transcutaneous, peripheral nerve,
    spinal cord and deep brain stimulation*
    R.B. North   281

11. *The place of neurosurgery in the treatment of intractable pain*
    B.S. Nashold, Jr., E. Bullitt and A. Friedman   305

12. *Radiotherapy, chemotherapy and hormone therapy in the relief of cancer
    pain*
    T. Bates   329

Appendix I   349

Appendix II   353

Subject index   355

List of contributors

Thelma D. Bates, M.B., Ch.B., F.R.C.R., M.C.R.A.
Consultant Radiotherapist and Oncologist, St Thomas's Hospial, Lambeth Palace Rd, London SE1 7EH, UK

Robert A. Boas, M.B., Ch.B., F.F.A.R.A.C.S.
Associate Professor of Anaesthetics, University of Auckland, School of Medicine, Auckland, New Zealand

David Bowsher, M.A., M.D., Ph.D., M.R.C.P.Ed., M.R.C.Path.
Reader, Department of Neurological Sciences, University of Liverpool; Director of Research and Postgraduate Studies, Pain Relief Foundation; Hon. Consultant in Pain Relief, Centre for Pain Relief, Walton Hospital, Liverpool L9 1AE, UK

Elizabeth Bullitt, M.D.
Division of Neurosurgery, UNC School of Medicine, Chapel Hill, NC, USA

Stephen H. Butler, M.D.
Department of Anesthesiology, Pain Center, University of Washington School of Medicine, Seattle, WA 98195, USA

J.Edmond Charlton, M.B.B.S., F.F.A.R.C.S.
Department of Anaesthesia, Pain Relief Clinic, Royal Victoria Infirmary, New-castle-on-Tyne, NE1 4LP, UK

Mark D. Churcher, M.B., B.S., F.F.A.R.C.S.
Consultant Anaesthetist, Pain Relief Unit, Derriford Hospital, Derriford Road, Plymouth, PL6 8DH, UK

Allan Friedman, M.D.
Division of Neurosurgery, Duke Medical Center, Durham, NC 27710, USA

Samson Lipton, M.B., Ch.B., F.F.A.R.C.S., D.A., O.B.E.
Medical Director, The Pain Relief Foundation, Walton Hospital, Liverpool L9 1AE, UK

Harold Merskey, M.A., D.M., F.R.C.P., F.R.C.P.(C), F.R.C. Psych.
Director of Research, London Psychiatric Hospital, London, Ontario, NGA 4H1, Canada

Terence M. Murphy, M.B., Ch.B., F.F.A.R.C.S.
Professor of Anesthesiology, Associate Director of Pain Center and Chief of Clinical Pain Service, University of Washington, Seattle, WA 98195, USA

Blaine S. Nashold, Jr., M.D.
Division of Neurosurgery, Duke Medical Center, Durham, NC 27710, USA

Richard B. North, M.D.
Department of Neurosurgery, Johns Hopkins University School of Medicine, Baltimore, MD, USA

Mark Swerdlow, M.Sc., M.D., F.F.A.R.C.S., D.A.
Former Director, Regional Pain Relief Centre, Hope Hospital, University of Manchester School of Medicine, Hon. Lecturer in Anaesthesia, University of Manchester, UK

Gordon M. Wyant, C.M., M.D., F.F.A.R.C.S., F.R.C.P.(C)
Former Director, Pain Management Service, University Hospital, University of Saskatoon, Saskatoon, Canada

Foreword

It gives me great pleasure to exchange my role as a 'part player' in the previous three editions of this monograph to that of a 'critic' in the present one. When Mark Swerdlow published the first edition of this monograph in 1974, there were only two or three books devoted to a comprehensive approach to the management of chronic pain. The fact that a fourth edition will now be published indicates that the third edition must be out of print, that the publishers think that there is a great demand for this monograph and that enough new information has accumulated since 1983 to warrant a new edition rather than a reprint. By inviting Dr. Ed Charlton to join him as co-editor, Dr. Swerdlow has ensured that future editions of this now classic volume will maintain the same high standard.

This edition shows a greater change in its contents and concepts than is apparent when earlier successive editions are compared. The present volume not only describes the current practice of the management of chronic pain, but it also attempts to evaluate critically the results obtained by the various modalities of treatment. There is a good balance between the basic science background and the clinical skills required for the optimal treatment of chronic pain. The illustrious contributors, selected from both sides of the Atlantic, all have a solid academic background in the scientific and clinical aspects of the investigation of the patient and the selection of the appropriate treatment modalities for chronic pain problems.

I am convinced that this new edition, like its predecessors, will continue to expand the horizon of those clinicians who are devoted to the concept that patients need and deserve the most up-to-date care available for the amelioration of their pain problem.

Before concluding this foreword, I would like to make a short sentimental journey into the past and take a brief look into the future. I have been interested in

the management of chronic pain since the late forties, long before the multidisciplinary approach to its management was developed by my good friend John Bonica. When Mark Swerdlow joined me at Mercy Hospital in Pittsburgh, Pennsyl-
vania, 30 years ago, we administered many hundreds of diagnostic and
therapeutic nerve blocks each year. We were also involved in clinical pharmacological studies with narcotics and narcotic antagonists. I would like to take a small
measure of credit for having aroused Dr. Swerdlow's interest in the treatment of
pain. I am also proud that I pointed out, early in our association, that 'sticking
long needles into patients' is not the whole answer to the treatment of chronic
pain. It is to his great credit that he saw far beyond my limited horizons and over
the years developed the comprehensive approach to chronic pain management so
practically and eloquently presented in this monograph.

What about the future of the relief of chronic pain? 'Navita de ventis de tauris
narrat arator'. For the benefit of those who did not 'enjoy' the privilege of 5
hours of Latin each week for eight years, may I translate: 'Sailors like to talk
about the winds, farmers about their oxen'. Being an amateur pharmacologist, I
feel that the greatest advances in the management of chronic pain will come from
the synthesis of drugs (of various kinds) with selective analgesic effect and little
or no side-effect liability. Combinations of such compounds (which will result
from advances in our knowledge of neuropharmacology and biochemistry), together with a caring approach to the psychological factors and demands on the
patient's mental and physical performance imposed by chronic pain will, one day,
greatly improve their wellbeing. I am sure that this much improved monograph
will receive the same enthusiastic reception as its predecessors.

FRANCIS F. FOLDES, M.D.

Preface to the first edition

Ideally, severe pain would be relieved by the removal or treatment of the cause and would never be allowed to become intractable. In reality, there are many conditions which are not at present amenable to such management and intractable pain is an all too common challenge in medical practice. Happily, there have been advances in the methods of treatment of the causative diseases, especially cancer, and progress has also been made in the development of pain-killing procedures and in the formulation of analgesic drugs. Recent advances in neurophysiology are producing a less purely anatomical approach to the interruption of the sensory pathway for relief of pain. Furthermore, the existence of an increasing number of Pain Clinics shows that there is a growing awareness of the problem of intractable pain and a willingness to try to tackle it.

The object of treatment is to provide the maximum relief of pain with the minimum of complications and disadvantages. The form of treatment which will offer the best prospects will differ from case to case and will depend, among other things, upon the aetiological condition, the age and fitness of the patient and his life expectancy. The management of patients with pain calls for a multidisciplinary approach, not only in arriving at a decision as to the cause and prognosis, but also in deciding on what is likely to be the most effective line of treatment and in carrying it out. However, there is nothing more harmful to the psychological welfare of the patient than diverging or conflicting statements by several physicians with different philosophical approaches to this problem.

This book is intended to give a concise but comprehensive picture of the methods and agents which are now of use in the relief of intractable pain. It should be of value not only to those who work in Pain Clinics, but also to family doctors and specialists of many kinds who have to deal with patients suffering chronic pain. It is hoped that the reader will gain a more profound knowledge of the part which his speciality can play, and also an increased awareness of the range of usefulness of the other disciplines in this field. The relief of pain is, however, only one contribution to the improvement of the patient's comfort and quality of life, just as the pain itself is only one of his many problems. The latter fact often becomes apparent after the pain has been removed, when many other therapeutic and rehabilitative services will still be required.

No attempt is made to give a detailed description of all the nerve blocks; these have been very adequately described and illustrated in the several text books expressly written on this subject and the reader is referred to these:

Bonica, J.J. (1953) *The Management of Pain*. Lea and Febiger, Philadelphia.
Erikssen, E. (1969) *Illustrated Handbook in Local Anaesthesia*. Lloyd-Luke, London.
Moore, D.C. (1965) *Regional Block, 4th Edition*. C.C. Thomas, Springfield.

M. SWERDLOW

Preface to the fourth edition

In this fourth edition of 'Relief of Intractable Pain', I welcome Dr. Edmond Charlton as co-editor.

The five years since the 3rd edition was published have seen many changes which merit a new edition of the book. We both felt that in this new version a serious attempt should be made to define as far as possible the quality of results which can be expected from the application of each of the treatment methods advocated. This taking stock of the present state of the art would give the reader a chance to judge which of the relevant therapies is most likely to be efficacious in each of the various pain syndromes.

Editing a new edition after a period of time inevitably involves a realisation and consideration of the changes which have taken place since the previous edition first appeared. Once again, it must be admitted that the greatest advances are apparent in the neurophysiological aspects of the subject. However, smaller but significant changes can be seen in most of the chapters. In the clinical field, not only have a number of new methods and agents been adopted, but consideration is now being given to the functions and value of the Pain Relief Clinic itself. The growth in the number of such clinics has continued apace worldwide, but now their cost-effectiveness has been called into question and some attempts are being made to measure their clinical and socio-economic value (as will be seen in Chapter 3). There is also some evidence that a start is being made to conduct controlled trials to assess the value of individual therapies more objectively. It is to be hoped that this element of self-inspection will be intensified, because this must result in advantage for the patient with chronic pain. Too often in the past there has been an unthinking acceptance of anecdotal studies that has led to the continued use of inappropriate or ineffective therapy.

As far as this volume is concerned, two chapters must be singled out as showing major change. The first is the introduction of a chapter on the assessment of the patient with chronic pain. In view of the fact that assessment and diagnosis of the cause of the pain are vital first steps in the management of the pain patient, the introduction of this chapter is timely and perhaps even overdue. The second major change is that the chapter on 'oncological methods' has been completely rewritten so that the account of this type of therapy is now related primarily to relief of pain rather than to the treatment of cancer. The latter has in the past been the approach of almost all articles on the place of oncology in pain relief. We feel sure that the present Chapter 12 will meet with the approval of all oncologists and pain workers.

The chapter on pharmacology represents an attempt to review the many and varied drugs and methods of delivery that are now available for the management of pain. The length of the chapter reflects the increasing importance of its contents. The subject of spinal opioids is now dealt with at some length and there is also an extended account of the membrane stabilizing drugs. The 'surgical' procedures of percutaneous cordotomy and pituitary injection of alcohol are no longer recent introductions requiring detailed description and these subjects have now been incorporated into the chapter on neurosurgery.

We are grateful to the chapter authors who have once again updated the material in their contributions and we welcome the new contributors, Drs Bates, Bullitt, Butler, Friedman, Nashold and North.

MARK SWERDLOW
J. EDMOND CHARLTON

M. Swerdlow and J.E. Charlton (eds.) *Relief of Intractable Pain*
© 1989, Elsevier Science Publishers B.V. (Biomedical Division)

1

Pain pathways and mechanisms

David Bowsher

INTRODUCTION

The physician working in a pain relief clinic commonly encounters two distinct varieties of pain. The commoner of the two is due to tissue damage caused by trauma or disease, and so may be called *noci*genic pain. Specific receptors (nociceptors) and their associated nerve fibres within the damaged region are stimulated, and if impulses generated in them eventually reach consciousness, pain is experienced. The second type of pain, more commonly encountered in the pain relief clinic than in the community, is due to a lesion in the peripheral or central nervous system, in the absence of nociceptor stimulation; such pain is known as *neurogenic*. It includes those pains which some authors call 'deafferation' and/or 'neuropathic' pains.

This chapter is devoted to the discussion of pain mechanisms, and in particular to an attempt to reconcile experimental findings in animals with clinical experience. It should however be pointed out at the very outset that there are two serious obstacles to this comparison:

. (1) Most experimental work has been performed on acute pain, often induced by high intensity electrical stimulation whose duration is measured in milliseconds, and which maximally activates every type of nerve fibre, without regard for receptor specificity. Such pain, even when more naturally caused by, for example, sharp objects, causes flexion withdrawal, which may indeed be used as the criterion to confirm that the stimulus is potentially 'painful'. Human subjects, on the other hand, do not complain to their doctors of pinpricks or hot water – they just withdraw from the offending stimulus! Chronic pain, causing immobilisation of part or all of the organism, is the form of nocigenic pain complained of by patients.

(2) Nearly (but not quite) all animal experiments have involved the noxious stimulation of skin, or of nerves leading from it; most chronic pain in man arises in structures deep to skin, whose innervation is, as we shall see, somewhat different.

Prior to the section specifically devoted to neurogenic pain, the following applies to the better-understood nocigenic pain.

PAIN THRESHOLDS AND PAIN MEASUREMENT

Pain perception threshold is defined as the lowest intensity of stimulation which causes a subject consciously to experience a sensation which is described as painful. Expressed in terms of heat applied to the skin, pain perception usually occurs at a temperature of 44–45°C, independent of the rate of temperature increase (Hardy et al., 1952). This threshold is remarkably constant, especially within the same individual, just as are other physiological thresholds, e.g., for mechanical force (= touch), light (= visual perception), sound (= hearing), etc.

The pain tolerance level (or threshold) is defined as the highest intensity of noxious stimulation which a subject is prepared to tolerate. Not only does this vary greatly from subject to subject, but can vary greatly within a single individual according to circumstances – we are all prepared to put up with much more pain when rescuing a child from a burning house than when it is gratuitously inflicted by altruistic seekers after physiological truth! The important point for the clinician to bear in mind is that patients do not come for medical advice until their pain is *beyond* tolerance threshold – in other words, when it has become *in*tolerable. It is because of the variability in tolerance that the tendency exists to say (wrongly) that subject A has a high pain threshold while subject B has a low one. As explained above, their threshold (which may be identical) isn't ever measured by the physician; it's their *tolerance* which differs. The next section will attempt to define the physiological correlates of perception threshold and tolerance threshold.

Many methods have been devised to measure pain. Most of them apply to experimentally inflicted pain, and are of little clinical value. Three may be retained in the medical context:

(1) The submaximum effort tourniquet test (Smith et al., 1966). This cumbersome and time-consuming test is very accurate and useful. A sphygmomanometer cuff is inflated to above systolic pressure on the elevated arm. A dynamometer is squeezed in rhythm with a metronome (to ensure constancy of force and rate); the time can then be measured to (*i*) pain perception, (*ii*) pain tolerance threshold and (*iii*) pain equal to that being experienced pathologically. Interestingly, most patients are able to analogise ischaemic cramp with whatever kind of pain they are experiencing as a result of injury or disease, so three objective measurements can be obtained from this test.

(2) The McGill Pain Questionnaire (Melzack 1975) can be diagnostic, by virtue of the categories of words chosen, while its intensity parameter, used at successive interviews, can measure the changing severity of the pain. It has the advantage that the patient can fill it in while waiting to be seen.

(3) The visual analogue scale (Bond and Pilowsky, 1966), consisting of a 10 cm line with 'no pain' written at one end and 'the worst pain ever felt' at the other, can be marked in a trice; and while it is of no value in comparing one patient with another, it is of enormous help in assessing the change in any given patient.

NOCICEPTORS

The technique of microneurography has made it possible to confirm that man has the same two types of pain receptor (nociceptor) as other mammals. The method makes it possible to record from, and more recently to stimulate, single nerve fibers in a fascicle penetrated across the skin by a needle electrode.

A category of small myelinated ($A\delta$) fibres are activated by high intensity mechanical (=pinprick) and sometimes also by noxious heat (> 44°C) stimuli. In the human median nerve (Torebjörk, 1985), stimulation of such fibres causes referral of pricking pain to a number of distinct points within a receptive field of about 2.5 cm^2.

$A\delta$ nociceptors are found in particular in the skin, including its infoldings at the two ends of the alimentary canal. They also occur in joints, where in anaesthetised animals they respond to degrees of hyperflexion or -extension which would be painful in conscious humans.

The great majority of unmyelinated (C) primary afferent fibres in man and other primates are constituted by *polymodal* nociceptors. These are so called because they respond to damaging stimuli whether mechanical, thermal or chemical. They are not truly polymodal, but rather, in keeping with the strict rule of receptor specificity, are activated by (a chain of?) chemical events resulting from tissue damage. They are therefore probably chemoreceptors, and in keeping with their evolutionary primitiveness, they are best considered as tissue-damage receptors. They are distributed throughout all tissues, with the notable exception of the central nervous system. They are, however, present in peripheral nerves as nervi nervorum, which may be responsible for the dull ache which can be accurately traced along the course of, e.g., the sciatic nerve in some cases of sciatica. In the human median nerve, stimulation of single C polymodal nociceptor fibres produces severe aching or throbbing pain, referred to a receptive field about ten times as big as that of $A\delta$ nociceptors. Co-activation of C polymodal nociceptors and heat receptors (also associated with a category of C fibre) may produce burning pain.

Many primary afferent C tissue-damage receptor fibres contain an 11-chain peptide known as Substance P (SP). When released at the central terminal of the primary afferent fibre in the spinal cord or brainstem, SP may act as a transmitter. However, it is also released at the peripheral end of active C fibres, where it appears to be involved in the inflammatory response. Unmyelinated nociceptors also contain calcitonin gene-related peptide (CGRP), and those coming from viscera in addition contain vasoactive intestinal peptide (VIP). The transmitter in $A\delta$ fibres remains unknown.

Pain responses

The two receptor types described above have been shown to underlie the phenomenon of double pain (fast and slow), first described by Goldscheider (1881), and which can be perceived by 80% of normal subjects (Sinclair, 1981). Given that they both signal the sensation commonly called pain, it may be useful here to compare and contrast them, and the fate of the information they carry (Bowsher, 1983).

Two points may be noted at this juncture:

(*i*) The very different segmental reflex responses must mean that separate and independent circuits are involved when either of the two fibre types is independently activated.

(*ii*) The very different responses to a therapeutic dose of morphine (e.g., 15 mg) suggests that impulses generated by the two types of nociceptor follow different pathways to consciousness within the CNS – one of which is morphine-sensitive and the other which is not.

TABLE 1.1

Comparison of responses to $A\delta$ and C stimulation

	First (fast) pain	Second (slow) pain
Adequate stimulus	Pinprick, phasic heat	Tissue damage
Fibre type	$A\delta$	C
Conduction velocity	5–15 m/s (11–34 mph)	0.75–1.5 m/s (1.5–3 mph)
Distribution	Tegument	All tissues except CNS
Sensation	Pricking, stinging	Aching, throbbing
Segmental reflex	Phasic Withdrawal	Tonic muscle contraction (Spasm, guarding, rigidity)
Biological value	Avoidance of damage	Promotion of natural healing; limitation of infection spread
Effect of morphine	Virtually none	Abolition of pain *and* muscle contraction

REFERRED PAIN

Reference of pain is usually from viscera to the body surface. It depends upon the fact that the segmental innervation of a viscus may be the same as a remote region of body surface. Most examples are well-known: uterus to low back, gall-bladder to shoulder blade, heart to upper limb. Other more recondite examples occur, for which the explanation can readily be found in any large textbook of topographical anatomy. Neurophysiologically, there are two mechanisms:

(1) Primary afferents from a viscus and from an area of body surface converge on the same central (dorsal horn) neurone.

(2) Two branches of the same primary afferent neurone supply (i.e., come from) both a viscus and an area of tegument.

These 'facts' do not however explain why pain is referred from a viscus to the body surface and not vice versa. It is usually assumed that an external body part of which the subject is aware, and which is much more frequently stimulated, is likely to pre-empt the input and thus the line to consciousness. A similar argument is used to explain the observation that phantoms of external body parts, but rarely of viscera, can occur following removal.

ENTRY INTO THE CNS (Fig. 1.1)

The 'pain' fibres with which this chapter is concerned enter the spinal cord through the spinal nerves (in the case of those coming from the neck, trunk and limbs) or the medulla oblongata of the brainstem through the trigeminal nerve. Since the arrangement within the medulla oblongata is similar to that in the spinal cord, the descending (caudal) nucleus of the medulla oblongata is frequently referred to as the 'medullary dorsal horn'. From this point on, the term 'dorsal horn' will therefore be taken to mean all the grey matter in the spinal cord or brainstem in which Aδ and C primary nociceptor afferents terminate.

Proximal to the dorsal root ganglion, at the point of entry into the spinal cord, there is a tendency for the dorsal root to separate into a medial part, containing the larger myelinated fibres, and a lateral part, containing the small myelinated (Aδ) and unmyelinated (C) fibres (Ranson, 1914; Sindou et al., 1975), thus making it possible for the surgeon to perform a functionally differential root section by the use of the operating microscope. However, the proximal axons of some 30% of C fibres, after leaving the dorsal root ganglion, double back to the junction of sensory and motor roots and enter the cord in the ventral root (Coggeshall et al., 1975) (Fig. 1.1). This phenomenon, in addition to the well-known segmental overlap in the peripheral distribution of the nerve, probably explains why dorsal rhizotomy is so rarely successful in relieving pain. Since all C fibres, however, have their cell bodies in the dorsal root ganglion, more may be achieved by dorsal root

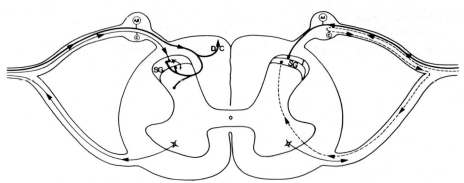

Fig. 1.1 Primary afferent terminations in the spinal cord. On the left, an unmyelinated (C) fibre enters through the lateral division of the dorsal root and ends in the substantia gelatinosa (SG). A large cutaneous myelinated fibre (Aβ) enters through the medial division of the dorsal root; its main axon passes without relay up the dorsal column (DC) while a collateral enters the medial aspect of the nucleus proprius of the dorsal horn and recurves up to the substantia gelatinosa where it ends in presynaptic relationship with the C terminal. This is the anatomical substrate of the presynaptic inhibition which is the basis of TNS and DCS.

On the right, a primary afferent C fibre has its cell body in the dorsal root ganglion (as do all primary afferents), but the central portion of its axon doubles back and enters the spinal cord through the *ventral* root. After passing up through the spinal grey matter, the axon ends in the substantia gelatinosa in exactly the same way as unmyelinated primary afferents entering through the lateral division of the dorsal root. The existence of these ventral root nociceptor afferents is one of the reasons why dorsal rhizotomy is so rarely effective in producing analgesia. The other primary afferent shown on the right-hand side of the diagram is a thin myelinated (Aδ) mechanical or thermal-mechanical nociceptor ending in the marginal zone (lamina I), which caps the substantia gelatinosa.

ganglionolysis (Nash, 1986). It may be noted that entry of a substantial portion of C primary afferents also occurs in the portio minor (motor root) of the trigeminal nerve (Young and Stevens, 1979).

When the lateral division of the posterior root penetrates the spinal cord at the tip of the dorsal horn, the small-diameter fibres which it contains mainly end in the most superficial part of the dorsal horn (Lamotte, 1977) – laminae I (marginal layer of Waldeyer) and II (substantia gelatinosa Rolandi) of Rexed; some nociceptor fibres also pass to end in circumcanalicular lamina X. Some fine myelinated (Aδ) nociceptors however penetrate more deeply to terminate in lamina V, in the neck of the dorsal horn. That third of C polymodal nociceptors which have entered through the ventral root pass up through the grey matter to end in the same way as those which have entered in the dorsal root, i.e., mainly in lamina II.

GATE CONTROL: INTRINSIC SPINAL MECHANISMS (Fig. 1.2)

Melzack and Wall put forward their theory of 'Gate Control' in 1965; it has

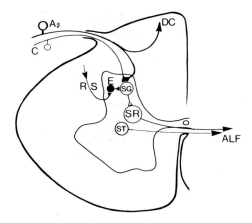

Fig. 1.2 Synaptic arrangements in the dorsal root entry zone. Unmyelinated nociceptor afferents (C) end in synaptic relationship with cells of the substantia gelatinosa (SG); these in their turn project (probably through several synapses) to spinoreticular neurons (SR) in the intermediate spinal grey matter (lamina VII). The axons of SR ascend on the opposite side of the cord, where they form the major component of the anterolateral funiculus (ALF); the minor component is formed by the crossed ascending axons of spinothalamic (ST) cells.

Collaterals of large low-threshold mechanoreceptor primary afferents (Aβ) end in presynaptic relationship to primary nociceptor afferents (C). When the Aβ peripheral fibres or their central stem axons ascending in the dorsal columns (DC) are activated, the collateral endings may presynaptically inhibit the C fibre terminals.

Also in the substantia gelatinosa are encephalinergic interneurones (E) whose short axons postsynaptically inhibit gelatinosal cells (SG). The encephalinergic interneurones can be supraspinally driven by descending raphe-spinal fibres (RS) (see Fig. 1.5), and perhaps also segmentally by impulses arriving through primary afferent Aδ (pinprick) fibres (see Fig. 1.3).

proved to be one of the most fruitful concepts of recent times, though its anatomical and physiological substrate has still not been completely worked out. The basic notion is that impulses in small ('pain') peripheral fibres push open a 'gate' to enter the nervous system and reach consciousness. Two things tend to close the gate (not necessarily completely): impulses in large ('touch') peripheral fibres and certain impulses descending from higher centres.

The most obvious example of the gate-closing action of large peripheral tactile fibres is the instinctive (and effective) action of 'rubbing a pain better'. This has been therapeutically exploited, first by high-frequency low-intensity electrical activation of large cutaneous fibres (Wall and Sweet, 1967), now known as Transcutaneous (Electrical) Nerve Stimulation (T(E)NS), and more recently by vibratory stimulation (Lundeberg, 1983), which may activate a slightly different set of Aβ fibres. It is now known that collaterals of the large primary afferent Aβ fibres, whose main axon passes up the dorsal columns, make contact in the superficial dorsal horn with GABA-ergic interneurones which presynaptically inhibit the cen-

8

tral terminals of primary afferent C polymodal nociceptors (Fig. 1.3), reducing their capacity to secrete transmitter substance and thus to pass on information. Because no opioid mechanism is involved, TNS- or vibration-induced analgesia is not naloxone-reversible (Sjölund and Eriksson, 1979).

The second mechanism (slamming the gate from the inside) comes into play when descending inhibitory fibres from the brainstem are activated, either by direct stimulation or by heterosegmental acupuncture (low-frequency high-intensity peripheral stimulation). In this case, the descending fibres activate encephalinergic interneurones in the superficial dorsal horn which postsynaptically inhibit gelatinosa cells, thus preventing them from transmitting information onwards.

OPIOID RECEPTORS AND MECHANISMS

It could have been deduced at any time in the past 75 years that the ability of morphine to block pain sensation without apparently affecting other sensations

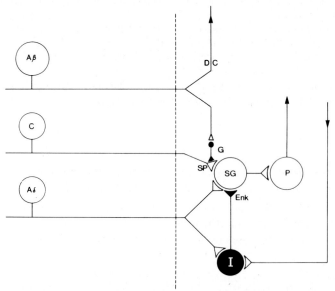

Fig. 1.3 Diagram to show gate mechanism in dorsal horn. Aβ and C primary afferents are as in Fig. 1.2. The transmitter substance in unmyelinated nociceptors is substance P (SP). Impulses from cells in the substantia gelatinosa (SG) reach projection neurones (P) whose axons ascend to supraspinal levels. Some SG cells may also be driven by primary afferent pinprick receptors (Aδ); some of these may have segmental collaterals which can excite inhibitory interneurones (I) in the substantia gelatinosa; these encephalin-releasing (Enk) terminals postsynaptically inhibit SG transmission neurones. Aβ primary afferent collatorals presynaptically inhibit C-fibre terminals (SP) through a GABA-ergic inhibitory interneurone (G). The inhibitory interneurones are also driven by descending supraspinal influences (see Fig. 1.5).

must mean that it acts only at particular synapses. Further thought would also have suggested that, as it is extremely unlikely that the mammalian nervous system specifically evolved neuronal membranes capable of binding extract of poppy. Thus, it was in 1973 that three research teams isolated the membrane sites to which morphine binds, and two years later that two groups discovered naturally occurring peptide substances which morphine imitates.

Pharmacologically, the membrane sites to which active molecules bind are known as 'receptors'. This is rather confusing since the same word is used by physiologists to describe nerve endings or other structures which transduce some form of physical or chemical energy into nervous impulses. In order to avoid such confusion as much as possible, pharmacological receptors will be referred to in this chapter by the name of 'binding sites'.

Several types of opioid binding site are now known to exist, each (virtually by definition) binding a different naturally occurring molecule, or ligand. Table 1.2 (from Kosterlitz and Paterson, 1985) shows the affinity of the various binding sites for natural ligands, morphine and the morphine antagonist naloxone.

Immunocytochemical studies have shown the greatest concentration of spinal opioid binding sites to be in the most superficial part of the dorsal horn of the spinal cord. Some μ receptors occur (non-synaptically) on the intraspinal terminals of primary afferent C fibres, as shown by the fact that there is a large reduction in the receptor population following dorsal rhizotomy (Lamotte et al., 1976). Their significance is revealed by the fact that morphine administration inhibits the release of Substance P (the probable transmitter of C polymodal nociceptors) from unmyelinated primary afferent nerve terminals. Other opioid binding sites are found on postsynaptic membranes in the substantia gelatinosa, where they are presumably the receiving areas for the axons of encephalinergic interneurones (referred to above) lying on the border of laminae I and II (Bennett et al., 1982).

TABLE 1.2

Percent binding affinity of receptors for opioids and naloxone

Substance	Receptor		
	μ	δ	κ
Morphine	97	2	1
Met-encephalin	9	91	0
Leu-encephalin	6	94	0
β-Endorphin	53	45	2
Dynorphin	5	6	89
Naloxone	85	6	9

These few data explain several phenomena of clinical importance:

(a) The fact that so many opioid binding sites are superficially situated in the spinal cord means that opiates can easily seep in from the surrounding cerebro-spinal fluid. Experimental observation (Yaksh and Rudy, 1976) of the direct spinal action of opiates led directly to their therapeutic use by intrathecal (Wang, 1977) and epidural (Bromage et al., 1980) administration.

(b) Because high-frequency low-intensity stimulation of peripheral (T(E)NS) nerves or of the dorsal column (DCS – Shealey et al., 1967) exerts its action through a GABA-ergic inhibitory interneurone, this form of pain relief is not reversed or blocked by the opiate antagonist naloxone (Abram et al., 1981; Sjölund and Eriksson, 1979).

(c) Low-frequency high-intensity (acupuncture) stimulation of peripheral nerves, on the other hand, activates $A\delta$ (pinprick) primary afferents which in their turn excite encephalinergic interneurones in the cord (Cervero et al., 1981). Thus, the (postsynaptic) inhibition of nociceptive input by segmental acupuncture is naloxone-reversible (Pomeranz and Chu, 1976; Mayer et al., 1977). This is also true of heterosegmental acupuncture, because the descending serotoninergic systems activated also impinge upon (the same?) local encephalinergic inhibitory interneurones (see below).

(d) Lastly, as we shall see later, the presence of high concentrations of opioid binding sites at higher levels in the ascending pathways responsible for conscious sensation of tissue-damage pain, and their paucity in 'pinprick' pathways, explains why systemic morphine abolishes tissue-damage pain but has little effect on pinprick sensation (Table 1.1).

ASCENDING PATHWAYS (Fig. 1.4)

It has, of course, long been known that the 'pain pathway' ascends in the antero-lateral funiculus of the spinal cord white matter contralateral to the side of entry of the noxious stimulus (Spiller, 1905). After three-quarters of a century, research is still continuing in order to establish the exact origin and termination of these fibres, though in broad outline they are sufficiently well known (Vierck et al., 1985). The destinations of ascending anterolateral fibres are:

(1) The medial brainstem reticular formation (Bowsher, 1957). This is quantitatively the major contingent of the ascending anterolateral tract (Bowsher, 1963). In the monkey, the cells of origin of these fibres are mainly in the neck of the dorsal horn (lamina V) and the deep spinal grey matter (laminae VII and VIII) (Kevetter et al., 1982) Spinoreticular impulses are mainly relayed on to:

(2) The intralaminar (medial) thalamus, where the smallest components of anterolateral fibres end (Bowsher, 1957; Mehler, 1962). Spinointralaminar or pa-

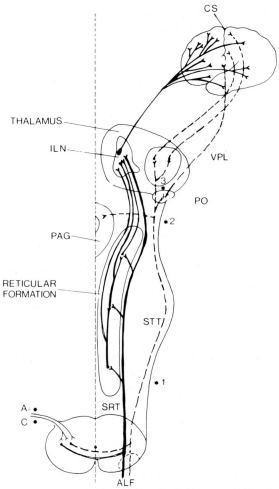

Fig. 1.4 Diagram to show pain pathways. Cells or origin of spinoreticular (SRT, solid line) and spin-othalamic (STT, interrupted line) tracts are excited by small myelinated (Aδ) and unmyelinated (C) primary afferents. Both tracts ascend in the anterolateral funiculus (ALF) of the spinal white matter. In the brain stem, STT remains in a lateral position and ends in the posterior group (PO) and ven-troposterolateral part (VPL) of the ventrobasal thalamic complex, having given off fibres or collaterals to the periaqueductal grey matter (PAG) in the midbrain. The spinoreticular fibres, on the other hand, swing medially in the brainstem, where they terminate at various levels within the reticular formation; a very few of them (the 'palaeospinothalamic fibres' of Mehler) go on to end in the intralaminar nuclei (ILN) of the thalamus. The ILN also receive the relayed output of the reticular formation. The ven-trobasal thalamus projects in a point-to-point fashion onto the postcentral gyrus and the second soma-tosensory area below the central sulcus, while the intralaminar nuclei project diffusely to the whole cortex, but with prefrontal predominance. *1 marks the level at which STT (but not SRT) may be dam-aged by occlusion of the medullary branches of the posterior inferior cerebellar artery. *2 is the level at which STT was surgically interrupted by the operation of mensencephalic tractotomy. *3 is where STT terminals are destroyed in the case of thalamic syndrome. All these lesions are capable of provok-ing 'spontaneous' central pain.

laeospinothalamic (Mehler, 1957) fibres originate, in the monkey, in mainly the same areas as spinoreticular axons, and also, to a lesser extent, in the most superficial lamina I (Willis et al., 1979). These palaeospinothalamic fibres are outnumbered by neospinothalamic axons ending in:

(3) The ventroposterior (ventrobasal) thalamic nucleus, in which somatotopically organised axons arise from cells in the marginal zone (lamina I) and neck of the dorsal horn (lamina V) (Willis et al., 1979).

This thalamic nucleus is also the target of axons in the medial lemniscus, conveying low-threshold mechanoreceptive information from the dorsal column nuclei. Recent research suggests that spinothalamic and medial lemniscal axons may even end on the same thalamic cell in the ventroposterior nucleus. Collaterals from lamina I spinothalamic axons end in the periaqueductal grey matter of the midbrain (Mantyh, 1982).

The above is somewhat of a simplification, since it is known that some spinal cord cells project collaterally to both medial and lateral thalamus, just as others project collaterally to both reticular formation and medial thalamus. However, the fact that in some instances different projections arise from the same lamina does not necessarily mean that they originate from the same cells, since each lamina in the human cord contains several (or even many) cell types (Abdel-Maguid and Bowsher, 1985).

Physiological analysis of spinal grey cells projecting into the anterolateral funiculus shows them to be of two types. The more superficial neurones tend to be nocispecific, that is to say, they respond *only* to high-threshold peripheral stimulation. Deeper cells, on the other hand, tend to be what is known as 'convergent' or 'wide dynamic range' (WDR) – they respond to virtually *all* peripheral stimuli, but with a different pattern of response according to the type of stimulus applied.

Since the reticular formation sends fibres upwards to the intralaminar (medial) nuclei of the thalamus, we are essentially concerned with the cortical destination of projections from the medial (intralaminar) and lateral (ventroposterior) thalamic nuclei, which are as follows.

(A) The postcentral gyrus (first somatic sensory area, SI) is the destination of the axons of cells in the ventroposterior thalamic nucleus, which also send fibres (mainly collaterally but also uniquely) to the small second somatic sensory area, which lies below the first, in the parietal operculum and retroinsular regions of the cortex.

Studies of thousands of discrete cortical injuries in both World Wars demonstrated that lesions in the postcentral gyrus virtually never cause loss of pain sensation, though they do cause somatotopically organised loss of low-threshold mechanoreceptive and thermal sensations, as well as pinprick sensation (Bowsher, 1975). Thus, it cannot be sufficiently emphasised that the direct spinothalamic tract and its cortical projection are *not* the 'pain pathway'.

Consonant with this is the clinical observation that a patient whose pain (e.g., biliary colic) has been relieved by a therapeutic dose of morphine is able to appreciate the pinprick sensation elicited by a further injection in much the same way as can an individual who has not been given an injection of morphine. The scientific correlates of this common but all too little thought about observation are that (*i*) there are few opioid binding sites at supraspinal levels of the direct spinothalamic pathway leading through the ventroposterior thalamic nucleus to the postcentral gyrus (Lamotte et al., 1978); and (*ii*) microinjection of morphine into the ventroposterior thalamic nucleus does not suppress pain behaviour in experimental animals (Pert and Yaksh, 1974).

Most nocispecific cells in the spinal cord project into this direct spinothalamic system.

(B) The intralaminar thalamic nuclei, receiving both direct and (mainly) relayed-through-the-reticular-formation information from the spinal cord, are at the origin of the so-called 'diffuse thalamo-cortical projection'. The highly branching axons of cells in these nuclei supply not only the corpus striatum (basal ganglia), but also reach the deepest and/or most superficial layers of the *whole* cortex (Bowsher, 1966; Jones and Leavitt, 1974), with prefrontal predominance in primates. In accordance with this, Lassen et al. (1978) have shown that while somatic stimuli such as touch cause an increase of blood flow in the region of the postcentral gyrus, painful stimulation in human volunteers brings about an increase of blood flow in prefrontal regions and *not* in the postcentral gyrus (Lassen et al., 1978). The cortical regions to which the intralaminar nuclei project are too widespread for injury to all of it to be compatible with any discrete loss of function. However, it is interesting in this context to note that prefrontal lobotomy may have an excellent effect in alleviating the suffering associated with pain from malignant disease (Freeman and Watts, 1946).

By the same token, supraspinal relays of the spino-reticulo-intralaminar thalamic pathway have high concentrations of opioid receptors (Lamotte et al., 1978), and microinjection of morphine into the reticular formation or intralaminar thalamus effectively abolishes pain reactions in experimental animals (Pert and Yaksh, 1974).

Most wide dynamic range cells in the spinal grey matter project into this system.

Thus, to summarise, the implication is that the pathway for tissue-damage pain is probably that from deep spinal grey → medial brainstem reticular formation → intralaminar thalamus → whole cortex with prefrontal predominance, while the pathway from more superficial spinal grey matter via the direct spinothalamic tract through the ventroposterior thalamic nucleus to the postcentral gyrus is responsible for thermal and pinprick sensations. However, the proviso must be borne in mind that the distinction between the two systems is in reality considerably less clear-cut than this simplified account may imply.

MODELS OF NOCIGENIC PAIN

Mention was made in the Introduction of the poor correspondence between chronic clinical pain and most stimuli used in physiological investigations of pain systems within the spinal cord and brain. Physiologists of course have not been unaware of this discrepancy, and there has been an intensive search for a reliable and verisimilitudinous model of chronic pain. The model on which most work has been done is rat polyarthritis induced by injection of Freund's adjuvant (Colpaert et al., 1982). While this may not be the right model for all types of nocigenic pain, it has revealed some interesting features which may be relevant at least to inflammatory pain.

Arthritic rats, like arthritic humans, have exquisitely tender joints. Light tactile stimuli, which would normally only activate Aβ primary afferents, are agonising. Recent work has shown that the thresholds of small-fibre nociceptors are so lowered that they are activated by low-intensity mechanical stimuli (Guilbaud et al., 1985), and so exhibit spontaneous activity (they are normally silent). It is believed that chemical changes resulting from inflammation (for example, the increase in Substance P content of synovial fluid) are responsible for the sensitisation of primary afferents; Heavey et al. (1985) have shown that aspirin reduces prostacyclin production in response to bradykinin injection. There is an increase in the proportion of ventroposterior thalamic units responding to stimulation of the inflamed joints (Guilbaud et al., 1981); might this correspond to increased somatic awareness of an inflamed joint? Kayser and Guilbaud (1984) have shown that a large number of cells in a thalamic intralaminar nucleus of arthritic rats respond to joint manipulation, while in normal animals they do not. This may be interpreted as evidence of the effect of lowering peripheral nociceptor thresholds, so that normally non-painful stimuli now excite nociceptive neurones throughout the CNS.

Another possibility, suggested both by Wall (1985) and by Morley (1985), is that a peptide neuromodulator passes up primary afferent C axons from damaged or inflamed tissue into the spinal cord and there sensitises nociceptive neurones. Such a possibility is particularly worthy of serious consideration because most of the spinal cord neurones at the origin of the spino-reticulo-diencephalototicortical pathway belong to the 'wide dynamic range' category; that is to say, they are cells which respond differentially to inputs from virtually all types of peripheral afferent. Sensitisation would therefore imply that they might respond with a noxious-type output to a normally sub-noxious input.

DESCENDING INHIBITORY CONTROL (Fig. 1.5)

The story of descending inhibition of noxious input began with two apparently

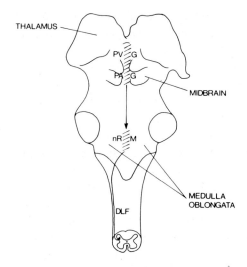

Fig. 1.5 Descending inhibitory systems. Fibres from the periventricular (PVG) and periaqueductal (PAG) grey matter descend to the nucleus raphe magnus (NRM) in the midline of the medullary reticular formation. Thence, serotoninergic fibres descend in the dorsolateral funiculus (DLF) of the spinal white matter, to terminate in the substantia gelatinosa of the dorsal horn, where they are believed to activate the encephalinergic interneurones shown in Fig. 1.2.

inexplicable findings. First, Tsou and Jang (1964) microinjected minute amounts of morphine into a large number of circumscribed brain sites and found that the most effective site by far, producing analgesia at the lowest concentration, was the periaqueductal grey matter (PAG) of the midbrain. Since the PAG was then known not to be a relay station in any ascending 'pain pathway', Tsou and Jang's strange finding was ignored. But only 5 years later, Reynolds (1969) found that electrical stimulation of the PAG produced profound analgesia, such that surgical procedures could be carried out on rats without any nocifensive reactions becoming apparent. When opioid receptors and naturally occurring opiates were discovered, it became clear that the PAG is in fact a relay station on a *descending* pathway capable of preventing noxiously generated information from being transmitted upwards to conscious levels of the brain.

The whole system, as now understood, may be described at this point. In the region of the arcuate nucleus in the hypothalamic infundibulum (itself under the control of the prefrontal cortex) is a group of cells which use β-endorphin as a transmitter. Axons from these cells pass through the periventricular grey matter in the wall of the third ventricle (where they may be surgically stimulated) to terminate in the PAG. Here they inhibit local inhibitory interneurones, thereby releasing from inhibition projection cells whose axons pass down to the region of the nucleus raphe magnus in the midline of the reticular formation of the medulla oblongata. Thence further neurones, mostly serotoninergic (i.e., having 5-hydroxy-tryptamine (5-HT) as their transmitter) send their axons down the dorsolateral funiculus (DLF) of the spinal cord to end in the superficial spinal dorsal horn. The most powerful inhibition, under experimental circumstances, is brought about by direct stimulation of the nucleus raphe magnus. However, because of its infratentorial location, this is not a practical possibility in the freely moving subject. In man, successful inhibition of pain has been brought about by the implantation of electrodes in a number of supratentorial locations in this descending inhibitory pathway; the periventricular grey (containing the periarcuate-PAG fibres) and the PAG itself have been the sites most frequently stimulated (Richardson, 1982).

Many of these raphe-spinal axons synapse with, and activate, the encephalinergic inhibitory neurones on the lamina I-II border (Glazer and Basbaum, 1984) which were described in an earlier section. However, some of these serotoninergic axons end freely within the neuropile (Maxwell et al., 1983; Hammond et al., 1985). The implication of this is that serotonin may act as a transmitter at synapses or as a local hormone which will act on any neurones with suitable specific receptors in the vicinity of its release. To this we may add the general release (into the bloodstream) of neurohormones such as β-endorphin from the hypothalamus (as well as its neurotransmitter role in infundibulo-PAG axons). Since β-endorphin seems to be the natural ligand for the non-synaptic μ binding sites on the intraspinal terminals of C polymodal primary afferent fibres, naturally occurring 'stress analgesia' could well be due to hormonally released and generally circulating β-endorphin acting at these and other μ sites.

Mention was made above of collaterals from spinothalamic axons originating in lamina I which terminate in the PAG (see Fig. 1.4). Since these nocispecific neurones are activated by stimuli such as pinprick, this connection may be at the origin of heterosegmental acupuncture effects (Bowsher, 1987) – especially as there is apparently some form of topical organisation within the PAG in experimental animals (Soper and Melzack, 1982), and therefore presumably in man.

Some raphe-spinal axons, and a greater number from reticular regions just lateral to the raphe, are noradrenergic. The largest number of noradrenergic fibres descending in the DLF, however, originate in the locus coeruleus in the upper pons. The inhibitory synaptic action of noradrenaline in the spinal cord is not apparently exerted through encephalinergic interneurones, but directly on cells in the nociceptive pathway.

The reuptake of both 5-HT and noradrenaline is inhibited by dicyclics and tricyclics, but not by tetracyclic antidepressants. This is the basis of the antinociceptive (analgesic) action of tricyclics, and is unrelated to their antidepressant action (Walsh, 1983; Feinmann, 1985). Serotoninergic inhibition is also believed to be facilitated to some extent by oral administration of its precursor, L-tryptophan (van Praag, 1981) (see also Chapter 5, p. 142).

NEUROGENIC PAIN

As stated at the beginning of this chapter, neurogenic pain may be defined as pain due to a lesion of the peripheral or central nervous system, and not to stimulation of nociceptor terminals. It has a number of features which set it apart, both clinically and pathophysiologically, from nocigenic (tissue damage) pain (Bowsher, 1988). These most notably include:

(1) Non-susceptibility to morphine and opiates in normally analgesic dosage. This clinically most important point also demonstrates that the mechanism of neurogenic pain must be quite different from that of opioid-sensitive nocigenic pain.

(2) In the vast majority of neurogenic pain conditions, there is a partial sensory deficit, pointing to sensory imbalance as being implicated in the pathophysiology.

(3) There is nearly always autonomic change, such as decreased blood flow and/ or hypo- or hyperhydrosis in the painful region; pain is also exacerbated (or brought on) by emotional disturbance or stress, including physical activity such as ejaculation. This phenomenon is doubtless related to the demonstration by Torebjörk and Hallin (1979) that the pain of causalgia is very severely exacerbated by the the intradermal injection of 1 μg of noradrenaline – a quantity which is entirely without effect in normal tissue. Although the basis of the phenomenon remains unknown, it at least provides some rationale for the effectiveness of sympathetic blockade in both peripheral and central (Loh, Nathan, and Schott, 1981) neurogenic pain.

(4) Allodynia commonly occurs – that is to say, a low-intensity, normally non-noxious stimulus is painful. This means that pain elicited by the stimulation of Aβ fibres such as touching or blowing in trigeminal neuralgia (Kugelberg and Lindblom, 1959), may excite WDR cells in the trigeminal nucleus or spinal cord to respond with a 'nociceptive discharge'. The fact that pain is produced by sudden on-off stimuli, such as brushing, and not by firm pressure demonstrates that allodynia is uniquely set off by rapidly adapting low-threshold mechanoreceptors, and not by the steady pressure which can elicit tenderness. This too points to a mechanism very different from that of nocigenic pain, in which tenderness is probably due to lowered threshold of Aδ and C nociceptor afferents. Indeed it was over a century ago that Trousseau (1877) drew attention to the similarity between paroxysmal shooting pains in trigeminal neuralgia and epileptic seizure discharge. Most of that century was to pass before trigeminal neuralgia was successfully treated with anticonvulsants; it is now known that all shooting neurogenic pains can be treated with anticonvulsants (Swerdlow, 1984).

(5) Although aching and/or throbbing is the commonest pain descriptor in the majority of neurogenic pain conditions, burning (often accompanied by coldness)* and/or shooting (see preceding paragraph) pains are frequently regarded as virtually pathognomonic of neurogenic pain. In this context, it must be recalled that many mixed pains, such as those involving nerve compression by a herniated intervertebral disc or tumour, include a burning or shooting neurogenic element. There is at present no explanation for these indisputable facts.

(6) Another unexplained but characteristic feature is the failure of even agonising neurogenic pain to prevent the patient from falling asleep 'normally'. Since the patients are often elderly, their 'normal' sleep pattern is frequently not that of younger people. Although the patient goes to sleep, he/she may awake in great pain.

Neurogenic pain takes many clinical forms. The commonest is postherpetic neuralgia, followed by trigeminal neuralgia. The latter is the 'odd man out' among neurogenic pain syndromes in that (i) the pain is uniquely shooting, with no burning element; and (ii) there is no partial sensory deficit, as in other neurogenic pain syndromes. A great deal of painful diabetic neuropathy is neurogenic in origin. Causalgia is classically due to subtotal peripheral nerve injury, particularly the median and ulnar. However, increasing numbers of cases involving the leg are seen following iatrogenic injury of lumbosacral nerve roots. The distal parts of the median or ulnar nerves are frequently damaged in fractures of the wrist, giving rise to causalgia minor, formerly known as reflex sympathetic dystrophy. Autonomic disturbance ('trophic changes') are particularly evident in causalgia, both major and minor. Neuromata occurring in amputation stumps can give rise to neurogenic pain. Work with experimentally produced neuromata in animals has shown that 'spontaneous' impulses arise from them; however it is far from certain that such a phenomenon 'explains' neurogenic pain. If it did, section of the nerve at a higher level would ineluctably abolish the pain; but it doesn't. Brachial plexus avulsion, due to trauma (commonly, motor cycle accidents) is a true 'deafferentation' syndrome, affecting the junction of the peripheral and central nervous systems – as does the now rare tabes dorsalis causing lightning pains and tabetic crises. Finally, neurogenic pain can be caused by lesions of the central nervous system, nearly always caused by a cerebrovascular accident. It is classically known as 'thalamic syndrome', though recent research has shown that the majority of cases have lesions in brain sites other than the thalamus (Bowsher et al., 1984).

With the exception of trigeminal neuralgia, the neurological signs and symptoms of all forms of neurogenic pain – peripheral, junctional and central – are

---

* The most articulate witnesses describe burning neurogenic pain as being like the paradoxical burning experienced when a hand is plunged in ice-water.

similar. Diagnosis is made on the basis of the history of the condition and the distribution of the pain. Reference has already been made to the treatment of the shooting element in neurogenic pain by anticonvulsants, as in the case of trigeminal neuralgia.

In addition to anticonvulsant therapy of epileptiform shooting or stabbing pains, the rational treatment of neurogenic pain is aimed at the reduction of sympathetic tone, for the pain is sympathetically maintained. Thus, tricyclic antidepressants reduce sympathetic outflow from the central nervous system (even though they may increase it peripherally because of their anticholinergic effect). Peripheral sympathetic ganglion blockade is frequently effective, as is depletion of noradrenaline in sympathetic terminals by guanethidine. Increase of peripheral parasympathetic tone by anticholinesterases may induce a relative decrease in sympathetic tone. For reasons as yet unknown, the longer a neurogenic pain has been established, the more difficult it is to relieve. This being so, precious time should not be wasted in attempting (unsuccessfully) to relieve neurogenic pain with conventional analgesics; antisympathetic treatment should be instituted at the earliest possible opportunity.

It must be remembered that many clinically encountered pains exhibit a mixture of nocigenic and neurogenic elements. Thus, for example, many tumours produce tissue damage *and* compress nerves; diabetic patients have nocigenic tissue damage from vascular disease and neurogenic pain due to neuropathy. In such cases, different treatments must be directed at the two totally different (from a pathophysiological and therefore therapeutic point of view) types of pain.

CONCLUSIONS

Two types of chronic pain should be recognised. The first is *nocigenic* essentially caused by tissue damage, which stimulates nociceptor nerve endings. This pain follows classical anatomical pathways, in which many synapses are sensitive to morphine and other narcotic analgesics. This pain can be controlled at a number of 'gates', of which the best-understood is now that at the entry to the CNS, in the spinal cord or brainstem. Non-opioidergic analgesic mechanisms, such as large fibre stimulation (TNS and DCS) are to be contrasted with descending opioidergic mechanisms originating in the forebrain and passing through the hypothalamus to the PAG, whence it relays through the midline of the lower brainstem reticular formation to the spinal cord. Ascending pathways may be interrupted or inhibitory mechanisms stimulated in the control of nocigenic pain.

Neurogenic pain (trigeminal neuralgia, central post-stroke pain ('thalamic syndrome'), partial plexus avulsion, causalgia, postherpetic neuralgia, etc.) occupies more than its fair share of pain relief clinic referrals, because it is resistant to narcotic analgesics (a point which cannot be too strongly emphasised when it comes to treatment of these conditions). It is due to dysfunction of the peripheral or central nervous systems in the absence of nociceptor stimulation, often resulting in partial sensory deficit; there may be a single or multiple pathophysiological mechanism(s). Many of these conditions also exhibit autonomic dysfunction, and can be relieved by sympathetic blockade; anticonvulsant therapy and pharmacological manipulation of non-opioidergic central (?) noradrenergic inhibitory mechanisms are also helpful.

REFERENCES

Abram, S.E., Reynolds, A.C. and Cusick, J.F. (1981) Failure of naloxone to reverse analgesia from transcutaneous electrical stimulation in patients with chronic pain. *Anaesth. Analg.*, 60, 81–84.

Abdel-Maguid, T.E. and Bowsher, D. (1985) The grey matter of the dorsal horn of the adult human spinal cord, including comparisons with general somatic and visceral afferent cranial nerve nuclei. *J. Anat.* (London), 142, 33–58.

Bennett, G.J., Ruda, M.A., Gobel, S. and Dubner, R. (1982) Enkephalin immunoreactive stalked cells and Lamina IIb islet cells in cat substantia gelatinosa. *Brain Res.*, 240, 162–166.

Bond, M.R. and Pilowsky, I. (1966) The subjective assessment of pain and and its relationship to the administration of analgesics in patients with advanced cancer. *J. Psychosom. Res.*, 10, 203–207.

Bowsher, D. (1957) Termination of the central pain pathway in man: the conscious appreciation of pain. *Brain*, 80, 606–622.

Bowsher, D. (1963) Les relais des sensibilités somethésique et douloureuse au niveau du tronc cérébral et du thalamus. *Toulouse Méd.*, 64, 965–984.

Bowsher, D. (1966) Some afferent and efferent connections of the parafascicular centromedian complex. in: *The Thalamus*, Editors: D.P. Purpura and M.D. Yahr. Columbia University Press, New York, pp. 99–108.

Bowsher, D. (1976) Role of the reticular formation in response to noxious stimulation. *Pain*, 2, 361–368.

Bowsher, D. (1983) A note on the distinction between first and second pain. pp. 3–6 In: *Anatomical, Physiological and Pharmacological Aspects of Trigeminal Pain*, Editors: B. Matthews and R.G. Hill, Excerpta Medica, Amsterdam, 1982.

Bowsher, D. (1987) Mechanisms of pain in man. ICI, Macclesfield, pp. 14.

Bowsher, D. (1988) Neurogenic pain. In: *Neurological Emergencies in Medical Practice*, Editor: D. Bowsher. Croom Helm, Beckenham, pp. 118–136.

Bowsher, D., Lahuerta, J. and Brock, L.G. (1984) Twelve cases of central pain, only three with thalamic lesions. *Pain* (Suppl. 2) 83.

Bromage, P.E., Camporesi, E. and Chestnut, D. (1980) Epidural narcotics for postoperative analgesia. *Anaesth. Analg.*, 59, 473–480.

Cervero, F., Schouenborg, J. and Sjölund, B.H. (1981) Effects of conditioning stimulation of somatic and visceral afferent fibres on viscero-somatic and somato-somatic reflexes. *J. Physiol. (London)*, 317, 84P.

Coggeshall, R.E., Applebaum, M.L., Frazen, M., Stubbs, T.B. and Sykes, M.T. (1975) Unmyelinated axons in human ventral roots, a possible explanation for the failure of dorsal rhizotomy to relieve pain. *Brain*, 98, 157–166.

Colpaert, F.C., Meert, T.H., De Witte, P.H. and Schmitt, P. (1982) Further evidence validating adjuvant arthritis as an experimental model of chronic pain in the rat. *Life Sci.*, 31, 67–75.

Freeman, W. and Watts, J.W. (1946) Pain of organic disease relieved by prefrontal lobotomy. *Lancet*, i, 953–955

Feinmann, C. (1985) Pain relief by antidepressants: possible modes of action. *Pain*, 23, 1–8.

Glazer, E.J. and Basbaum, A.I. (1984) Axons which take up [³H]serotonin are presynaptic to enkephalin immunoreactive neurons in cat dorsal horn. *Brain Res.*, 298, 386–391.

Goldscheider, A. (1881) Zur Lehre von den specifischen Energien der Sinnesorgane. Schumacher, Berlin.

Guilbaud, G., Gautron, M. and Peschanski, M. (1981) Réponses électrophysiologiques des neurones du complexe ventrobasal du thalamus à des stimulations cutanées et articulaires chez des rats présentant une polyarthrite inflammatoire. *C.R. Acad. Sci. (Paris)*, 292, 227–230.

Guilbaud, G., Iggo, A. and Tegner, R. (1985) Sensory receptors in ankle joint capsules of normal and arthritic rats. *Exp. Brain Res.*, 58, 29–40.

Hammond, D.L., Tyle, G.M. and Yaksh, T.L. (1985) Effects of 5-hydroxytryptamine and noradrenaline into spinal cord superfusates during stimulation of the rat medulla. *J. Physiol. (London)*, 359, 151–162.

Hardy, J.D., Wolff, H.G. and Goodell, H. (1952) *Pain Sensations and Reactions.* Williams and Wilkins, Baltimore.

Heavey, D.J., Barron, S.E., Hickling, N.E. and Ritter, J.M. (1985) Aspirin causes short-lived inhibition of bradykinin-stimulated prostacyclin production in man. *Nature (London)*, 318, 186–188.

Jones, E.G. and Leavitt, R.Y. (1974) Retrograde axonal transport and the demonstration of non-specific projections to the cerebral cortex and striatum from thalamic intralaminar nuclei in the rat, cat, and monkey. *J. Comp. Neurol.*, 154, 349–378.

Kayser, V. and Guilbaud, G. (1984) Further evidence for changes in the responsiveness of somatosensory neurons in arthritic rats: a study of the posterior intralaminar region of the thalamus. *Brain Res.*, 323, 144–147.

Kevetter, G.A., Haber, L.H., Yezierski, R.P., Chung, J.M., Martin, R.G. and Willis, W.D. (1982) Cells of origin of the spinoreticular tract in the monkey. *J. Comp. Neurol.*, 207, 61–74.

Kosterlitz, H.W. and Paterson, S.J. (1985) Types of opioid receptors: relation to antinociception. *Philos. Trans. Royal Soc. Lond.*, 303B, 291–298.

Kugelberg, E. and Lindblom, U. (1959) The mechanisms of pain in trigeminal neuralgia. *J. Neurol. Neurosurg. Psychiatr.*, 22, 36–43.

Lamotte, C.C. (1977) Distribution of the tract of Lissauer and the dorsal root fibers in the primate spinal cord. *J. Comp. Neurol.*, 172, 529–562.

Lamotte, C.C., Snowman, A., Pert, C.B. and Snyder, S.H. (1978) Opiate receptor binding in rhesus monkey brain: association with limbic structures. *Brain Res.*, 155, 374–379.

Lassen, N.A., Ingvar, D.H. and Skinhøj, E. (1978) Brain function and blood flow. *Sci. Am.*, 239, 50–59.

Loh, L., Nathan, P.W. and Schott, G.D. (1981) Pain due to lesions of the central nervous system removed by sympathetic block. *Br. Med. J.*, 282, 1026–1028.

Lundeberg, T.C.M. (1983) Vibratory stimulation for the alleviation of chronic pain. *Acta Physiol. Scand.*, 523, (Suppl.), 1–51.

Mantyh, P.W. (1982) The ascending input to the midbrain periaqueductal gray of the primate. *J. Comp. Neurol.*, 211, 50–64.

Maxwell, D.J., Leranth, Cs. and Verhofstad, A.A.J. (1983) Fine structure of serotonin-containing axons in the marginal zone of the cat spinal cord. *Brain Res.*, 266, 233–260.

Mayer, D.J., Price, D.D. and Rafii, A. (1977) Antagonism of acupuncture analgesia in man by the narcotic antagonist naloxone. *Brain Res.*, 121, 368–372.

Mehler, W.R. (1957) The mammalian 'pain tract' in phylogeny. *Anat. Rec.*, 127, 332.

Mehler, W.R. (1962) The anatomy of the so-called 'pain tract' in man: an analysis of the course and distribution of the ascending fibers of the fasciculus anterolateralis. In: *Basic Research in Paraplegia*, Editors: J.D. French and R.W. Porter. C.C. Thomas, Springfield, pp. 26–55.

Melzack, R. (1975) The McGill Pain Questionnaire: Major properties and scoring methods. *Pain*, 1, 277–299.

Melzack, R. and Wall, P.D. (1965): Pain mechanisms: A new theory. *Science*, 150, 971–979.

22

Morley, J.S. (1985) Peptides in nociceptive pathways. In: *Persistent Pain: Modern Methods and Treatment, Vol. 5.* Editors: S. Lipton and J.B. Miles. Academic Press, London, pp. 65–91.

Nash, T.P. (1986) Percutaneous radiofrequency lesioning of dorsal root ganglia for intractable pain. *Pain*, 24, 67–74.

Pert, A. and Yaksh, T.L. (1974) Sites of morphine-induced analgesia in the primate brain: relation to pain pathways. *Brain Res.*, 80, 135–140.

Pomeranz, B. and Chiu, D. (1976) Naloxone blocks acupuncture analgesia; Endorphin implicated. *Life Sci.*, 19, 1757–1762.

Ranson, S.W. (1914) The tract of Lissauer and the substantia gelatinosa Rolandi. *Am. J. Anat.*, 16, 97–126.

Reynolds, D.V. (1969) Surgery in the rat during electrical analgesia induced by focal brain stimulation. *Science*, 164, 444–445.

Richardson, D.E. (1982) Analgesia produced by stimulation of various sites in the human β-endorphin system. *Appl. Neurophysiol.*, 45, 116–122.

Shealey, C.N., Mortimer, J.T. and Reswick, J.B. (1967) Electrical inhibition of pain by stimulation of the dorsal columns: Preliminary clinical report. *Anesth. Analg.*, 46, 489–491.

Sinclair, D.C. (1981) *Mechanisms of Cutaneous Sensation.* Oxford University Press, London.

Sindou, M., Quoex, C. and Baleydier, C. (1975) Fiber organization in the posterior spinal cord-rootlet junction in man. *J. Comp. Neurol.*, 153, 15–26.

Sjölund, B.H. and Eriksson, M.B.E. (1979) The influence of naloxone on analgesia produced by peripheral conditioning stimulation. *Brain Res.*, 173, 295–302.

Smith, G.M., Egbert, L.D., Markowitz, R.A., Mosteller, R. and Beecher, H.K. (1966) An experimental pain method sensitive to morphine in man: The submaximum effort tourniquet technique. *J. Pharmacol. Exp. Ther.*, 154, 324–332.

Soper, W.Y. and Melzack, R. (1982) Stimulation-produced analgesia: evidence for somatotopic organization in the midbrain. *Brain Res.*, 251, 301–312.

Spiller, W.G. (1905) The occasional clinical resemblance between caries of the vertebrae and lumbothoracic syringomyelia and the location within the spinal cord of the fibres for the sensations of pain and temperature. *Uni. PA Med. Bull.*, 18, 147–154.

Swerdlow, M. (1984) Anticonvulsant drugs and chronic pain. *Clin. Neuropharmacol.*, 7, 51–82.

Torebjörk, H.E. (1985) Nociceptor activation and pain. *Trans. Royal Soc. Lond.* B, 308, 227–234.

Torebjörk, H.E. and Hallin, R.G. (1979) Microneurographic studies of peripheral pain mechanisms in man. *Adv. Pain Res. Ther.*, 3, 121–131, Raven Press, New York.

Trousseau, A. (1877) Clinique médicale de l'Hôtel-Dieu de Paris. Baillière et Fils, Paris, 1877.

Tsou, K. and Jang, C.S. (1964) Studies on the site of analgesic action of morphine by intracerebral microinjection. *Sci. Sinica*, 13, 1099–1109.

Van Praag, H.M. (1981) Management of depression with serotonin precursors. *Biol. Psychiatr.*, 16, 291–310.

Vierck, C.J., Greenspan, J.D., Ritz, L.A. and Yeomans, D.C. (1985) The spinal pathways contributing to the ascending conduction and the descending modulation of pain sensations and reactions. In: *Spinal Systems of Afferent Processing* Editors: T.L. Yaksh. Plenum Press, New York, pp. 1–42.

Wall, P.D. (1985) Future Trends in Pain Research. *Philos. Trans. R. Soc. Lond.*, 308B, 393–402.

Wall, P.D. and Sweet, W.H. (1967) Temporary abolition of pain in man. *Science*, 155, 108–109.

Walsh, T.D. (1983) Antidepressants in chronic pain. *Clin. Neuropharmacol.*, 6, 271–295.

Wang, J.K. (1977) Analgesic effect of intrathecally administered morphine. *Reg. Anesth.*, 4, 2–3.

Willis, W.D., Kenshalo, D.R. and Leonard, R.B. (1979) The cells of origin of the primate spinothalamic tract. *J. Comp. Neurol.*, 188, 543–574.

Yaksh, T.L. and Rudy, T.A. (1976) Analgesia mediated by a direct spinal action of narcotics. *Science*, 192, 1357–1358.

Young, R.F. and Stevens, R. (1979) Unmyelinated axons in the trigeminal motor root of human and cat. *J. Comp. Neurol.*, 183, 205–214.

M. Swerdlow and J.E. Charlton (eds.) Relief of Intractable Pain
© 1989, Elsevier Science Publishers B.V. (Biomedical Division)

2

The psychological treatment of pain

Harold Merskey

'By Hill 60...everything I could see seemed to be made of jelly. I bit the end of my tongue, and then shot over the debris of no-man's land like a clockwork man. My feet seemed to be six inches off the ground most of the way. The spike of a barbed wire strand stuck in the back of my knee and I pulled it out with the flesh hanging to it. But couldn't feel any pain. It seemed like someone else's leg.' (Newspaper account of a man's experiences in the First World War.)

'...whoever has read Hippocrates or Dr. James Mackenzie, and has considered well the effects which the passions and affections of the mind have upon the digestion (why not of a wound as much as a dinner?) may easily conceive what sharp paroxysms and exacerbations of his wound my Uncle Toby must have undergone upon that score alone.' (from *Life and Opinions of Tristram Shandy Gent*, by Laurence Sterne.)

As in the previous editions, the two quotations at the head of this chapter illustrate the observations that extreme fear may prevent pain from arising when we would expect it, whilst, at other times, anxiety or emotional change may provoke or exacerbate pain. There is much evidence (Beecher, 1959; Merskey and Spear, 1967; Sternbach, 1968) that emotions may make pain worse, or alternatively, reduce the severity with which it is felt. Apart from the fact that pain may be thus modified by the emotions, it is also recognized that pain may originate from psychological illness. Thus, the psychological state of the individual may produce pain, increase the severity with which it is felt, or diminish that severity. It is currently thought that emotion may sometimes abolish pain altogether, even though the individual is suffering from severe trauma to the body and is conscious. This means that no discussion of the relief of pain can be complete without consideration of the psychological illnesses which alter pain or the mechanisms which promote it. It would be unusual to find anyone working in a pain clinic or in the treatment of pain who did not support this view. The extent to which such considerations apply will be considered shortly.

The treatment of illnesses often proceeds without complete knowledge of their causes. The management of oedema with diuretics may be helped by some knowledge of kidney function but probably depends more upon the ingenuity and resourcefulness of pharmacologists and organic chemists than upon the appraisal of glomerular permeability. Effective treatment of endogenous depressive illness likewise began with ECT, and with drugs affecting brain amine metabolism, and then, subsequently, biological evidence appeared in regard to possible mechanisms of depletion of brain amines underlying the various depressive syndromes. Similarly, psychological techniques such as suggestion, relaxation, faith healing and placebo responses were known to relieve pain before anyone formally defined what is meant by pain. Narcotic drugs and surgery are sometimes effective, especially where an organic cause for pain is recognizable. Nevertheless, failures in the management of pain often occur and some of them may result from a wrong or poor appraisal of the reasons why people have pain. This in turn may be due to a failure to appreciate exactly what ought to be understood by the word 'pain'.

THE NATURE OF PAIN

Difficulty in defining pain was noted by Beecher (1959), who found that many distinguished authorities were unable or unwilling to specify in words what they meant by it. The difficulty seemed to this writer to arise because people tended to forget that pain, whether mild or severe, is always a conscious experience. Some authors seemed to think of pain as happening in nerve endings or nerve tracts. Even if they recognized it was something people felt consciously, they were liable to deny its presence unless physiological or pathological changes could be demonstrated. On the other hand, they seemed ready, as we all sometimes are, to suppose that a patient was in pain because he groaned, even though he was anaesthetized and could presumably have no conscious experience. These difficulties are avoided if one insists that the definition of pain must be a psychological one and that it should be based on an individual's awareness of his experience. This is not to deny at all the importance of physical or organic changes in promoting pain. But it is to insist that what we regard as pain must, in the last resort, be what somebody has in his conscious awareness and not what we might detect with a cathode-ray tube and a pair of electrodes. Pursuing this line of thought, the International Association for the Study of Pain settled on the following definition of pain: 'An unpleasant sensory and emotional experience associated with actual or potential tissue damage or described in terms of such damage' (IASP, 1979). We first learn to use the word pain from the knocks or bangs or blows which we suffer as young children and which are then associated with the word in the descriptions or language of other people around us. The child learns that pain is an experience associated with damage to the body and it is ordinarily, and sometimes extraordinarily, unpleasant. If it is not unpleasant it is not pain, and unpleasant experiences which are associated with illness but not with evident damage to the body may be classified separately. For example, nausea is not at all pleasant but is not usually regarded as a necessary sign of physical injury occurring in some organ or region. On the other hand, the unpleasant experience which is typical of pain does not necessarily depend on the presence of tissue damage even though we first learn to identify it from its association with trauma.

If this definition is accepted it becomes relatively easy to avoid the pitfalls of telling patients that they do not have pain or that their pain is not bad when they say it is severe, and so forth. Even in cases with intractable pain it is possible, especially for the doctor who is failing to relieve the patient's suffering, to suppose that because he has recently not confirmed the presence of an active organic cause, the man or woman is not really suffering. A continual insistence on putting the patient's experience first helps to preserve a perspective which is useful and helpful in treating the patient.

THE INCIDENCE OF PAIN

Table 2.1 shows the frequency of pain and psychiatric illness in some reports from different sources which include general practice, general (internal) medicine, a large general hospital out-patient service and several psychiatric centres. It cannot be assumed that diagnostic practices or methods of data collection were identical in even two of these reports and the estimates for the frequency of psychiatric illness are based on this writer's interpretation of the different authors' material. Nevertheless, two obvious points emerge. The first is that pain is a common symptom; the second is that pain is often attributed to psychological causes. We know both of these conclusions already from clinical experience. We are often less ready to acknowledge Stengel's observation that pain is a common sign of psychiatric illness (Stengel, 1960).

The exact meaning of these figures is uncertain, however. They do not distinguish between acute and chronic pain: selection factors are unquestionably important in channelling patients with psychological illness and organic complaints to hospital and some of the psychological illness might be a consequence of pain, rather than its cause. Nevertheless, they reinforce the point that psychological factors are likely to be abundant in any hospital or clinic population with pain.

This evidence also gives us no epidemiological guidelines as to the frequency of either acute or chronic pain. It only tells us what is found in certain settings.

If we look for epidemiological evidence we can learn that, according to Waters (1975), almost all young adult females suffer from headache, the exception being

TABLE 1

Some reports on the frequency of pain

Authors	No. of patients	Source: type of patient	Overall proportions with pain (%)	Overall frequency of psychiatr. illness (%)	Probable frequency of pain, no. of relevant lesions and psychiatric illness (%)
Douglas-Wilson	810	Medical clinic – neurotic patients	87	29	87
Friedlander and Freyhoff	50	Effort syndrome	88[b]	100	88
Apley	100	Children with abdominal pain	100	56–67[a]	56–64[a]
Bain and Spaulding	4000	Toronto General Hospital medical outpatients	37[d]	22–53+	22–53[c]
Devine and Merskey	182	Medical outpatients	75	39	38
Gomez and Dally	96	Medical surgical outpatients with abdominal pain	100	84	84
Kirk and Saunders	358	Neurol. clinic psychiatr. cases	40–47[d]	100	100
Baker and Merskey	276	General practice	65	28	17
Klee et al.	150	Psychiat. clinic outpatients	61	100	?61
Spear	180	Psychiatric outpatients	65.6	100	44.6
Delaplaine et al.	227	Psychiatric hospital	38	100	22
Weider et al.	1000	Potential military recruits/headache	8.7	–	>8.7
Weider et al.	113	Rejected cases headache	35.4	?100	>35

[a] Depending on criteria used.
[b] Precordial pain or chest pain.
[c] According to site.
[d] Percentage of complaints.

Reprinted with acknowledgements from *Pain*, edited by John J. Bonica (1980) Raven Press, New York.

only some 3% approximately of women of that age, whilst among young males, similarly aged from 21–34, 80% suffer from headaches. With increasing age the frequency of headache as a complaint declines and at 55 or over slightly less than half of all males have mild or severe headache and slightly more than half of all females have such complaints. Low back pain is also very common. According to one report, 21% of adults had experienced back pain in the preceding 14 days (Dunnell and Cartwright, 1972). Although most of that may not be clinically important, chronic back pain is a major cause of disability. According to Wood and Badley (1980), 'On any one day about ten thousand insured persons in Britain, something like 0.05% of the work force, have been off sick with their back troubles for more than 6 months, and 45% of these have been incapacitated for more than 2 years.'

Crook et al. (1984) undertook a community survey of chronic pain. They found that 11% of the adults surveyed had chronic pain and 5% had had acute pain within the previous 2 weeks. The low back was the commonest site for chronic pain and the head for acute pain. The Nuprin Pain Report (Taylor and Curran, 1985), a telephone survey in America, is already out of print but is summarized by Sternbach (1986). It showed that 9% of the representative sample of adult Americans had had backache on 101 or more days in the previous 12 months. Twelve percent of all the people in this survey had a pain which occurred on more than 101 days in 12 months (Sternbach, 1987).

In general practice, in psychiatric work and in neurological practice the head is the commonest site of the pain. In pain clinics, the low back is usually if not always the commonest. Whatever the exact prevalence of chronic pain, it cannot be denied that Bonica and Albe-Fessard (1976) are right when they say that chronic pain is one of the most disabling disease states.

Selection factors

In view of the widespread occurrence of pain, its frequently disabling characteristics and the many reports which testify to its association with psychiatric illness, it would be easy to conclude as is often done that emotional changes may cause pain, that pain may itself cause emotional disturbance and that frequently the pain of lesions is made far worse by emotional difficulties. All authors in this field have made such points repeatedly. Nevertheless, there is another important consideration which was noted briefly above and which deserves to be taken into account. It is the significance of the selection process.

In a study in general practice, Banks et al. (1975) asked patients to keep a sickness diary of all the incidents of sickness or ill health which they experienced. Sore throat, coryza, dizzy spells, headache, gastrointestinal disturbances, swollen feet, and numerous other ordinary symptoms were noted by the patients. Only 3% of sickness symptoms or incidents actually resulted in a general practice consultation. Upper respiratory tract infections often led patients to seek consultation but many headaches occurred which were not brought to physicians. Thus, whilst pain may occur for physical reasons, it is perhaps only reported to the doctor if the patient is emotionally concerned or realistically aware that it carries some important hazard.

Another observation in the same direction is to be found in the work of Pond and Bidwell (1959). They studied patients in general practice who had epilepsy and discovered that practitioners referred the patients to neurologists twice as often if they had a psychological disturbance associated with the epilepsy. The referral to the neurologist was thus apparently for an organic disease, but was really for help in the management of a psychological condition. The influence of processes like this on hospital samples is immeasurable. Thirdly, we can note that as clinics become more and more specialized, so the personality features of the individual patient become more and more stereotyped or characteristic for that clinic. Patients with migraine attending famous clinics were reasonably enough reported to be of a certain personality type which was called the migraine personality (Touraine and Draper, 1934; Wolff, 1948). Rees and Henryk-Gutt (1973) showed that migraine clinic patients had more evidence of neuroticism and hostility than did a group with migraine found by a survey of postoffice workers. The migraine patients in the clinic showed higher scores than controls but the meaning of this is open to question since there was only a 54% return rate for questionnaires distributed. We can very reliably conclude that clinic patients are highly selected and one should therefore be cautious about making generalisations in regard to the psychological significance of hospital patients' pain. On the other hand, one should be continuously aware that the very presence of patients at hospital with a chronic complaint may reflect a personality problem!

We also know now that patients in pain clinics are different from patients in a family practice sample with chronic pain. Crook and Tunks (1985) demonstrated that the former more often attributed their pain to injury at work, were more often unemployed because of the accompanying disability (38% compared with 2%) and had longer and more frequent attacks of pain. The pain clinic patients had many more medical attendances, more pain on activity, more limitation of their activities, more depression and anxiety and a greater incidence of job changes, law suits, disability claims and addiction to drugs or alcohol. They thought their pain worse than did patients in family practice and they did less or could do less to avoid, prevent or reduce pain. Crook and Tunks (1985) have also found that among family practice patients who had had pain for less than 3 years initially, 50% were free of pain problems after 2 years; in pain clinic patients, this figure fell to 25%. For those who initially had had pain for more than 3 years, the family practice patients were 33% improved, and the pain clinic patients 9%.

29

Psychiatric illness and chronic pain

It has to be accepted in all cases that the many reports on patients with psychiatric illness and pain come from selected samples. At present, there is no exception to this rule. Nevertheless, for those involved in treating the samples it makes perfect sense to try to understand their nature. The largest series of psychiatric patients with pain of all types is reported by Walters (1961), who described 430 cases seen privately for intractable pain. In analysing his cases, Walters distinguished three separate ways in which psychological factors can evoke pain: (1) psychogenic magnification of physical pain; (2) psychogenic muscular pain (as a result of tension); and (3) psychogenic regional pain. He proposed this last term in place of the older one of hysterical pain because these patients did not show the traditional picture of happy or contented acceptance of their symptoms; they were often anxious and depressed, though many might have some sort of conversion symptom. This writer prefers to keep the term 'hysteria' and has dropped the use of the word 'psychogenic'. Nevertheless, Walter's article demonstrates phenomena which are still found repeatedly.

Working within a psychiatric clinic in a general hospital service at Sheffield University, the present writer examined 100 patients with persistent pain without any prima facie evidence of physical causes for their illness. In these patients, who represent a fairly chronic and intractable psychiatric population, certain patterns of diagnosis and life style emerged, rather in accordance with the suggestions made previously by Engel (1951, 1959). It was found that the commonest association of persistent pain in psychiatric illness was with hysteria, anxiety neurosis and neurotic depression. These were the principal forms of psychological disturbance in which pain was a persistent and intractable problem. Although there were patients with endogenous depression and with schizophrenia who had persistent pain, the symptom was relatively less common with those diagnoses. There were also, apart from these diagnostic characteristics, a marked tendency for patients with pain to be married, to come from large families, to be engaged in relatively unskilled or semiskilled work and to be very persistent in seeking additional consultations. Within marriage, the patients with persistent pain tended to have a poor sexual adjustment and, in addition, these patients at all times showed relatively more resentment towards other people than did a comparable group of psychiatric patients without pain. There was a greater emphasis in them on bodily complaints in general and an increased history of painful illness in the past. Some similar patterns of findings emerge from a study of Pilling et al. (1967) of psychiatric patients with pain as a presenting symptom. On the Minnesota Multiphasic Personality Inventory (MMPI), these patients, when compared with controls, were found to have less depression and anxiety as presenting symptoms but much more hypochondriasis. Hysterical personality characteristics and a history of conversion symptoms were also more common in the patients with pain.

Subsequent studies from various sources have confirmed that in specialized centres the common associations of chronic pain are a hypochondriacal hysterical pattern (Smith et al., 1969; Sternbach et al., 1973; Sternbach, 1974; Wiltse and Rocchio, 1975; Blumetti and Modesti, 1976; Jamison et al., 1976; Waring et al., 1976; Pilowsky et al., 1977; Cummings et al., 1978; Kudrow and Sutkus, 1979; Chapman et al., 1979) and depression (Romano and Turner, 1985; Gupta, 1986). The reviews emphasize the importance of distinguishing between symptoms and a syndrome. Many patients with chronic pain have some symptoms of depression, such as mild irritability, fatigue or changes in mood (Pelz and Merskey, 1982). Formal studies emphasize the finding of a proportion of patients who have a depressive state which fulfills the criteria for a well-defined syndrome, such as a major affective disorder in the DSM-III-R (Diagnostic and Statistical Manual, Revised, of the American Psychiatric Association). To comply with the latter, a patient must have had at least five of the following symptoms during the same 2 week period and they must represent a change from previous functioning: depressed mood; markedly diminished interest or pleasure; significant weight loss or gain; insomnia or hypersomnia; psychomotor agitation or retardation; fatigue or loss of energy; feelings of worthlessness, etc.; diminished ability to think or concentrate or indecisiveness or recurrent thoughts of death or suicidal ideation. Of these, at least one of the symptoms must be either depressed mood or loss of interest or pleasure. These are not all the criteria or conditions for making the diagnosis but they indicate the degree of change which has to be considered in making a diagnosis of depression. By those standards, it appears that in most pain clinics the frequency of clinically recognizable depression in terms of the DSM-III-R or the International Classification of Diseases (ICD-9) will range between 30 and 65%. By contrast, the range of frequency for major affective disorder and other affective disorders in three American communities is between 2.7 and 4.6% for adult men and between 4.6 and 6.5% for adult women overall (Myers et al., 1984). The more chronic the pain, the more often the hysterical problems appear (Merskey and Spear, 1967; Crown and Crown, 1973; Sternbach et al., 1973; Kudrow and Sutkus, 1979). Also, the more highly selected the pain clinic, the more it appears that depression will be a frequent finding. This allows at least three hypotheses to be formulated, each of which is probably correct for some patients. They are: (1) the psychiatric state often causes or promotes the pain; (2) patients with hysterical or dependent personalities seek treatment most often for the pain and (3) chronic pain from lesions causes a change in personality or mood or both.

It should also be emphasized that much pain which has been called hysterical in the past could have another explanation in dysfunction arising in soft tissue. This is discussed further below.

MECHANISMS OF PAIN

The discussion of diagnosis is relevant to the understanding of the mechanisms by which pain may arise. From the physiological aspect it is possible to suppose that anxiety and depression, states of altered vigilance in the nervous system, and switching of attention will have a physiological influence ultimately translated into changes at the spinal cord level as postulated by Melzack and Wall (1965). However, it is difficult to believe from the psychiatric evidence that modification of all types of pain can be understood in terms of ascending and descending influences upon the spinal cord, although that hypothesis is undoubtedly valuable. In particular, the production of pain by psychological mechanisms other than those of depression and anxiety is hard to see in the same way as the production of pain through fluctuations at the 'gate' in response to cutaneous stimulation or activity in descending pathways from the reticular system. Some pain, indeed, much pain, almost certainly arises from an anxiety-tension mechanism of the conventional type which is often propounded. It is often suggested that excessive contraction of muscles because of tension gives rise to the accumulation of metabolites which are not carried away sufficiently quickly by the circulation, and thence to the stimulation of susceptible nerve endings which give rise to the experience of pain. This experience in turn makes patients who are already anxious more anxious, and they then become more tense and their pain increases, and so forth. This vicious-circle theory of chronic-tension pain or pain due to anxiety almost certainly has some truth in it, but is not the whole truth. Many clinical instances arise in which the tension theory is inadequate to account for continuing pain for which there is no organic basis. For example, instances occur in which patients experience pain which one can apparently see as deriving directly from their mental processes. Moreover, the frequency with which hysterical symptoms are seen to occur in relation to chronic pain of psychological origin makes it likely that the tension mechanism is relatively less important than is often supposed in perhaps the majority of patients with chronic pain due to psychological illness.

Thus, there is only a small correlation between muscle tension and anxiety and a similar small correlation between anxiety and pain (Sainsbury and Gibson, 1954). There is more muscle tension in migraineurs than in tension headache patients (Bakal and Kaganov, 1977) and the association of frontalis tension with headache accounts for as little as 5% of the variance (Martin and Mathews, 1978; Epstein et al., 1978); further, headache intensity correlates with a hysterical pattern of response rather than with muscle tension (Harper and Steger, 1978). With the foregoing qualifications, the two main acceptable mechanisms of psychological causation of pain are thus: first, anxiety tension and second, hysterical conversion, or at least pain due to the patient's thoughts, even if one does not wish to say that the mechanism is always a hysterical one. A third mechanism is that of hallucinations, but this is rare and not often of practical importance even to psychiatrists.

One other mechanism which has not been well explained may be postulated on the basis of the gate theory. It is frequently observed that patients who have a state of anxiety experience much greater pain from lesions than would otherwise be expected. This sometimes happens in circumstances when the tension pain mechanism is not applicable. A reduction of anxiety also leads to a considerable reduction in pain. Perhaps this is the situation where the gate theory type of explanation may be most relevant to pain due to psychological causes. It is plausible to suppose that pain which is related to some existing activity in peripheral nerve pathways and in the spinal cord may be greatly increased as a result of heightened arousal in the patient, so that an effect is transmitted through descending pathways to the spinal cord, thus increasing the abnormal activity which itself is ultimately the basis for the experience of pain consciousness. This explanation remains speculative, but it is certainly a fact that pain in clinical practice is frequently much relieved by measures which ease the patient's anxiety about his condition.

Soft tissue pain

A number of pains which affect regions of the body have been regarded as hysterical, but they might be soft tissue pain, particularly when the pain is as diffuse as in fibrositis, which may be assumed to have an organic basis. In the past, many of these conditions have been regarded as hysterical, particularly if they were related to a claim for compensation. There are some problems that emphasise the need for caution in the diagnosis of hysteria. First it should be pointed out that the mere absence of physical evidence for the cause of the pain does not justify a diagnosis of hysteria, which should always be made on the basis of positive evidence. In cases of paralysis and some other types of loss of function, neurological examination has revealed positive evidence that the patient is able to do things which he or she thinks are not feasible. In the case of pain itself, that opportunity does not exist. On the contrary, there are probably certain signs which are traditionally taken to be evidence of hysteria and which are misleading in regard to patients with pain. These signs include unwillingness to use a limb (which may be due to a conscious recognition that it hurts to do so) and so-called non-anatomical complaints of pain or impaired sensitivity. Wall (1984) summarized evidence that at least some cells in the dorsal horn may, on occasion, serve to receive input from the whole of the limb. Thus, as Fishbain et al. (1986) point out, the issue of non-dermatomal sensory abnormalities and their significance may need more research. Pain arising from parts of a limb not directly affected by a lesion may nevertheless be a form of referred pain due to the involvement of adjoining parts by an irritable focus. Impaired sensation in the region of pain may also be a result of increased threshold due directly to the actions of noxious stimulation or due indirectly to the effects of distraction because of noxious stimulation.

Problems with hysteria also exist because of misdiagnoses. Several conditions which are basically physical have been mistaken for hysteria or diagnosed as malingering or as a psychiatric disorder. The writer has known mistakes of this sort to occur with pain from ectopia cerebelli, facial pain with dyskinetic movements, brain tumour, thoracic outlet syndrome, muscular dystrophy and prechronic paroxysmal hemicrania. A number of conditions which were regarded as hysterical, such as dyskinesias, hemi-facial spasm, spasmodic torticollis, globus hystericus in many instances and some cases of vertigo, are rarely considered now to be hysterical.

Further, there is increasing reason to believe that fibrositis or fibromyalgia may provide a diagnosis, and consistent evidence for this has been brought forward by Smythe and his colleagues (Smythe, 1985). Moreover, localized myofascial syndromes have also been recognized increasingly (Littlejohn, 1986; IASP, 1986). Such relatively subtle syndromes, which depend for their recognition on advances or improvements in clinical methods, may often have been misdiagnosed as hysteria in the past, and the possibility still exists of such a misdiagnosis. We thus have to consider that a number of the soft tissue pains which were previously classed as hysteria may be more correctly attributable to subtle organic syndromes which are being increasingly recognized, such as fibrositis.

Even if fibrositis has a physical basis, it has an interesting interaction with the psychological state. Moldofsky and his colleagues have obtained evidence that patients with pain, stiffness and disturbed sleep show simultaneous occurrence of alpha rhythms with delta in non-REM sleep.

Similar pain and stiffness were produced in normal controls by wakening them repeatedly. Moldofsky et al. (1975) postulated an alteration of serotonin metabolism both in the sleep disorder and in the 'fibrositic' symptoms. Moldofsky and Warsh (1978) also found an inverse relationship between free plasma tryptophan and subjective pain in the syndrome. Findings of this sort point to an obscure but potentially important link between emotional disturbance, arousal and pain.

Factors modifying pain

With these causes of pain in mind it is now convenient to consider the other known circumstances which will alter or reduce pain. Many of these have been described repeatedly and noteworthy reviews are those by Barber (1959), Beecher (1959) and Sternbach (1968). A detailed discussion of these factors also appears in Merskey and Spear (1967). Beecher has particularly emphasized the way in which the circumstances of wounding give rise to more or less pain. Those to whom the pain has some advantage – as for example soldiers able to leave the battlefield – may have less pain than those to whom the wound is a wholly unwarranted interruption of their normal life. The latter is the situation which prevails in civilians undergoing routine surgery. Anxiety is generally recognized as increasing pain and, therefore, factors which diminish anxiety may be expected to diminish pain and, on the other hand, excitement or aggression may leave subjects oblivious of gross trauma. Football players, soldiers in battle and other men engaged in active occupations are often observed not to notice pain from quite severe blows until the match or the battle is over. These comments on mortal combat and on the battles of footballers require qualification. The types of injury in the soldiers whom Beecher studied may have been somewhat different from the types of injury experienced by civilians. Most of the soldiers' wounds could have been from high velocity missiles. Further, there is reason to believe that acute trauma, even in civilian life, is not necessarily painful initially. Thus, Melzack, Wall and Ty (1982) studied new cases of trauma presenting at an emergency department and found that as many as one-third did not complain of pain despite the occurrence of substantial physical lesions. The pain may, however, have developed later in most or all of these cases.

Placebo techniques in pharmacology have repeatedly been shown to reduce pain (Beecher, 1959) and supportive and suggestive measures such as psychotherapy, psychoprophylaxis in childbirth and the use of hypnosis are regularly associated with reports that pain is lessened. The exact significance of the effects in hypnosis will be considered shortly. Egbert et al. (1964) showed that demands for postoperative analgesia were halved in patients who had been given suitable preoperative encouragement compared to the control group. Jellinek (1946) found over 30 years ago that 52% of patients with headache were relieved by placebos. Certain sorts of psychiatric treatment, for example, phenothiazines, antidepressants, ECT and even leucotomy, have all been reported at times as being effective in the treatment of pain. Accepting that these relationships do exist, we can consider the effects of particular individual treatments. Before doing so, however, the psychodynamics of pain and the effect of chronic pain of physical origin on the emotional state require attention.

Psychodynamic aspects

A chapter by Blumer (1975) gives a vivid account of the more profound psychodynamics of pain of psychological origin. He builds upon the ideas previously developed by a number of analysts and by Engel (1951, 1959) which were evaluated by Merskey and Spear (1967). Patterns of denial and sadomasochistic relationships appear prominent in his patients, as well as a self-sacrificing life-style combined with dependent attitudes and relentless activity. Patients of this sort include a number who seek inappropriate surgery and are often very difficult to manage. An example of one of Blumer's patients is a 33-year-old farmer's wife who had neck pain for 10 years. The onset of the pain coincided with divorce from an abusive first husband and remarriage to a 'wonderful' second husband. Despite two operations on her neck, she continued to practice horseriding and shooting. Another of his patients with pain had three husbands, none of whom treated her well and two of whom were violent. Her own father was an alcoholic who beat her mother frequently. She was constantly selfless for others: parents, husbands, children.

The occurrence of denial is perhaps one of the most frequent of these dynamic mechanisms. One of my own patients who had transvestite interests never declared them to me, despite a number of attempts to persuade him to discuss the topic. It is likely, although there is as yet no proof by controlled investigations, that there is a significant association between character traits such as those mentioned above and the development of persistent pain. Cases of this sort differ somewhat from patients with other hysterical symptoms in that the pain rarely solves an acute conflict but seems to arise because of more long-standing personality problems or environmental stress, particularly in regard to relationships with other people. Their tendency to deny any current maladjustment makes it important to enquire particularly carefully into the marital and social background of all patients with chronic pain who do not have an obvious physical cause and for whom operative intervention is being considered. Such enquiry will normally commence with a psychiatric interview and extend to interviews with a spouse or a near relation. The difficulty of persuading such patients to accept referral for psychiatric opinion may be great but has to be weighed against the hazards of intervention without the benefit of such highly relevant information. Pain clinics which operate with a psychiatrist as a normal part of the team generally find it possible to explain to patients that the interview is a routine matter on the grounds that all possible aspects of such a long-standing illness need to be considered and that no matter what the psychiatrist finds, both he and the rest of the team will still regard the pain as 'real'. If psychological factors are so important in the production of chronic pain then personality testing or psychiatric help ought to be valuable to the surgeon in selecting appropriate patients who will or will not respond to surgery for pain. Psychiatrists have little experience in such work and without it might well not be as successful as surgeons who operate intuitively. However, systematic psychiatric work ought, in theory, to assist in the choice of candidates for surgery. One brief report which supports this idea is provided by Wiltse (1975), who describes significant discrimination with the MMPI hysteria and hypochondriasis scales between patients who had a good result and patients who had a bad result from low back surgery. Smith and Duerksen (1979) have likewise demonstrated some predictive value for the MMPI in relation to surgery for low back pain.

Emotional effects of continued pain

Regardless of whether pain originates for psychological or physical reasons, it is likely that its continuation will cause secondary disturbances in the lives of the patients affected. There is in general an impression that severe chronic pain of physical origin disturbs the individual's life more. Indeed, if one sees pain of psychological origin as contributing to the solution of some problems, this is hardly surprising, since pain of physical origin will usually produce fresh problems without any accrued benefit to the individual. It is suggested that the condition which arises in patients referred for psychiatric opinion, but who already have a physical cause for their pain, is thus somewhat different from patients who have no physical cause. In the author's experience, such patients tend not to have hysterical symptoms; there is much more often a lack of evidence of previous neuroticism, but there is a good deal of current emotional disturbance manifesting itself as anxiety and depression with some resentment perhaps and, if the pain is severe, demanding attitudes. Many of these effects must be seen as secondary to the continuation of unsolved, unpleasant illness for which adequate relief has not been provided. Swerdlow (1972) notes that the persistence of pain produces psychological changes in the patient which are very difficult to reverse. For example, patients with postherpetic neuralgia are often worn out and very depressed by the intractable nature of the pain. Taub (personal communication, 1972) observes similarly that patients in a neurological clinic with pain of physical origin tend to present a picture initially of anxiety and depression.

The resentment that some patients with pain feel has been shown to be significantly increased in psychiatric patients with pain (Merskey, 1965) and is also notable in some of those with physical causes for their pain; it may be understood as having certain obvious causes: first of all, doctors who have failed to cure patients become more offhand or are themselves disappointed, and difficulties arise between them and the individual who still seeks relief. More important probably is the fact that pain itself gives rise to irritability and resentment. It has been noted with rats (O'Kelly and Steckley, 1939) that if an electric current is put across the bars of the floor of the cage the rats may turn round and bite each other. Aggression is one of the main responses which occur in the presence of trauma that gives rise to pain. The substantial evidence on this is reviewed by Ulrich (Ulrich et al., 1965; Ulrich, 1966). Aggression in response to pain is presumably part of the 'fight or flight' mechanism, the alternative being retreat. It is not surprising then that people with chronic pain become irritable and perhaps resentful and difficult. Woodforde and Merskey (1972) collected some evidence that patients with pain of physical origin actually become more anxious, more depressed and more subject to signs of neuroticism than patients whose pain has no physical cause and who are known to have psychiatric illness. These patients with physical causes for their pain do, however, tend to see themselves as being persons who in the past were well adjusted, stable, successful and well controlled. They have a high score on the 'L' scale of the Eysenck personality inventory. This scale was at first thought to indicate a tendency to falsify the account of the individual's previous personality by 'faking good'. Other evidence (Morgenstern, 1967; Bond, 1971) indicates that high 'L' scores are associated with physical disability. In the light of these findings, Woodforde and Merskey (1972) suggested that high 'L' scores in patients with pain of organic origin, accompanied by raised neuroticism scores, have the following explanation: they represent a compensatory favourable evalua-tion of their own personalities by individuals struggling to keep themselves stable in the face of damage already done to their personalities and in the face of increas-ing anxiety and depression as a result of their suffering. Weir Mitchell (1872) noted mood changes after nerve injuries, and emotional changes may be anticipat-ed in almost anyone who suffers from chronic pain (Bonica, 1967). This is true both on common-sense grounds and in practice. Occasionally these changes will take the form of increased drive and persistence whilst making the best possible adjustment; more often some increased neurotic responses will be evident.

Because of the impressive reasons which have accumulated in the literature to justify the view that pain may result primarily from emotional maladjustment, the alternative possibility that the emotional changes are consequent upon the organic illness has been somewhat neglected. However, further work emphasises the need to take both situations into account. For example, Sternbach et al. (1973) showed that chronic pain patients had increased hysteria, depression and hypochondriasis scores on the MMPI compared with patients with acute (back) pain, suggesting (although not proving) that persistence of the unpleasant disability may give rise to emotional change. Kertesz and Kormos (1976) noted as much or more evidence of neurosis in patients with back pain and relevant physical signs as in those with less convincing evidence of physical disease. Sternbach and Timmermans (1975) conversely showed a reduction in neuroticism in patients whose pain was relieved by back surgery.

A change of view has also occurred with respect to rheumatoid arthritis, an ill-ness in which chronic pain is common. It was formerly held that a special person-ality contributed to the development of the illness, but Wolff (1971) concludes from a review that this concept is unwarranted and Crown and Crown (1973) have shown that patients with early rheumatoid arthritis are not particularly neurotic. It seems reasonable to conclude that the tendency for patients with chronic pain to have emotional changes is attributable to a significant extent to the physical disturbance from which they suffer.

It is not surprising that many such patients see themselves as having been for-merly fit and able and may react with depression or protest to their current, never-ending plight. We have tended in the past to ignore this and the fact that pain

38

can provoke irritability or aggressive responses which are quite important biologically. To continue to accept pain quietly when it is due to an internal lesion causing disease is probably helpful. To continue to accept it quietly when it has an external agent in the form of an aggressor will often be unhelpful in the preservation of the individual or species. Flight or, not infrequently, aggression may thus be considered appropriate responses to chronic pain, and since flight is not easy to arrange, aggression is the more common outcome. The management of patients with pain obviously requires an understanding of this matter.

ASSESSMENT

The range of psychiatric illnesses and the diagnostic possibilities are such that no attempt will be made here to offer a comprehensive guide to the assessment of psychological factors in relation to pain. However, some simple principles can be stated and should prove useful to the practising clinician. The first issue is to establish the presence or absence of a psychiatric diagnosis. The conditions with which the practitioner in the pain clinic should be most familiar are depression and personality disorder. The former is usually quite easy to diagnose. Personality disorder is often difficult for practising psychiatrists as well as for other specialists or general practitioners.

In looking for evidence of depression, the physician will seek to establish whether there is an altered mood and then whether there are changes in the above-mentioned features, such as the ability to concentrate and remember, a tendency to blame oneself or to dwell upon suicidal thoughts and alterations in the vegetative state of the individual, such as retardation and change of weight and the pattern of sleep. Effects on the latter two items should not be confused with the effects of pain, and one can only say that disturbed sleep is a sign of depression after establishing that it is not a secondary effect of pain.

Establishing evidence of personality disorder is much more complex. In general, individuals who have led a stable and effective life will either be free of the obvious patterns of dependency and attention-seeking, which are sometimes held to characterize patients with chronic pain, or will merely show obsessional phenomena with marked conscientiousness and sometimes concern over relatively trivial detail. The degree of psychological evidence should be such that it can be appraised by anyone with a modicum of experience as proportionate to the pain with which it is associated. If it is proportionate, the question arises as to which effect is primary and which one secondary. A simple examination of the date of onset of two conditions can be revealing and must be taken very seriously. Individuals who were always upset and troubled prior to developing their pain may well have developed it as a result of their emotional state, particularly if there was a major stress just prior to the onset of the pain. On the other hand, individuals who were free from maladjustment and who develop a significant physical illness can be expected to show emotional changes in due course, and those changes will be secondary.

Of course, the most difficult instances arise where the individual is hypochondriacal or dependent prior to the onset of the current main symptom pattern but also sustains some physical change which may have contributed to the pain. In these cases, the evaluation of the state of the individual may indeed require specialist support or help. At other times, it can be attempted at least on a pragmatic basis by any moderately experienced practitioner.

In assessing psychologically patients with pain, the practitioner should go through the usual diagnostic process that is employed by psychiatrists or by general practitioners. He should first of all establish the significant and troublesome complaints and then proceed to establish information about the individual's past life and adjustment. The family history and particularly evidence of deprivation or ill-treatment in childhood are relevant. There is an increased tendency for patients to have psychiatric illness with pain as a consequence if they have experienced deprivation of care in childhood, marked separation from parents or ill-treatment by foster parents or other early psychological traumata. The level of achievement at school and social adjustment, the number of marriages or sexual relationships, the frequency and nature of past illness and the level of achievement at work and consistency of employment all help in estimating the premorbid features of the individual who is now affected by pain.

With regard to current symptoms, the psychological assessment will take note of the use or abuse of drugs, as will the general physical assessment. It will also look at the frequency of signs of depression and of hysterical complaints (which are relatively hard to identify) and the way the patient uses symptoms to solve problems. Information can often be obtained from a member of the family which will be helpful and assist in making decisions as well. At a later phase, interaction with members of the family may be important in treatment.

TREATMENTS

Some specific treatments

Before considering the general psychiatric approach to patients, some specific psychiatric treatments will be reviewed. It needs to be said that the application of such treatments is only appropriate after all proper steps have been taken to establish the diagnosis, whether physical or psychiatric. Further, some psychiatric illnesses respond to specific treatments and the treatment of pain due to them is thus the treatment of the basic disorder.

HYPNOTHERAPY

Hypnosis, as already mentioned, is sometimes thought of as being an important treatment which might be helpful in the management of chronic pain. It is more likely that it is unsatisfactory because it is insufficiently effective as a specific measure. This judgement depends partly upon experience in the use of hypnosis and the reports thereon and partly upon one's appraisal of the nature of hypnosis (Merskey, 1971). The reports are quite straightforward. There are a few limited accounts of the use of hypnosis in the management of pain from neoplasms (e.g., Dorcus and Kirkner, 1948; Sacerdote, 1962, 1965, 1966). It is clear from these reports that relief is rarely complete where there is an important physical cause of pain and frequently it is of only modest proportions. For the relief to be helpful, treatment has to be continued frequently, and at least one report (Dorcus and Kirkner, 1948) indicates that this is more than a little strain upon the hypnotist. This is not surprising if one looks with a critical eye at the claim that hypnosis can relieve severe pain of organic origin. Barber (1959), who has carefully reviewed the reports of operations performed under hypnosis, provides a convincing series of illustrations to suggest that the effects of hypnotism are rarely, if ever, to abolish completely pain from operations. What seems to happen is that most patients undergoing operations under hypnosis experience discomfort which is evidenced by groans or even by occasional statements at the time of the operation. After the operation, when asked to recount their experience, they either deny pain or say that it was 'not too bad'. At other times, people who produce this type of story about their experience can be made to admit that they experienced much pain but did not wish to disappoint the doctor (as in natural childbirth) (Mandy et al., 1952). In a sympathetic and careful review of the literature on operations under hypnotic analgesia, Hilgard and Hilgard (1975) note that claims for the successful use of hypnosis as the sole anaesthetic agent range from an unlikely maximum of 10% to a more cautious estimate of 1%. Reports, therefore, of the effective relief of severe pain by hypnosis ought to be treated with considerable reserve.

It is not part of our purpose here to explain the nature of hypnotism, but the observations quoted above fit very well with the analysis of hypnotism that has been made on an experimental basis over a number of years by Barber (1959). This analysis has been summarized as follows: 'Hypnosis is a manoeuvre in which the subject and hypnotist have an implicit agreement that certain events (e.g., paralysis, hallucination, amnesia) will occur, either during a special procedure or later in accordance with the hypnotist's instructions. Both try hard to put this agreement into effect and adopt appropriate behavioural roles and the subject uses mechanisms of denial to report on the events in accordance with the implicit agreements. This situation is used to implement various motives, whether therapeutic or otherwise, on the part of both participants. There is no trance state, no detectable cerebral physiological change, and only such peripheral physiological responses as may be produced equally by non-hypnotic suggestion or other emotional changes' (Merskey, 1971).

In the light of this summary of available evidence, it is understandable that reports of the effective relief of severe pain by hypnotism are treated with reserve. On the other hand, any procedure involving suggestion will relieve moderate pain at least to a moderate extent on occasion, and hypnotism is no less effective than other methods of suggestion and encouragement in inclining people to be less anxious, more calm and therefore less subject to pain from modest degrees of noxious stimulation. For practical purposes, the writer does not regard hypnotism as worth using in anyone with pain of physical origin and very rarely in patients with pain that is psychological in origin. In general, it is also true that the more severe and overwhelming the pain of physical origin, the less likely it is to be amenable to relief by methods employing suggestion.

Investigations of the relief of severe pain tend to be somewhat more reliable than those of the relief of mild or moderate pain, since the possibility of placebo mechanisms is more relevant in the latter instances. To be able to discount a placebo mechanism is harder when patients are treated for mild pains than when they are treated for severe ones. The more intense the stimulus, the less relief is usually available by placebo methods.

BIOFEEDBACK

In recent years there has been growth in the use of behaviour therapy techniques in psychiatry. Such techniques have, so far, not been found to be of much value for pain, but out of this has arisen a growing and promising interest in the possibility of using biofeedback to treat a variety of somatic conditions, ranging from spasticity to migraine.

Another factor encouraging the trial of biofeedback in conditions such as migraine has been the work of Neal Miller (1974) and his school, who have produced evidence to support the view that autonomic conditioning, e.g., of heart rate, blood pressure and vascular mechanism, might occur. Anyone interested in exploring these topics in detail should consult Miller (1974) for a general survey of their place in psychiatry and medicine. The annual manual on biofeedback published by the Aldine Press and the publications of the Biofeedback Research Society are also valuable sources of information, as well as the usual psychosomatic and psychological journals.

At its simplest, the idea of biofeedback implies knowledge of results, a concept which Miller points out was known to Thorndike, and which has always been used by good teachers. Applied to a state of muscle tension, it means using the instrumentation which is now readily available to show a patient when he is relaxing or contracting a particular group of muscles. With electronic amplification, it is now easy to demonstrate muscle contraction as variable noise, proportionate to the amount of contraction, and many people have learned how to contract or relax individual muscles. Relaxation of single, neuromuscular units has even been reported, with a concomitant decline in the activity of neighbouring units (Smith et al., 1974).

Muscular relaxation has long been established, at least since the work of Jacobson (1929), as a possible method for the relief of tension headache. Benson et al. (1974) report an apparent, albeit limited use in some migraine patients of relaxation achieved by transcendental meditation. It has always been hard, however, to disentangle any specific effects of relaxation, transcendental meditation and other procedures like overt suggestion from those of calming and the relief of anxiety, not to mention placebo responses. Biofeedback in theory offers a way to improve muscular relaxation techniques, although it is clearly difficult to provide it with 'blind' controls.

The past literature on biofeedback tended to suggest that it could be used to enable the individual to gain control over unconscious or autonomic functions. This is now relatively little believed. Miller (1974) was unable to replicate some of his earlier work on which this belief was based. This is not to say that the pulse rate or blood pressure might not be somewhat conditioned with the help of biofeedback, but this may be more by learning tricks of relaxation than by a direct interaction between the autonomic state and some subjective awareness of it and the biofeedback information.

As for pain, at least three reviews concur in the view that, in general, biofeedback is no more effective than relaxation (Jessup et al., 1979; Turk et al., 1979; Neuchterlein and Holroyd, 1980). Sovak and colleagues (1978) presented evidence which suggests that some subgroups of patients provided with the hand-warming technique for migraine may benefit relatively more than from other measures, and Sternbach (1980) argued that studies of biofeedback should focus on well-defined symptoms and groups of patiens in which case the treatment might be more effective than other methods. Some evidence in favour of this view has been produced by Blanchard and his colleagues (Blanchard et al., 1980; Blanchard and Andrasik, 1982; Blanchard et al., 1983), who showed that if those who fail at relaxation training are studied, biofeedback can help to produce a further significant improvement in something more than one-third of patients with headache. Stenn (1987) points out that biofeedback may still be working in these cases by its motivational impact.

OPERANT CONDITIONING

The covert motives of some pain patients and the pain therapist have been wittily discussed by Sternbach (1974), who, taking up the examples of Szasz (1968) and Berne (1964), shows how certain pain patients use their pain as a form of interpersonal manipulation. This may happen, amongst others, in those patients who have strong masochistic needs, those who seek relief by narcotics and those who have an incentive to be regarded as disabled, e.g., those who have, for unconscious reasons, adopted the sick role and those who are in receipt of compensation payments.

Sternbach points out that, after analysis of the situation, such patients must be offered realistic and potentially gratifying alternatives to the pain life-style, or they have no reason to get well. An alternative which he advocates (Sternbach and Rusk, 1973) is to set a treatment contract with goals. He draws attention in this context to the substantial differences known to exist between ethnic groups in tolerating or inhibiting pain complaints and argues that this offers to the therapist the opportunity to intervene in the learned behaviour patterns which cause or exacerbate the pain. For this purpose, Fordyce (Fordyce et al., 1968; Fordyce, 1974, 1976) and Greenhoot and Sternbach (1974) have described behavioural modification techniques based upon operant conditioning. The essence of these approaches is to encourage ('reinforce') behaviour such as activity which is held to be desirable but is associated by the patient with pain and to discourage ('negatively reinforce') complaints of pain and the resort by the patient to rest. Group therapy which deals with the patient's 'games' is also recommended.

A number of reports give estimates of success with behavioural approaches. Cairns et al. (1976) use the operant approach in the second phase of treatment of patients with chronic low back pain. In the first phase, orthopaedic assessment takes place, regional blocks may be given and narcotic and psychotropic drugs are prescribed if necessary. Patients are asked to set goals for their lives, including vocational, domestic and recreational objectives. The patients are regularly involved in group discussions which family members attend. These patients came from a severely disabled group with a mean of 1.5 surgical operations, 37 months off work, and 8.7 years of illness. Personality testing disclosed MMPI, Hs, and Hy scores all elevated above 70, i.e., by more than 2 standard deviations. A postal survey of 100 patients carried out at an average of 10 months after discharge elicited replies from 90, of whom 70% were improved and 74% had not sought further treatment. Seventy-five percent were working at follow-up and were involved in a training programme. Ignelzi et al. (1977) reported on 54 patients who had been treated in a multidisciplinary programme which included vocational rehabilitation, physical therapy, operant conditioning, relaxation therapy and group treatment. Three years after discharge, the patients' pain estimate and analgesic intake were still significantly below the levels on admission and their degrees of activity were still increased. As in the report by Cairns et al. (1976), these patients who were first described in 1974 (Greenhoot and Sternbach, 1974) had MMPI elevations over 70 for the first three scales when they entered the programme. Roberts and Reinhardt (1980) report the only comparative study using operant treatment. Twenty-six treated patients were compared with 20 who were rejected for treatment by a clinic team and with 12 who refused treatment. These three groups had similar MMPI score patterns but there were significant initial differences between them and other patients in the same clinic. The three groups scored lower on depression and hypochondriasis scales and higher on the ego strength scale than the remainder. The 26 patients in the treated group had 4.5 operations and the other groups had 2.8 and 2.6 operations on average. The treated group was using an average number of four drugs, the others average numbers of 2.6 and 4.8 drugs. In contrast to this pattern of more previous treatment in the group of 26, those who were rejected for treatment had a shorter history of pain than the treated patients or those who refused treatment. The spouses of successfully treated patients, interestingly enough, had lower scores at baseline on the hypochondriasis and hysteria scales of the MMPI than did the spouses of unsuccessfully treated patients. At follow-up ranging from 1 to 8 years, 77% of the treated participants were leading normal lives without medication for pain compared with one patient in the other two groups. The program of treatment includes a contingency contract, identification of pain behaviours which are ignored by the treatment team, physical therapy, occupational therapy and nursing service exercises, reduction of pain-related medications through a 'pain cocktail' and work opportunities as similar as possible to those expected to follow discharge. In addition, the family is taught how to identify pain behaviours, to consistently ignore them and to reinforce activity and other 'well' behaviours. As a result of this programme, striking results were obtained, as already mentioned, and there were also many improvements in indices of disturbance, such as the use of other medications, resort to hospital care, and scores on the hypochondriasis depression and hysteria scores of the MMPI.

The groups overall which were compared had been selected from a total population of 124 patients. These very good results were evidently obtained in a sub-set of the total population which was considered for treatment. In fact, only 20 of the original number can be regarded as having improved and only 26 of the original number were treated so that the real success rate in the total population considered is relatively small. Of course, no treatment should be expected to apply to all patients indiscriminately. However, it appears so far from the pilot studies of operant treatment in selected populations that they have been applied only to a very small group of the total of patients with chronic pain who are apparently untreatable in other respects. Moreover, even in this last excellent study, the report describes the simultaneous use of multiple approaches even though it is called a pure operant programme. Such a practice is in line with the first priority of medicine which is to do all one can for the patient. However, it seems that there is no evidence that operant conditioning works alone, without the support of other treatments. The same probably also applies to many other treatments in medicine and makes assessment of this matter extremely difficult (Sternbach, 1981).

Aronoff et al. (1983) have compared the results from multidisciplinary units for chronic pain and concluded that there were many difficulties with their reports. These include variations in the samples, the instruments employed for measurement, the times of follow-up and dependence on memory of events other than assessments at the appropriate time. There was also a problem in finding adequate comparison groups. The findings by Aronoff and his colleagues quoted earlier have an obvious message in this context: the source of the patients is extremely important.

Perhaps the major problem with operant conditioning is that it seems to neglect the experience of the patient. There need be no objection to recognizing that for the patient and his family to dwell on or cherish his (or her) sufferings is unhelpful and leads in the wrong direction, i.e., away from attempts at rehabilitation. When, however, an individual is continuously aware of unpleasant sensations which are related to his movements, which attack him whether or not he is thinking about them and which come on whenever he tries to make a step forward or a fresh movement, it is hard to suppose that this pain is likely to respond in itself to a program which ignores it. Unwanted behaviour may be diminished but it seems very unlikely that the pain itself will go away. There is always the risk of the patient feeling, quite rightly, that his pain persists but he is not allowed to talk about it. This is as much true in patients with back pain for whom this approach is most often recommended, as with others. On the other hand, some patients with back pain whom I have studied find sustained sitting difficult and indeed are more willing to be up and about than may be recognized. To me, the least acceptable aspect of the operant conditioning approach is the belief that the pain in question is both learnt and unlearnt. This view, which characterizes the stronger components of the method, is perhaps only of theoretical significance and yet it is highly undesirable to accept a theoretical position which leads one into erroneous clinical judgements. For several years, there has been a view that pain might in certain circumstances be learned. For example, Melzack and Scott (1957) demonstrated that puppies experience difficulty in appreciating noxious stimulation if they are deprived of sensory experience of the world around them in the first year of life. Nathan (1967) presented evidence that mnemic traces for pain might exist, particularly for direct and specific injuries. Much of this evidence was based upon the work of Reynolds and Hutchins (1948) on dental fillings with general anaesthetic or with local anaesthetic, when it became clear that people who had had dental fillings under a general anaesthetic were much more liable to experience pain related to those fillings subsequently than people who had had the dental fillings under a local anaesthetic. I argued myself that there was some modest evidence for the development of the ability to feel pain (Merskey, 1970). However, none of this comes anywhere near the proposition that major continuing pains can be learnt and unlearnt as a result of manoeuvres in the adult environment. Apart from the fact that it is highly questionable that such learning has ever been demonstrated, it is also easy to suppose there are alternative and probably more appropriate formulations to deal with the matter. On other occasions (Merskey, 1974, 1979), I have described a patient who developed pain as a result of an emotional conflict. Such cases occur in clinical practice quite often, although they are not the commonest form of pain of psychological origin. Many other authors have described them, e.g., Engel (1959). His patient had pain which was sustained by specific unconscious difficulty and when the latter was removed her pain was easily relieved with hypnosis. The notion of learnt pain takes no notice of the whole idea of pain which is due to motives. It is of course possible for learning theorists, if they wish, to include the idea of a drive in their hypotheses. Their notion of reward of which the individual may not be overtly aware is actually very close to that of psychodynamic theories. Nevertheless, the current theories of operant conditioning for the treatment of pain do not take these possibilities into account, and seem to ignore them almost wilfully.

For theoretical and practical reasons, the operant conditioning approach, as currently stated, thus seems to be unsatisfactory, partial and limited to a small population. It is, however, important to recognize that what the operant pain theorists are talking about is something which is known to other clinicians by different names. To Walters, it is at times 'psychogenic regional pain', to the writer, it is a mixture of anxiety and hysteria as soft tissue pain, to others it is 'compensationitis' and so forth. The proposition which is significant and relevant to all practitioners is that patients with these sorts of characteristics will not get better with conventional physical treatments, except as part of a placebo response. Many of them will also not do well with antidepressants or psychotropic medication and they are best suited by a rehabilitative approach which minimizes the production of dependent attitudes.

On the surface, the conditioning element of this approach appears mechanical and unsympathetic. In practice, it seems to do good in terms of rehabilitation but the reported benefits cannot be linked to it alone. Moreover, despite the skill and perception with which it has been applied, it can rarely, indeed only sometimes fortuitously, remove the fundamental motives which such patients may have to persist in their illness. One benefit of the emphasis on the occurrence of 'pain games', however, is the reminder to the doctor not to persist with potentially dangerous remedies; in other words, not to be out-manoeuvred into prescribing either drugs or surgery. In addition, Fordyce et al. (1981) have shown systematically that exercise helps to reduce pain or the behaviour related to it. It has long been recognized that exercise could be beneficial in some cases of pain, just as increased activity in the presence of stiffness which itself was produced by over-activity may help to abate the aching discomfort and incapacity. In clinical practice it remains very difficult at times to know which patients are going to benefit from exercise and which will be made worse. It is certainly true, and has been recognized since the days of John Hilton (1863), that rest is also beneficial for pain.

The patients with whom we are concerned at this point are undoubtedly therapeutically intractable and the approaches described provide an alternative repertoire of counter-responses by therapists to patients. However, there is no evidence that they are any more helpful than less elaborately stated schemes of management which implicitly make use of the same principle by encouraging patients to take up alternative interests, discouraging inactivity or brooding over symptoms and frowning upon claims for medication whilst responding favourably to efforts at occupational rehabilitation.

COGNITIVE THERAPY

Cognitive approaches to the management of pain have been much studied lately. Beck (1976) and others have demonstrated an attractive approach to the management of mood disorders, particularly depression, the theory of which depends in essence upon teaching the patient to revise his thoughts, after which, if the treatment is successful, he will feel different. There is evidence that in the management of mild or moderate depression this approach is as effective as the use of antidepressants (Rush et al., 1977; Blackburn et al., 1981). Accordingly, it deserves to be taken seriously and has begun to be applied to pain. So far, the great majority of the work on the cognitive treatment of pain has been done in the experimental laboratory. The theoretical basis of these approaches for pain is reviewed by Chaves and Barber (1974) and by Meichenbaum and Turk (1976) and some of the results to date are evaluated by Tan (1982), Turner and Chapman (1984) and Turk et al. (1984). In general, cognitive therapy emphasizes ways of handling the subjective experience and seeks to offer 'coping strategies'. In a very interesting pilot study, Khatami and Rush (1978) provided three major types of treatment to each of six patients. The first section of the treatment involved relaxation, biofeedback and autohypnosis; the second part involved cognitive treatment; the third part was based on management of the patient's relationships with his family to prevent secondary gain. It was nicely demonstrated that each phase contributed to the final results, with some patients responding particularly to one element of the package and others to one of the remaining elements. Formal trials of cognitive therapy for pain have been reported by Rybstein-Blinchik (1979) and by Holroyd et al. (1977); both provide controlled evidence in its favour. The next phase of psychological work on pain patients is thus likely to be marked by the spread of clinical studies of cognitive therapy.

It has long been known that both attention and distraction may modify pain, for example, Morgenstern (1964). It will be valuable to see how treatments which combine or contrast thinking about the pain, distraction from the pain, distancing oneself from it and so forth will affect chronic pain. The writer's guess is that mild to moderate pain will respond best as was found by Melzack et al. (1963) in their study of sound and pain; patients in whom psychological factors are important may well only respond at a placebo level, whilst those with definite lesions will probably get most benefit, even if the latter is limited.

AMOUNTS OF BENEFIT FROM THERAPY

All the psychological treatments carry a so-called 'non-specific' benefit. This is often confused with a placebo response. The latter, strictly speaking, is only that part of the non-specific benefit which is attributable to faith or trust in the therapist and the treatment or attention received. The natural resolution of illnesses and spontaneous healing or improvement constitute another element of supposedly non-specific responses, and changes in the environment can be very relevant also to psychological improvement, e.g., a difficult boss leaves, financial worries abate, a spouse recovers from illness or alters in attitude, and the patient responds accordingly.

Most psychological illnesses which promote chronic pain (depression, anxiety, hysteria) have a useful spontaneous rate of recovery. Most respond also to measures adapted to the individual case, be it counselling in one instance or relaxation treatment in another. The best results are usually for depression, the worst for chronic personality disorders. Chronicity is also the strongest predictor of a poor response in all psychiatric illnesses. Further, considerations such as age, the availability of employment, past operations for pain and the extent of previous treatment all influence prognosis. Hence, it is much easier to compare treatments with each other than to give quantitative statements of their usefulness overall. For every treatment, the psychological, social and physical features of the group of patients to be treated must be defined as well as specific diagnoses whenever possible. The features of improvement being examined must also be comparable, including symptoms and their change, altered activity for better or worse, the reduction of narcotics and the possibility of return to employment. The length of the follow-up has to be taken into account.

Bearing the above strong qualifications in mind, we can note the following quantitative estimates. Almost all measures of support, encouragement and counselling will produce some symptomatic response in one-half to two-thirds of those pain patients whose illness is principally due to psychological causes. The rate will be highest in those with clear psychological difficulties which can be resolved, and least in those with personality disorders and chronic maladjustment. Complete recovery will be obtained in a few, varying perhaps from 5–20% in specialist practice to 30–50% in general practice. Useful improvement will be obtained in comparable additional numbers in both specialist and general practice, although probably never more than 70–80% in total will get worthwhile benefit overall. Antidepressants (discussed below) will normally provide up to an 80% response rate for combined remission and improvement in appropriate cases with well marked depressive illness. Such benefits are rare, however, in pain clinics and similar selected populations.

Hypnosis has been said to help 50% of terminal cancer patients to some extent (Hilgard and Hilgard, 1975). That does not mean complete relief and the same figure could probably apply to all types of psychological intervention including cognitive therapy, supportive psychotherapy and biofeedback. The best results reported in biofeedback appear to be those cited earlier of one-third benefit for those with headache who have already failed with relaxation treatment alone (Blanchard and Andrasik, 1982; Blanchard et al., 1983). Operant conditioning at best has been claimed to provide good benefits for 77% as discussed above with respect to Roberts and Reinhardt (1980). This finding reflects the outcome, however, in a very highly selected group. Another chronic sample treated by Corey et al. (1987) using a comprehensive and intensive cognitive behavioural program obtained 71% good results with return to full or part-time work among 72 patients initially with good maintenance of their response (69%) at 18 months. It should be emphasized that this is a comprehensive and multimodal approach.

Cognitive therapy alone is not known to provide high rates of return to work. Indeed, very few of these treatments have or can be applied in a pure form. However, an improvement of about one-third in the estimates of pain may be anticipated from cognitive treatment of moderately severe and mild pain. Cognitive therapy seems less likely to work well in the long term with more severe chronic pain.

Even if the patients cease to seek further care and even if they return to work, their subjective complaints may remain unchanged (Newman et al., 1978). Perhaps one of the most realistic results with a truly intractable population is reported by Swanson et al. (1979), who used a comprehensive multimodal program. At 3–6-months follow-up, 30% were improved and 10% were employed.

These reports give some idea of the considerable range of variation in the response to treatment depending on selection factors, criteria for admission for treatment, the combination of different treatments and the length of follow-up.

PSYCHOTROPIC MEDICATIONS

It has been well known for some years that certain psychotropic drugs have additional therapeutic uses in the management of patients with chronic pain. It is not the case that any drug used in psychiatry will relieve any patient with pain; only certain types of drug work. The evidence for this has been reviewed in some detail by Merskey and Hester (1972), but Taub and Collins (1974) also report benefit from a combination of phenothiazines and antidepressants and the same approach has been used in Continental Europe (see Kocher, 1976). As already indicated, certain depressive illnesses with which pain is associated respond extremely well to antidepressant medication and to little else. These are generally illnesses in which the presence of depression can be recognized and the response either to antidepressants drugs or to ECT is regarded by the psychiatrist as appropriate; in such cases, the pain is also relieved because it is part of a psychological illness. On the other hand, some antidepressants have been credited with independent analgesic effects. Because of the frequent association of depression with pain, this has been hard to demonstrate, but Watson et al. (1982) managed to show that amitriptyline was effective in a double-blind placebo-controlled trial in patients with postherpetic neuralgia who did not have evidence of concomitant depression, at least as measured by the Beck Depression Scale. Subsequent studies by other authors including Sharav et al. (1987) and Max et al. (1987) have supported this effect for amitriptyline. It might be thought that amitriptyline acts as an analgesic because of its serotoninergic characteristics. This is not believed to be the case. Other serotoninergic drugs such as chlomipramine and trazodone have not been shown to have any special analgesic features. An open label study of zimelidine, a more serotoninergic drug than amitriptyline, comparing it with amitriptyline, was very much in favour of the latter (Watson and Evans, 1985). Amitriptyline may have calcium channel-blocking effects or it may have other actions (e.g., adenosinergic ones) which may contribute to its analgesic potency (Salter, 1987). Be that as it may, the two drugs for which most controlled trials show an analgesic effect are amitriptyline and imipramine (Monks and Merskey, 1989). Other antidepressants do not necessarily share these characteristics.

In addition to responding to antidepressants, certain pain syndromes such as postherpetic neuralgia, causalgia, thalamic pain and other pains due to lesions affecting the nervous system, which may all be classed as neurogenic pain, respond somewhat to phenothiazine drugs. It has been recognized for some years that chlorpromazine is effective in this respect and it has a respectable and established place in anaesthesia and analgesia. The maintenance use of chlorpromazine and non-narcotic analgesics for patients with chronic pain has been described in some detail by Merskey and Hester (1972). Other phenothiazines in addition to chlorpromazine are also useful in the treatment of pain (Sigwald et al., 1957; Chavanne, 1960; Lasagna and Dekornfeld, 1961; Paradis, 1962; Montilla et al., 1963; Bloomfield et al., 1964), and antihistamines too have been reported as being similarly effective for some patients with chronic neurogenic pain (Rosner, 1957). The effects of phenothiazines and other psychotropic medication on pain are also reviewed by Monks and Merskey (1989).

Bearing in mind the possible analgesic effects of phenothiazines, the present writer developed a treatment regime, based upon phenothiazines and other drugs, for patients with pain due to organic lesions. In this regime, phenothiazines are regularly supplemented by antidepressant drugs. One reason for this is that, as mentioned, the antidepressants are thought to have perhaps some separate analgesic effect apart from their use in depression. The second, as became clear in clinical practice and as was discussed earlier, is that several of the patients who were presenting with these pain syndromes had both physical lesion and depression. The third reason which appears to be of some importance is that if the phenothiazines are used alone, they may at times provoke depressive states (De Alarcon and Carney, 1969; Merskey and Hester, 1972; Johnson, 1981). It is therefore quite important in treating patients with pain by means of phenothiazines to use antidepressants, either as adjuvants or prophylactically, whilst the administration of the phenothiazine is being continued.

The writer's preference at the present time is to initiate treatment with amitriptyline for pain if it is thought that the pain has not responded adequately to nonnarcotic analgesics and also if it is thought that it is due to a physical lesion. If the pain is primarily due to a psychiatric illness, an alternative antidepressant with fewer side effects may be preferred. Having, if possible, established a satisfactory dose of amitriptyline, the use of a phenothiazine can then be considered if further treatment is needed to relieve pain. It is best to settle on one phenothiazine which the therapist prefers to use. In the case of the present writer, the current favourite drug is methotrimeprazine, given with an antidepressant and if necessary, with an antihistamine. However, fluphenazine, perphenazine, pericyazine and chlorpromazine have all been used. The method of administration of these drugs tends to vary according to whether the patients are in-patients or out-patients. There is no fixed dose of any one of these substances. The dose must be adjusted in relation to the emergence of side effects and the quantity of drugs which the patient can tolerate. It is, however, a good rule of thumb to start by giving the patient most of his medication at night with the aim of ensuring that first and foremost he has a good night's sleep. This alone reduces the impact of chronic pain upon patients and is much appreciated by them. So often patients who are in pain all day and woken by pain at night degenerate to a miserable condition until at least normal sleep is provided. The procedure used, thus, is to prescribe most of the phenothiazine at night starting with a fairly substantial dose with in-patients and a smaller dose with out-patients and to give this together with an established tricyclic antidepressant. Barbiturates, narcotic drugs if possible, and alcohol are all forbidden. The main reason for the restriction is that these drugs tend to induce hepatic enzymes and consequently reduce the effectiveness of other medication which one is attempting to use. Benzodiazepines are also best avoided. A careful explanation of what is intended has to be given to the patient or he will not readily accept the necessary manoeuvres and reduction of medication which have to be gone through. If he is convinced that only barbiturates enable him to have even a few hours rest from his intolerable pain he will not relinquish them without a careful discussion of the reason why. Nevertheless, we have not failed to be able to provide adequate sleep for any patient who is prepared to take the treatment regime which we recommended, without using barbiturates or narcotic drugs. In helping the patient to sleep, promethazine may be useful. Despite the reports mentioned of the use of antihistamines to relieve pain, the writer's impression is that they are at best weak analgesic agents, but may be valuable for night sedation with nitrazepam, tricyclic antidepressants and phenothiazines, when insomnia from pain is a major problem. Having established good overnight sleep, patients then find that some of the benefit may carry over to the next day. This is particularly so if the phenothiazine is continued in reduced doses during the day. In addition, although it is not part of the purpose of this chapter to describe the use of minor analgesic drugs, it is important to use such analgesics liberally. The writer's present favourite is paracetamol (acetaminophen), but one of the new anti-inflammatory drugs such as floctafenine or diflunisal may ultimately prove more satisfactory. The relevant advice to the patient is to take these drugs in substantial doses regularly, without waiting for the pain to become strong before resorting to the medication. Patients who wait for pain to become intolerable before they take enough to ease it, find the pain much harder to control than those who regularly, by the clock, take a fixed dosage of minor analgesics.

Unfortunately, many minor analgesics cause indigestion when taken regularly. Sometimes, one has to consider removing all minor analgesics such as acetaminophen or the non-steroidal anti-inflammatory drugs and prescribing a limited stable dose of codeine alone. Whilst it is not the writer's practice to prescribe codeine except in very rare instances, some patients who are taking it regularly in the form of compound preparations do not appear to increase the dose beyond a fixed level and it is not practical to try and withdraw from codeine all patients who are taking it.

The reduction in anxiety which is brought about by a confident approach from the doctor, the use of tranquillizing drugs and the gradual control of pain is not infrequently effective in producing a substantial reduction in the severity of the chronic pain. However, it is rare for the writer to find that his patients lose their pain altogether if it has an organic cause, and psychological improvement alone is never enough to abolish causalgia or central pain. Interestingly, Weir Mitchell noted that causalgia sometimes remitted spontaneously over a period of months or years (Mitchell, 1872), but this, of course, is not a common experience in current practice. Indeed, unfortunately these patients rarely obtain spontaneous relief, and when relief is provided which they at first acknowledge, they tend later to say that the pain is just the same, even though they may have been very grateful a month or two before for the benefit of the new drugs. Sometimes as a result they drop their medication by way of experiment; the invariable effect then is for the pain to come back, not in extra force but to the pretreatment level. At this point they recognize, as a rule, that they are in need of maintenance medication.

PSYCHOTROPIC EFFECTS OF DRUGS

The extent of benefit to painful syndromes from antidepressants may be gauged from a survey of papers on this topic provided by Monks and Merskey (1989). Out of 46 reports in which there were adequate data, 41 showed that more than 50% of the patients had moderate pain relief or better on follow-up at 1–3 months. In postherpetic neuralgia, Watson et al. (1982) showed that good to excellent pain relief was obtained in 16 out of 24 patients given amitriptyline, double-blind, irrespective of whether or not the patients had depression. Formal figures of the benefits of phenothiazines are harder to find. It is the writer's clinical impression that after the use of amitriptyline, another 10–20% of patients may gain worthwhile benefit from the addition of a phenothiazine.

Side effects

The drugs recommended here have several side effects which are not always easy to tolerate. Obstinate constipation is one of them, but it may be overcome either by ordinary laxatives or by the combined use of purgatives and cholinergic medication, for example, prostigmine. If the phenothiazines are used alone, they tend to cause depression, and, with the tricyclic group, a dry mouth. Almost all psychotropic drugs tend to cause a dry mouth but the patients will normally tolerate this as an alternative to the pain from which they previously suffered. A brief case history may indicate some of the effects of these types of medication and the problems encountered in practice.

Case history. Mrs. T. is a married professional woman born in 1924 – the breadwinner of her family, with a much older invalid husband and two sons aged 14 and 8 years, handicapped by congenital illness and in receipt of private education. Her childhood was unhappy and she was nervous but she served in the women's air force as a sergeant during the war and was mentioned in despatches. Her marriage was happy. In July 1964 she sustained a partial right median nerve lesion which produced causalgia which persisted despite settlement of a legal claim in March 1970. Combined antidepressants in the form of trimipramine at night and phenelzine by day and chlordiazepoxide produced only temporary improvement. She was first seen by us in December 1970 when she had severe pain, sometimes extending to the elbow and shoulder. She said it wore her out and she would have committed suicide were it not for her children. She held her right hand slightly abducted and was tense and tearful. At the time of referral she was having trimipramine 150 mg nocte, phenelzine 15 mg t.d.s. and chlordiaze-poxide 10 mg t.d.s. She was asked to continue these drugs adding promethazine 25 mg nocte. No improvement having occurred after 1 week, she was then told to try pericyazine 5 mg midday and 10 mg nocte, rising to 10 mg midday and 20 mg nocte. A further increase of pericyazine to 25 mg b.i.d. and 50 mg nocte abolished her pain altogether within 3 weeks of starting treatment. She remained well for 2 weeks when oedema of the legs developed, a complication sometimes noted with combined antidepressants and phenothiazines, and she was advised to reduce the pericyazine, which she did, whereupon pain recurred. She was therefore asked to stop the phenelzine and restore the pericyazine. Within 2 days the pain was again abolished and after 10 days the oedema resolved. Some drowsiness was noted with the pericyazine but she was able to continue with all her responsibilities and remained free from pain.

In February 1971, a programme was commenced to reduce drugs which might not be required and she dispensed successfully with promethazine and chlordiazepoxide. Pericyazine was also reduced to 87.5 mg daily, then her trimipramine was also gradually reduced to 50 mg nocte.

In May 1971 she returned for an urgent consultation because of severe depression which had developed insidiously as her drugs were reduced. There was no pain but she was unable to cope with her work and she spent her time sitting around, lacking energy. She was deluded that it was impossible to help her and that she had spent extravagantly, that she could not afford the rail fare for her NHS appointments and that she would not recover. Physically she had a mask-like face, cog-wheel rigidity in the limbs combined with akathisia and involuntary movements of the tongue at rest. Conjugate deviation on upward gaze was lost.

She was thought to have a drug-induced syndrome of Parkinsonism and endogenous depression. She would only agree to reduce her pericyazine (whereupon her pain recurred in part) but not to stop it. The restoration of trimipramine 150 mg nocte and the use of orphenadrine 50 mg t.d.s. resolved her depression and Parkinsonism within 3 weeks (i.e., by June 1971) and she has remained well since that time taking 150 mg of trimipramine, 150 mg of orphenadrine and 100 mg of pericyazine daily, the latter two in divided doses.

In this case, repeated reductions in pericyazine were accompanied by a return of pain, and restoration of pericyazine was needed to control the pain. The analgesic effect of pericyazine was apparently specific in this patient. However, when TENS became available she made a very good response to it and could discontinue medication.

This case emphasizes some of the problems of the use of phenothiazine medication continuously in patients with chronic pain. Constipation was mentioned earlier as a troublesome side effect of this medication. Depression and Parkinsonism and possibly oedema may also present difficulty at times. Nevertheless, the relief obtained can be so considerable that patients will willingly tolerate these very tedious and unpleasant side effects for the sake of relief from pain or from the depression which accompanies it, or both.

It might be argued that any sort of psychiatric treatment which reduced anxiety would contribute to the abatement of pain and indeed this is probably true. However, it also seems likely that the phenothiazine group and, to some extent, the antidepressants and antihistamines may be having more specific analgesic effects. Comparable degrees of relief of pain are not procured by the use of those tranquillizers which are most effective in states of pure anxiety. Diazepam or chlordiaze-poxide are not as valuable for the reduction of pain as the phenothiazine group and yet they are more effective in the reduction of anxiety. It is reasonable to suppose that there is a specific analgesic action, possibly upon the multisynaptic small cell system, which is thought to be involved in the causation of chronic pain (Cassinari and Pagni, 1969).

FAMILY AND GROUP TREATMENT APPROACHES

The influence of some aspects of the family pattern on patients with pain was noted by Freud (1893–1895). Apley (1959), Merskey (1965), Mohamed et al. (1978) and Shanfield et al. (1979) have all noted evidence of the importance of disturbed family or marital relationships in patients with pain. The involvement of family members in discussion and management is a normal part of the work of a good clinic, e.g., Swanson et al. (1979). The writer has not used group treatment for pain. Several reports from Greenhoot and Sternbach (1974), Pinsky (1975), Cairns et al. (1976) and Newman et al. (1978) describe group treatment as management of patients in a pain clinic. Herman and Baptiste (1981) describe a sensitive group approach and the management of patients within a pain clinic. The approaches range from psychodynamic (Pinsky, 1975) through transactional analysis (Greenhoot and Sternbach, 1974) to supportive. Families may be involved in the group treatment (Swanson et al., 1979) and manipulation of the patient or his environment may follow. Back pain education programs (Robinson, 1980) also involve group presentations. At the present state of the art, group treatment seems to serve a useful role in those clinics which have incorporated them into a larger programme.

A general psychiatric approach to the relief of pain

Drawing on what has been said so far it is evident that the writer thinks well of relaxation treatment and of drug treatment when indicated, has some cautious hopes from cognitive therapy, is disappointed in the outcome of biofeedback, sees no point in hypnosis and deprecates some aspects of operant conditioning as well as being doubtful about its usefulness. These viewpoints need to be incorporated in an overall statement of how to look after patients with chronic pain.

If the pain is due to psychological illness then the techniques used to relieve the pain must be those which are appropriate to the particular illness. Depressive illness, especially if it has an endogenous pattern, is often very satisfying for the psychiatrist to treat since, unless the environmental causes which promote it are intractable, it usually can be expected to respond very well to a combination of medical measures, such as drugs and ECT, with psychological management in the form of interviews with the patient and his relations, guidance in adjusting to difficulties in his environment and so on. Anxiety states, unless chronic, similarly tend to respond relatively well, although not invariably so, to medication and psychological treatments. The latter may be more prolonged and at times, pain of psychological origin may respond to psychotherapy. There are all grades and intensities of psychotherapy available for the management of patients but the emphasis need not usually be on intensive detailed frequent interviews. The patients who have ascertainable psychological problems can usually disclose these in about half a dozen interviews and a reorientation of their attitudes and relationships can often be obtained over the course of 10 or 12 interviews of moderate length, certainly not exceeding an hour.

In general, if psychotherapy does not work within the sort of time schedule outlined, the benefits from subsequent efforts are low in proportion to the time expended or the cost to the patient. Nevertheless, a chronic pain syndrome due to emotional conflict and potentiated by anxiety can be greatly helped by psychological measures. Where intensive psychotherapy is not appropriate, nor even brief analytic psychotherapy, patients may nevertheless be helped by supportive interviews. One or two such interviews which review life problems and give the individual some backing and encouragement from the doctor may be extremely useful in enabling him to deal with the circumstances which are helping to cause his illness. Where the altered circumstances and distress are partly due to physical illness, this type of interview assists the patient to accept his situation better and to maintain a more useful and effective adjustment thereafter. Once this is done, subsequent interviews need not be frequent or prolonged, but can be brief and supportive, yet still valuable.

If the chronic psychological illness mainly involves hysterical mechanisms, then radical treatment has little to offer, but again a supportive relationship with psychiatrist, physician or general practitioner may be beneficial and should be attempted. If the hysterical mechanisms are only part of a wider psychiatric illness in which there are some elements of depression, conflict with others and anxiety, then the emphasis should not be on the hysterical mechanisms but more upon the general difficulties which the individual faces. In this situation as with more severe hysterical illnesses, two things help the patient particularly. The first is the recognition by the doctor that his or her pain or problems are real and not 'imaginary', and the second is the support and guidance given in managing day-to-day affairs and problems. It is often held that demanding patients with hysterical symptoms are difficult to treat but this is not wholly correct. Many respond to a combination of sympathy and support with a diminution in the pressure of their symptoms and then they demand less help and less inappropriate treatment from their medical advisers and the people around them. It should not be expected that they will cease to have hysterical personality characteristics, or that all their symptoms will necessarily resolve, or that the pain will be removed altogether. But understanding guidance, a willingness to accept the symptoms as troublesome and unpleasant for the patient, even though not amenable to analgesic treatment, and sometimes the use of minor tranquillizers or antidepressants will often help these patients to achieve more satisfactory relationships both in their ordinary life and in the clinic.

Other approaches can also be utilized against this background of tolerant support. Family interviews and cognitive therapy are tried when indicated, and often when they are not clearly required, out of hope that may be beneficial. Group treatment also is always worth considering if it is available. It is perhaps worth emphasizing that in treating these patients a willingness to review the physical situation from time to time and to consider whether or not fresh evidence for an organic symptom is emerging, is of great importance. This does not mean that repeated investigation is necessary. It is always a problem to strike a balance between investigating excessively on the one hand and missing significant organic disease on the other. The safest approach is to be open with the patient and to say that reasonable investigations have been conducted, the symptoms are typical of psychological illness, there is no certainty that they are absolutely due to psychological troubles, but that the appropriate way is to regard them as such and to review the matter if they do not improve with psychiatric treatment or if any further development gives rise to a suspicion of physical illness. In the writer's own practice, this approach seems to be accepted by most patients. It is an important precaution if treatment does not progress well, however, and if the response is not as good as anticipated, to consider after, say, a period of six months, whether an organic review may be indicated and to seek this fairly readily. In this respect, the opinion of one's physician or surgeon colleague and his attention to the patient is more important than extra investigations. Patients find this approach reassuring and understand that they are being handled with tolerance and without dogmatism. Summarising these views, it can be said that pain of psychological origin deserves treatment for the appropriate psychiatric illness. When this is done, it will resolve if the psychological illness resolves. It is worth emphasising, however, that pain in association with psychological illness does not always recover with it. Bradley (1963) showed that if the pain appeared before the onset of other signs of psychological disturbance it tended to persist after the psychological illness had recovered. If the problem is mainly linked to a personality disorder and difficulties in personal relationships there is some scope for treatment in a proportion of patients. No figure can be given for the precise proportion, since the selection of patients will vary significantly according to the types of clinics or other practitioners with whom the psychiatrist is associated. In my own experience during a period of 9 years' work in association with neurologists and neurosurgeons, less than one-third of these particularly difficult patients were helped significantly by psycho-

58

therapy, although there were some very pleasant, occasional surprises.

Some psychological or psychiatric techniques, e.g., cognitive therapy, phenothiazines and antidepressants are also useful for pain from lesions, without any presumption that the emotional state is the cause of the pain. Moreover, all patients with chronic pain need understanding in regard to its emotional concomitants and social consequences.

CONCLUSIONS

It can be seen that the management of pain normally involves taking account of psychological factors. The first essential in any case of chronic pain is to establish whether or not there is a physical lesion and secondly, if there is a psychological disturbance, what is its nature. It is relevant to know whether the pain is primarily psychological in origin or whether it is complicated by pathological disturbances. Fear itself may be promoting the psychological trouble and making the pain worse, or chronic pain because of its severity and intolerable quality may be reducing the patient to psychological illness. Appropriate treatments are available for patients in these different circumstances. Some of them require skilled psychiatric help but others may be made available by the careful use of medication and normal understanding, sympathy and support. Of course, serious emotional problems giving rise to chronic pain require the help of qualified psychiatrists. It is worth emphasizing that a number of psychotropic drugs in common use have analgesic effects which are at least to some extent independent of their use in the management of psychiatric illness and independent of their effect in reducing anxiety. Some recent developments which include more use of relaxation treatment, cognitive therapy and attention to the family and social situations are also advocated.

REFERENCES

Apley, J. (1959) *The Child with Abdominal Pains*. Blackwell Scientific Publications, Oxford.
Aronoff, G.M., Evans, W.O. and Enders, P.L. (1983) A review of follow-up studies of multidisciplinary pain units. *Pain*, 16, 1–11.
Bakal, D.A. and Kaganov, J.A. (1977) Muscle contraction and migraine headache: Psychophysiologic comparison. *Headache*, 17, 208–215.
Banks, M.H., Beresford, S.H.A., Morrell, D.C., Waller, J.J. and Watkins, C.J. (1975) Factors influencing demand for primary medical care in women aged 20–40 years; a preliminary report. *Int. J. Epidemiol.*, 4, 189–255.
Barber, T.X. (1959) Toward a theory of pain: Relief of chronic pain by pre-frontal leucotomy, opiates, placebos and hypnosis. *Psychol. Bull.*, 56, 430.

Beck, A.T. (1976) *Cognitive Therapy and the Emotional Disorders*. International Universities Press, New York.

Beecher, H.K. (1959) *Measurement of Subjective Responses. Quantitative Effects of Drugs*. Oxford University Press, New York.

Benson, H., Klemchuck, H.P. and Graham, J.R. (1974) The usefulness of the relaxation response in the therapy of headache. *Headache*, 14, 49–52.

Berne, E. (1964) *Games People Play*. Grove Press, New York.

Blackburn, I.M., Bishop, S., Glen, A.I.M., Whalley, L.J. and Christie, J.E. (1981) The efficacy of cognitive therapy in depression: A treatment trial using cognitive therapy and pharmacotherapy, each alone and in combination. *Br. J. Psychiatry*, 139, 181–189.

Blanchard, E.B., Andrasik, F. and Silver, B.V. (1980) Biofeedback and relaxation in the treatment of tension headaches. *J. Behav. Med.*, 3, 227–232.

Blanchard, E.B. and Andrasik, F. (1982) Psychological assessment and treatment of headache: recent developments and emerging issues. *J. Consult. Clin. Psychol.*, 50 (6), 859–879.

Blanchard, E.B., Andrasik, F., Neff, D.F., Saunders, N.L., Arena, J.G., Pallmeyer, T.P., Teders, S.J., Jurish, S.E. and Rodichok, L.D. (1983) Four process studies in the behavioural treatment of chronic headache. *Behav. Res. Ther.*, 21 (3), 209–220.

Bloomfield, S., Simard-Savoie, S., Bernier, J. and Tetreault, L. (1964) Comparative analgesic activity of levomepromazine and morphine in patients with chronic pain. *Can. Med. Assoc. J.*, 90, 1156.

Blumer, D. (1975) Psychiatric considerations in pain. In: *The Spine, Vol. 2*. Editors: R.H. Rothman and F.A. Simeone. W.B. Saunders Co., Philadelphia.

Blumetti, A.E. and Modesti, L.M. (1976) Psychological predictors of success or failure of surgical intervention for intractable back pain. In: *Advances in Pain Research and Therapy, Vol. 1*. Editors: J.J. Bonica and D. Albe-Fessard. Raven Press, New York, pp. 323–325.

Bond, M.R. (1971) The relation of pain to the Eysenck personality inventory. Cornell Medical Index and Whiteley Index of Hypochondriasis. *Br. J. Psychiatry*, 119, 671–678.

Bonica, J.J. (1967) Management of intractable pain. In: *New Concepts in Pain and Its Clinical Management*. Editor: E.L. Way. Davis, Philadelphia.

Bonica, J.J. and Albe-Fessard, D. (1976) Introduction to First World Congress on Pain. In: *Recent Advances in Pain Research and Therapy, Vol. 1*, Proceedings of the First World Congress on Pain. Editors: J.J. Bonica and D. Albe-Fessard. Raven Press, New York, pp. 27–39.

Bradley, J.J. (1963) Severe localized pain associated with the depressive syndrome. *Br. J. Psychiatry*, 109, 741.

Cairns, D., Thomas, L., Mooney, V. and Pace, J.B. (1976) A comprehensive treatment approach to chronic low back pain. *Pain*, 2, 301–308.

Cassinari, V. and Pagni, C.A. (1969) *Central Pain: A Neurological Survey*. Harvard University Press, Cambridge.

Chapman, C.R., Sola, A.E. and Bonica, J.J. (1979) Illness behaviour and depression compared in pain center and private practice patients. *Pain*, 6, 1–17.

Chavanne, J. (1960) Treatment of pain with a group of phenothiazine amines. *Presse Med.*, 68, 2347.

Chaves, J.F. and Barber, T.X. (1974) Cognitive strategies, experimenter modelling and expectation in the attenuation of pain. *J. Abnorm. Psychol.*, 4, 356–363.

Corey, D.T., Etlin, D. and Miller, P.C. (1987) A name-based pain management and rehabilitation programme: an evaluation. *Pain* 29, 219–229.

Crook, J., Rideout, E. and Brown, G. (1984) The prevalence of pain complaints in a general population. *Pain*, 18, 229–314.

Crook, J. and Tunks, E. (1985) Defining the 'Chronic Pain Syndrome': an epidemiological method. In: *Advances in Pain Research and Therapy, Vol. 9*. Editors: H.L. Fields, R. Dubner and F. Cervero. Raven Press, New York, pp. 871–877.

Crown, S. and Crown, J.M. (1973) Personality in early rheumatic disease. *J. Psychosom. Res.*, 17, 189–196.

Cummings, C., Evanski, P.M., DeBenedetti, M.J. and Waugh, T.R. (1978) Use of the MMPI in a low back pain treatment program. *Pain Abstracts, Vol. 1*. Second World Congress on Pain, p. 247.

DeAlarcon, R. and Carney, W.M.P. (1969) Severe depressive mood change following slow intramuscular fluphenazine injection. *Br. Med. J.*, 3, 564.

Dorcus, R.M. and Kirkner, F.J. (1948) The use of hypnosis in the suppression of intractable pain. *J. Abnorm. Soc. Psychol.*, 43, 237.

Dunnell, K. and Cartwright, A. (1972) *Medicine Takers, Prescribers, and Hoarders*. Routledge and Kegan Paul, London.

Egbert, L.D., Battit, B.E., Welch, C.E. and Bartlett, M.K. (1964) Reduction of postoperative pain by encouragement and instruction of patients. A study of doctor-patient rapport. *N. Engl. J. Med.*, 270, 825.

Engel, G.L. (1951) Primary atypical facial neuralgia. An hysterical conversion symptom. *Psychosom. Med.*, 13, 375–396.

Engel, G.L. (1959) 'Psychogenic' pain and the pain prone patient. *Am. J. Med.*, 26, 899–918.

Epstein, I.H., Abel, G.G., Colline, F., Parker, L. and Cinciripini, P.M. (1978) The relationship between frontalis muscle activity and self-reports of headache pain. *Behav. Res. Ther.*, 16, 153–160.

Fishbain, D.A., Goldberg, M., Meagher, B.R., Steele, R. and Rosomoff, H. (1986) Male and female chronic pain patients categorized by DSM-III psychiatric diagnostic criteria. *Pain*, 26, 181–197.

Fordyce, W.E., Fowler, R.S., Lehmann, J.E. and De Lateur, B.J. (1968) Some implications of learning in problems of chronic pain. *J. Chron. Dis.*, 21, 179–190.

Fordyce, W.E., (1974) Pain viewed as learned behaviour. In: *Advances in Neurology, Vol. 4*. Editor: J.J. Bonica. Raven Press, New York, pp. 415–422.

Fordyce, W.E. (1976) *Behavioral Methods in Chronic Pain and Illness*. C.V. Mosby, Co., St. Louis, p. 236.

Fordyce, W.E., McMahon, R., Rainwater, G., Jackins, S., Questad, K., Murphy, T. and De Lateur, B. (1981) Pain complaint-exercise performance relationship in chronic pain. Research Report. *Pain*, 10, 311–321.

Freud, S. (1893–1895) (1955) *Studies in Hysteria. Complete Psychological Works. Standard Edition, Vol. 2*. Hogarth, London.

Greenhoot, J.H. and Sternbach, R.A. (1974) Conjoint treatment of chronic pain. In: *Advances in Neurology, Vol. 4*. Editor: J.J. Bonica. Raven Press, New York, p. 595.

Gupta, M.A. (1986) Is chronic pain a variant of depressive illness? A critical review. *Can. J. Psychiatry*, 31, 241–248.

Harper, R.C. and Steger, J.C. (1978) Psychological correlates of frontalis EMG and pain in tension headache. *Headache*, 18, 215–218.

Herman, E. and Baptiste, S. (1981) Pain control: Mastery through group experience. *Pain*, 10, 79–86.

Hilgard, E.R. and Hilgard, J.R. (1975) *Hypnosis in the Relief of Pain*. William Kaufmann Inc. Los Altos, California.

Hilton, J. (1863) *Rest and Pain*. Editors: E.W. Walls and E.E. Philipp. G. Bell, London, 1950.

Holroyd, K.Q. Andrasik, F. and Westbrook, T. (1977) Cognitive control of tension headache. *Cogn. Ther. Res.*, 2, 121–133.

Ignelzi, R.J., Sternbach, R.A. and Timmermans, G. (1977) The pain ward follow-up analyses. *Pain*, 3, 277–280.

International Association for the Study of Pain (Subcommittee on Taxonomy) (1979) Pain terms: A list with definitions and notes on usage. *Pain*, 6, 249–252.

International Association for the Study of Pain (1986) Classification of chronic pain: Descriptions of chronic pain syndromes and definitions of pain terms. Editor: H. Merskey. Monograph for the Sub-Committee on Taxonomy. *Pain* (Suppl. 3), Elsevier Science Publishers, Amsterdam.

Jacobson, E. (1929) *Progressive Relaxation*. University of Chicago Press, Chicago.

Jamison, K., Ferrer-Brechner, M.T., Brechner, V.L. and McCreary, C.P. (1976) Correlation of personality profile with pain syndrome. In: *Advances in Pain Research and Therapy, Vol. 1*. Editors: J.J. Bonica and D. Albe-Fessard. Raven Press, New York, pp. 317–321.

Jellinek, E.M. (1946) Clinical tests on comparative effectiveness of analgesic drugs. *Biomed. Bull.*, 2, 87–91. Cited by Beecher (1959).

Jessup, B.A., Neufeld, R.W.J. and Merskey, H. (1979) Biofeedback therapy for headache and other pain: An evaluative review. *Pain*, 7, 255–270.

Johnson, D.A.W. (1981) Studies of depressive symptoms in schizophrenia. I. The prevalence of depression and its possible causes. II. A two-year longitudinal study of symptoms. III. A double-blind trial of orphenadrine against placebo. IV. A double-blind trial of nortriptyline for depression in chronic schizophrenia. *Br. J. Psychiatry*, 139, 89–101.

Kertesz, A. and Kormos, R. (1976) Low back pain in the workman in Canada. *Can. Med. Assoc. J.*, 115, 901.

Khatami, M. and Rush, A.J. (1978) A pilot study of the treatment of out-patients with chronic pain: Symptom control, stimulus control and social system intervention. *Pain*, 5, 163–172.

Kocher, R. (1976) Use of psychotropic drugs for the treatment of chronic severe pain. In: *Advances in Pain Research and Therapy, Vol. 1*. Editors: J.J. Bonica and D. Albe-Fessard. Raven Press, New York, pp. 579–582.

Kudrow, L. and Sutkus, B.J. (1979) MMPI pattern specificity in primary headache disorders. *Headache*, 19, 18–24.

Lasagna, L. and DeKornfeld, T.J. (1961) Methotrimeprazine: A new phenothiazine derivative with analgesic properties. *J. Am. Med. Assoc.*, 178, 887.

Littlejohn, G.O. (1986) Repetitive strain syndrome: An Australian experience. (Editorial). *J. Rheum.*, 136, 1004–1006.

Mandy, A.J., Mandy, T.E., Farkas, R. and Scher, E. (1952) Is natural childbirth natural? *Psychosom. Med.*, 14, 431.

Martin, P.R. and Mathews, A.M. (1978) Tension headaches: Psychophysiological investigation and treatment. *J. Psychosom. Res.*, 22, 389–399.

Max, M.B., Culnanae, M., Schafer, S.C., Graceley, R.H., Walther, D.J., Smoller, B. and Dubner, R. (1987) Amitriptyline relieves diabetic neuropathy pain in patients with normal or depressed mood. *Neurology* (NY) 37, 589–596.

Meichenbaum, D. and Turk, D. (1976) The cognitive-behavioral management of anxiety, anger and pain. In: *The Behavioral Management of Anxiety, Depression and Pain*. Editor: P.O. Davidson. Brunner/Mazel, New York.

Melzack, R. and Scott, T.H. (1957) The effects of early experience on the responses to pain. *J. Comp. Physiol. Psychol.*, 50, 155–161.

Melzack, R., Weisz, A.Z. and Sprague, L.T. (1963) Strategems for controlling pain: Contributions of auditory stimulation and suggestion. Exp. Neurol., 8, 239–247.

Melzack, R. and Wall, P.D. (1965) Pain mechanisms: A new theory. *Science*, 150, 971–979.

Melzack, R., Wall, P.D. and Ty, T.C. (1982) Acute pain in an emergency clinic: Latency of onset and descriptor patterns related to different injuries. *Pain*, 14, 33–43.

Merskey, H. (1965) Psychiatric patients with persistent pain. *J. Psychosom. Res.*, 9, 299–309.

Merskey, H. and Spear, F.G. (1967) *Pain: Psychological and Psychiatric Aspects*. Bailliere, Tindall & Cassell, London.

Merskey, H. (1970) On the development of pain. *Headache*, 10, 116–123.

Merskey, H. (1971) An appraisal of hypnosis. *Postgrad. Med. J.*, 47, 572.

Merskey, H. and Hester, R.N. (1972) The treatment of chronic pain with psychotropic drugs. *Postgrad. Med. J.*, 48, 594–598.

62

Merskey, H. (1974) The contribution of the psychiatrist to the treatment of pain. In: *Advances in Neurology, Vol. 4*. Editor: J.J. Bonica. Raven Press, New York, pp. 605–609.

Merskey, H. (1979) The role of the psychiatrist in the investigation and treatment of pain. Research Publications, Vol. 58. Ass. Res. Nerv. Ment. Dis. In: *Pain*. Editor: J.J. Bonica. Raven Press, New York, pp. 249–260.

Miller, N. (1974) Applications of learning and biofeedback to psychiatry and medicine. In: *Comprehensive Textbook of Psychiatry, 2nd Edition*. Editors: A.M. Freedman, M.I. Kaplan and B.T. Sadock. Williams & Williams, Baltimore.

Mitchell, S.W. (1872) *Injuries of Nerves and Their Consequences 1965 Edn.*, Dover, New York.

Mohamed, S.N., Weisz, G.M. and Waring, E.M. (1978) The relationship of chronic pain to depression, marital adjustment and family dynamics. *Pain*, 5, 285–292.

Moldofsky, H., Scarisbrick, P., England, R. and Smythe, H. (1975) Musculoskeletal symptoms and non-REM sleep disturbance in patients with 'fibrositis syndrome' and healthy subjects. *Psychosom. Med.*, 37, 341–351.

Moldofsky, H. and Warsh, J.J. (1978) Plasma tryptophan and musculoskeletal pain in non-articular rheumatism. *Pain*, 5, 65–71.

Monks, R. and Merskey, H. (1989) Treatment with psychotropic drugs. In: *Textbook of Pain, 2nd Edn.*, Editors: P.D. Wall and R. Melzack. Churchill Livingstone, London pp. 702–721.

Montilla, E., Frederik, W.S. and Cass, L.J. (1963) Analgesic effect of methotrimeprazine and morphine: A clinical comparison. *Arch. Int. Med.*, 111, 725.

Morgenstern, F.S. (1964) The effects of sensory input and concentration on post-amputation phantom limb pain. *J. Neurol. Neurosurg. Psychiatry*, 27, 58–65.

Morgenstern, F.S. (1967) Chronic Pain. D.M. Thesis, Oxford.

Myers, J.K., Weissman, M.M., Tischler, G.L., Holzer, C.E., Leaf, P.J., Orvaschel, H., Anthony, J.C., Boyd, J.H., Burke, J.D., Jr., Kramer, M. and Stoltzman, R. (1984) Six-month prevalence of psychiatric disorders in three communities: 1980–1982. *Arch. Gen. Psychiatry*, 41, 10, 959–967.

Nathan, P.W. (1967) When is an anecdote? *Lancet*, 2, 607.

Nuechterlein, K.M. and Holroyd, J.C. (1980) Biofeedback in the treatment of tension headache – current status. *Arch. Gen. Psychiatry*, 37, 866–873.

Newman, R.I., Seres, J.L., Yospe, L.P. and Garlington, B. (1978) Multidisciplinary treatment of chronic pain: Long-term follow-up of low-back pain patients. *Pain*, 4, 283–292.

O'Kelly, L.E. and Steckley, L.C. (1939) A note on long enduring emotional responses in the rat. *J. Psychol.*, 8, 125. Cited by Ulrich et al. (1965).

Paradis, B. (1962) Analgesic and anaesthetic properties of levomepromazine (Nozinan). 17044 R.P. *Can. Anaesth. Soc. J.*, 9, 153.

Pelz, M. and Merskey, H. (1982) A description of the psychological effects of chronic painful lesions. *Pain*, 14, 3, 293–301.

Pilling, L.F., Brannick, T.L. and Swenson, W.M. (1967) Psychological characteristics of patients having pain as a presenting symptom. *Can Med. Assoc. J.*, 97, 387–394.

Pilowsky, I., Chapman, C.R. and Bonica, J.J. (1977) Pain, depression and illness behavior in a pain clinic population. *Pain*, 4, 183–192.

Pinsky, J.J. (1975) Psychodynamics and psychotherapy in the treatment of patients with chronic intractable pain. In: *Pain: Research and Treatment*. Editor: B.L. Crue, Jr. Academic Press, New York, pp. 383–398.

Pond, D.A. and Bidwell, B.H. (1959) A survey of epilepsy in 14 general practices. II. Social and psychological aspects. *Epilepsia (Amsterdam)*, 1, 285.

Rees, W.L. and Henryk-Gutt, R. (1973) Psychological aspects of migraine. *J. Psychosom. Res.*, 17, 141–154.

Reynolds, C.E. and Hutchins, H.C. (1948) Reduction of central hyperirritability following block anaesthesia of peripheral nerve. *Am. J. Physiol.*, 152, 158.

Roberts, A.H. and Reinhardt, L. (1980) The behavioral management of chronic pain: Long-term follow-up with comparison groups. *Pain*, 8, 151–162.

Robinson, G.E. (1980) A combined approach to a medical problem. *Can. J. Psychiatry*, 25, 138–142.

Romano, J.M. and Turner, J.A. (1985) Chronic pain and depression: Does the evidence support a relationship? *Psychol. Bull.*, 97, 18–34.

Rosner, S. (1957) The potentiating effects of diphenydramine hydrochloride (Benadryl). *J. Nerv. Ment. Dis.*, 125, 229.

Rybstein-Blinchik, E. (1979) Effects of different cognitive strategies on chronic pain experience. *J. Behav. Med.*, 1, 93–101.

Rush, A.J., Beck, A.T., Kovacs, M. and Hollon, S.D. (1977) Comparative efficacy of cognitive therapy and pharmacotherapy in the treatment of depressed out-patients. *Cogn. Ther. Res.*, 1, 17–37.

Sacerdote, P. (1962) The place of hypnosis in the relief of severe protracted pain. *Am. J. Clin. Hypn.*, 4, 150.

Sacerdote, P. (1965) Additional contributions for the hypnotherapy of the advanced cancer patient. *Am. J. Clin. Hypn.*, 7, 308.

Sacerdote, P. (1965) Hypnosis in cancer patients. *Am. J. Clin. Hypn.*, 9, 100.

Sainsbury, P. and Gibson, J.G. (1954) Symptoms of anxiety and tension and the accompanying physiological changes in the muscular system. *Psychosom. Med.*, 17, 216–224.

Salter, M. (1987) Personal Communication.

Shanfield, S.B., Heiman, E.M., Cope, N. and Jones, J.R. (1979) Pain and the marital relationship: Psychiatric distress. *Pain*, 7, 343–351.

Sharav, Y., Singer, E., Schmidt, E., Dionne, R.A. and Dubner, R. (1987) The analgesic effect of amitriptyline on chronic facial pain. *Pain* 31, 199–209.

Sigwald, J., Hebert, H. and Quentin, A. (1957) The treatment of herpes and post-herpetic pain (and other persistent forms of pain) with phenothiazine derivatives. *Sem. Hop. Paris*, 33, 1137.

Smith, A.M., Jr., Basmajian, J.V. and Vanderstoep, S.F. (1974) Inhibition of neighbouring motoneurons in conscious control of single spinal motoneurons. *Science*, 183, 975.

Smith, D.P., Pilling, L.F., Pearson, J.S., Rushton, J.G., Goldstein, N.P. and Gibilisco, J.A. (1969) The psychiatric study of atypical facial pain. *Can. Med. Assoc. J.*, 100, 286–291.

Smith, W.L. and Duerksen, D.L. (1979) Personality in the relief of chronic pain: Predicting surgical outcome. In: *Pain: Meaning and Management*. Editors: W.L. Smith, H. Merskey and S.C. Gross. Spectrum, New York.

Smythe, H.A. (1985) Fibrositis and other diffuse musculoskeletal syndromes. In: *Textbook of Rheumatology*. Editors: W.N. Kelley, E.D. Harris, Jr., S. Ruddy et al. W.B. Saunders, Philadelphia, pp. 481–489.

Sovak, M., Kunzel, M., Sternbach, R.A. and Dalessio, D.J. (1978) Is volitional manipulation of hemodynamics a valid rationale for biofeedback therapy of migraine? *Headache*, 18, 197–202.

Stengel, E. (1960) *Pain and the Psychiatrist*. Medical Press, 243, 28–30.

Stenn, P. (1987) Personal Communication.

Sternbach, R.A. (1968) *Pain: A Psychological Analysis*. Academic Press, New York.

Sternbach, R.A. and Rusk, T.N. (1973) Alternative to the pain career. *Psychother. Theor. Res. Pract.*, 10, 321.

Sternbach, R.A., Wolf, S.R., Murphy, R.W. and Akeson, W.H. (1973) Traits of pain patients: The low-back 'loser'. *Psychosomatics*, 14, 226–229.

Sternbach, R.A. (1974) *Pain Patients. Traits and Treatment*. Academic Press, New York.

Sternbach, R.A. and Timmermans, G. (1975) Personality changes associated with reduction of pain. *Pain*, 1, 177–181.

Sternbach, R.A. (1980) Letter to the Editor. *Pain*, 9, 111–113.

64

Sternbach, R.A. (1981) A search for the neurochemical basis of hypnotic analgesia. Paper presented at the International Association for the Study of Pain, Proc. 3rd. World Congress, Edinburgh, Scotland. *Pain* Suppl., 1, S162.

Sternbach, R.A. (1986) Survey of pain in the United States: The Nuprin Pain Report. *Clin. J. Pain*, 2, 49–53.

Sternbach, R.A. (1987) Personal Communication.

Swanson, D.W., Maruta, T. and Swenson, W.M. (1979) Results of behavior modification in the treatment of chronic pain. *Psychosom. Med.*, 41, 55–61.

Swerdlow, M. (1972) The pain clinic. *Br. J. Clin. Pract.*, 9, 403.

Szasz, T.S. (1968) The psychology of persistent pain. A portrait of l'homme douloureux. In: *Pain*. Editors: A. Soulairac, J. Cahn and J. Charpentier. Academic Press, New York.

Tan, S.Y. (1982) Cognitive and cognitive-behavioural methods for pain control: A selective review. *Pain*, 12, 201–228.

Taub, A. (1972) Personal Communication.

Taub, A. and Collins, W.F. (1974) Observations on the treatment of denervation dysaesthesia with psychotropic drugs: Post-herpetic neuralgia, anaesthesia dolorosa, peripheral neuropathy. In: *Seattle Symposium on Pain. Advances in Neurology, Vol. 4*. Editor: J.J. Bonica. Raven Press, New York.

Taylor, H. and Curran, N.M. (1985) The Nuprin Pain Report. Louis Harris & Associates, New York.

Touraine, G.A. and Draper, G. (1934) The migrainous patient. *J. Nerv. Ment. Dis.*, 81, 1–23, 182.

Tunks, E. (1987) Personal Communication.

Turk, D.C., Meichenbaum, D.H. and Berman, W.H. (1979) Application of biofeedback for the regulation of pain: A critical review. *Psych. Bull.*, 86, 1322–1338.

Turk, D.C., Meichenbaum, D.H. and Genest, M. (1984) *Pain and Behavioral Medicine*. Guildford Press, New York.

Turner, J.A. and Chapman, C.R. (1982) Psychological interventions for chronic pain: A critical review. I. Relaxation training and biofeedback. *Pain*, 12, 1–21.

Ulrich, R.E., Hutchinson, P.R. and Azrin, N.H. (1965) Pain-elicited aggression. *Psychol. Rec.*, 15, 11.

Ulrich, R.E. (1966) Pain as a cause of aggression. *Am. Zool.*, 6, 643.

Wall, P.D. (1984) The dorsal horn. In: *Textbook of Pain*. Editors: P.D. Wall and R. Melzack. Churchill Livingstone, Edinburgh, pp. 80–87.

Walters, A. (1961) Psychogenic regional pain alias hysterical pain. *Brain*, 84, 1–18.

Ward, N.G., Bloom, V.L. and Friedel, R.D. (1979) The effectiveness of tricyclic antidepressants in the treatment of coexisting pain and depression. *Pain*, 7, 331–342.

Waring, E.M., Weisz, G.M. and Bailey, S.I. (1976) Predictive factors in the treatment of low back pain by surgical intervention. In: *Advances in Pain Research and Therapy, Vol. 1*. Editors, J.J. Bonica and D. Albe-Fessard. Raven Press, New York, pp. 939–942.

Waters, W.E. (1975) Epidemiology of migraine. In: *Modern Topics in Migraine*. Editor: J. Pearce. William Heinemann Medical Books Ltd., London, pp. 8–21.

Watson, C.P.N., Evans, R.J., Reed, K., Merskey, H., Goldsmith, L. and Warsh, J. (1982) Amitriptyline versus placebo in postherpetic neuralgia. *Neurol.* 32, 671–673.

Watson, C.P.N. and Evans, R.J. (1985) A comparative trial of amitriptyline and zimelidine in postherpetic neuralgia. *Pain*, 23, 387–394.

Wiltse, L.L. (1975) Predicting the success of low-back surgery by the use of preoperative psychological tests. *J. Bone Jt. Surg.*, 57-B, 259.

Wiltse, L.L. and Rocchio, P.D. (1975) Preoperative psychological tests as predictors of success of chemonucleolysis in the treatment of low-back syndrome. *J. Bone Jt. Surg.*, 57-A1, 478–483.

Wolff, H.G. (1948) *Headache and Other Head Pain*. Oxford University Press, London.

Wolff, B.B. (1971) Current psychosocial concepts in rheumatoid arthritis. *Bull. Rheum. Dis.*, 22, 161–167.

Wood, P.H.N. and Badley, E.M. (1980) Back pain in the community. In: *Clinics in Rheumatic Diseases*. W.B. Saunders, London, pp. 3–16.

Woodforde, J.M. and Merskey, H. (1972) Personality traits of patients with chronic pain. *J. Psychosom. Res.*, 16, 167–172.

M. Swerdlow and J.E. Charlton (eds.) Relief of Intractable Pain
© 1989, Elsevier Science Publishers B.V. (Biomedical Division)

3

The structure and functions of a pain relief clinic

Stephen H. Butler and Terence M. Murphy

INTRODUCTION

The resurgence of interest in pain started when the 'Gate Theory' of Melzack and Wall (1965) led to the formation of the International Society for the Study of Pain in 1975. As a sequel to this, the number of pain relief clinics has increased dramatically. The stimulus for their foundation has varied from the crassly commercial to the most altruistic, based on patient care and research.

Pain relief centres are difficult to quantify and categorize. The number of them has risen without doubt since the survey by the American Society of Anesthesiologists and the International Association for the Study of Pain published in 1979, which identified 430 clinics worldwide, with 288 in the United States and 19 in the United Kingdom (Carron et al., 1979). A new survey is now underway, but no data are available at present. The development of pain relief clinics in Europe has been described by Swerdlow (1986).

In the United States of America enthusiasm for pain clinics is being dampened somewhat by current politics and the economics of patient care and research. Conservatism and cost accounting are thus decreasing the number of active centres. To counter this tendency an evaluation of pain clinics in the U.S.A. is being undertaken under the auspices of a private organization, the Commission on Accreditation of Rehabilitation Facilities (CARF). To date, 85 multidisciplinary pain relief clinics in America have been evaluated and approved by this organization. CARF has produced a monograph to assist in the evaluation of pain clinics and as an attempt to address some of the concerns being expressed by health insurance agencies. As an example, the Washington State Department of Labor and Industries, a state-run workman's compensation organization, is now requiring CARF accreditation for approved centres of treatment for injured workers.

In previous editions of this book, the chapter on pain relief clinics dealt primarily with the structure of the multidisciplinary clinic at the University of Washington Medical School, Seattle, Washington. This chapter attempts to address a broader picture of structure, function, purpose and problems over a variety of clinics. The information is presented from an evolutionary point of view, starting with the simplest form of practice and proceeding to the structure and function of a full multidisciplinary in-patient/out-patient centre. The perspective is that of an anaesthetist, but the developments and problems are really generic and any other medical discipline can be substituted for the most part, but bearing in mind the need for a diagnostic facility.

SETTING UP A PAIN CLINIC

The simplest form of pain clinic is an out-patient unit run by a single practitioner using a single treatment modality for a single problem, e.g., biofeedback for headache, active/passive physical therapy for low back pain. This simplified clinic is ideal for its limited purpose, in that there is no ambiguity over patient selection and treatment and there are impressive opportunities for accurate prospective research into treatment outcome. However, such clinics are rare and the majority seem to have little interest in research. Elaboration on this simple organization may take several forms. Originally, most clinics in North America, Western Europe and the Antipodes based their practice firmly on the medical model. This implies identifying a disease or structural abnormality which can be treated in a 'hands-on' way through nerve block, surgery and/or medications. This is still the trend, despite the early insistence of Bonica (1953) and others (Melzack and Wall, 1965; Sternbach, 1974; Fordyce, 1976) that learning and psychosocial factors and psychiatric problems may be equally or more important in maintaining the chronic pain state. The acceptance of psychosocial factors as important in chronic pain has produced a minority of psychiatry/psychology-based clinics polarized against the medical model with the obvious deficiencies of a different sort of 'tunnel vision'.

The small clinic

Many physicians begin pain treatment practice as part of a general medical practice, but it is not usually appreciated how a small interest can overwhelm one's major practice. The chronic pain population may be very difficult to manage and can require tremendous resources in time and manpower from the health care system. 'Pain relief clinic' can equate to 'dustbin' in the eyes of colleagues, and a new face in the arena may quickly find himself the managing physician, treating everyone else's failures. Beginning a solo pain practice part-time requires ground rules for self-protection:

(1) Referral is for consultation only and does not imply assumption of total care.

(2) A single treatment modality may be offered and if one has the expertise or desire for a limited involvement only, then this should be made clear to one's colleagues as part of (1).

(3) Chronic non-malignant pain is not an emergency; patients will be seen expeditiously, but not immediately. As a corollary, cancer patients with pain should be seen as soon as possible.

(4) A block of time should be set up to see pain patients and this service should not encroach upon one's regular activities. It may be necessary to modify this when dealing with patients in hospital or with pain arising from cancer.

(5) A clinical area with privacy and some staff support for record keeping is advisable for most practitioners and mandatory for others who wish to pursue research or treatment outcome.

(6) Careful documentation of evaluation, treatment and its immediate effects should be recorded. The primary and referring physician must be kept fully informed. Word of mouth is not adequate, even in the most casual of practices, although it is a good public relations approach and gives a more personal touch to the subsequent correspondence.

The larger clinic

Expansion to a full-time practice with chronic pain patients is more difficult than starting part-time and should be a carefully weighed professional and economic decision. It may require a break from one's previous professional direction and interest, and a change in practice environment or geography. An increase in administrative responsibilities must be anticipated. For some, this decision is made during their postgraduate training years when education in a pain relief clinic may lead to a full-time career. Training posts in pain treatment are very rare and only a minority of practitioners follow this route. Most clinicians still begin with a part-time interest.

A decision must be made about the type of practice to be pursued and consideration of the ground rules [1–6] outlined earlier is advisable for successful practice. Involvement in a pre-existing multidisciplinary practice requires many other considerations. Again, full-time or part-time commitments are possible and this decision may direct one to one kind of facility rather than another depending upon their make-up and requirements. Some 'multidisciplinary' clinics in effect are no such thing; each specialist works as an individual and patients are passed from one specialist to another without much communication and without decisions about treatment being made through discussion and mutual consent. This format is really a group of solo clinics, although the loose 'multidisciplinary' organization theoretically facilitates more rapid evaluation and triage. In this environment, the individual physician may function in a limited capacity seeing a specific patient population and providing a limited evaluation or treatment function. Conversely, the practice can be as a primary health care provider coordinating evaluation and treatment. In either capacity, administration, teaching and research are strong possibilities and clear decisions concerning practice need to be made with these options in mind when choosing or creating a multidisciplinary facility.

The multidisciplinary clinic

The multidisciplinary clinic as originally espoused by John Bonica (1953) involves several disciplines with equal input and responsibility: Those representing the medical model (i.e., anaesthesia, medicine, neurology, neurosurgery, physical medicine, etc.) and those representing the behavioural model (i.e., psychiatry, psychology). Clinical decisions are made at the time of evaluation, when a mutually acceptable diagnosis, prognosis and treatment plan are formulated. This information should be presented to the patient and spouse by one or more representatives of the medical and behavioural disciplines together so that it is clear that decisions have been made after assessing all aspects of the problem. If more data are necessary to complete the evaluation, this must be obtained so that all concerned can be satisfied that the investigation has been complete. Too often, when behavioural/psychological factors are discussed, the impression given is that the pain problem is considered to be 'all in the head'. Pejorative connotations are too frequently perceived, and the patient and family feel abandoned by the medical community. Equally, a referring physician who had felt that neurolysis somewhere in the pain transmission system was the solution to the patient's problem may be upset if it is not obvious that appropriate medical evaluations have been made if a behavioural modification approach to treatment is chosen.

The combined approach on ward rounds and out-patient visits is necessary to discuss problems and therapeutic options. Thus, the patient always deals with 'the team' when important issues appear. This mutual cooperation and responsibility between medical and behavioural practitioners requires some open-mindedness not found in all. It also requires a degree of mutual understanding of the other's disciplines and a sound basic knowledge of the 'puzzle of pain'.

STRUCTURE AND FUNCTION OF AN ACADEMIC MULTIDISCIPLINARY PAIN RELIEF CLINIC

In an effort to be all things to all people, this section will outline what may be a somewhat biased description of an 'ideal' academic pain relief clinic. This facility uses many specialists from a wide variety of medical, surgical and behavioural backgrounds to provide the optimum in patient care for chronic non-malignant pain as well as pain in the cancer patient. This facility should also be an effective teaching resource, both basic and clinical science for undergraduates in medicine and related disciplines and for postgraduate training in pain evaluation and treatment on a formal and informal basis.

This type of Pain Centre must also conduct and foster research, both clinical and basic, to advance treatment and patient care and to assess therapeutic outcome.

Director

This unenviable position calls for multiple talents. Obviously administrative experience and expertise is a necessity. In some centres, financial concerns necessitate some business flair, but it is less of a prerequisite in our theoretical academic clinic.

An extensive knowledge of the pathophysiology of pain states and their investigation and treatment is another necessity to provide leadership in clinical and research activities. Finally, tact, diplomacy and a sense of humour are qualities that are strongly recommended to deal with the variety of personalities and their interactions.

Personnel

Physicians involved in evaluation and treatment can come from any clinical background. The only primary qualification is that they should have an interest in, knowledge of, and tolerance for, patients with pain problems. As more training programmes appear, more practitioners with special education in pain management become available. By default and historical peculiarity, these 'pain specialists' tend to be anaesthetists, but this is not the exclusive province of this speciality. Indeed, it is an advantage to have representatives from neurology, neurosurgery, orthopaedic surgery, physical medicine and dentistry as part of the physician team. Anaesthetists with expertise in regional anaesthesia and pain may be an integral part of the team, especially if treatment of cancer pain is a high priority.

Psychiatric/psychological personnel represent the other half of the evaluation and treatment team. Interest in pain relief is often greater in behavioural and cognitive psychologists, although some behavioural psychiatrists are becoming members of pain relief clinics. Psychiatric consultation is necessary because of the prevalence of organic psychiatric disease, particularly depression, in pain patients.

72

Nurses

Nursing personnel are needed for both in-patient and out-patient areas, and preferably these individuals should be comfortable in either setting as part of the team. Special interest and training is necessary as the duties are different to those for standard medical/surgical ward nursing. Their skills must include in-depth psychological support, familiarity with analgesic drugs and comfort in the invasive ambience of the procedure room helping with nerve blocks, etc.

Other specialists

Physiotherapists and occupational therapists play a large part in treatments on an in-patient and out-patient basis. Again, those with a strong interest in and a high tolerance for chronic pain patients are needed.

 With the increasing emphasis on the economic aspects of treatment plans, vocational rehabilitation counsellors are a necessity. For psychological as well as financial reasons, return to productive employment is a necessary goal for most pain relief programmes dealing with chronic non-malignant pain. Evaluation by these counsellors can help with setting these goals prior to acceptance for treatment. The transition from treatment to the workforce is difficult physically, psychologically and also administratively, given the complexities of workman's compensation organizations. Vocational rehabilitation counsellors are adept at negotiating patients through the system to maximise long-term effectiveness of treatment.

 Ancillary technical staff are obviously a necessity. Receptionists, secretaries and

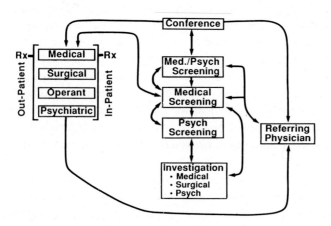

Fig. 3.1. Pain relief clinic flow-chart.

coordinators for arranging the patient's route from referral through the maze of the evaluation and treatment programs hold the system together.

Ancillary research staff may also be a part of a multidisciplinary pain relief clinic, but their backgrounds and function vary so greatly from organization to organization that they will not be identified here.

Function

Again, using an ideal scenario, let us follow a patient through the organization as indicated by the scheme in Fig. 3.1. As stated in the guidelines, it should be mandatory for all patients to be referred by a physician who knows their medical background and is willing to resume responsibility for health care following discharge from any level of the process.

Step 1

The letter of referral is evaluated by a physician in the clinic. More information may be needed before deciding on the appropriate evaluation process that should be requested. For medically circumscribed problems (e.g. acute or chronic herpes zoster pain, early sympathetic dystrophy, trigeminal neuralgia, or pain associated with cancer), an urgent or routine medical consultation is arranged. For less clear problems (e.g., low back pain, headache), then a multidisciplinary evaluation by a physician, psychiatrist/psychologist and, if indicated, by a vocational rehabilitation counsellor is arranged. Appropriate documentation of previous evaluations, i.e., radiological, electrodiagnostic, surgical reports, medical reports, will be requested to be present at the time of evaluation. Certain behavioural/psychological and demographic forms may be sent to the patient for completion, or they may be completed in the clinic prior to evaluation.

Step 2

Step 2a. Those patients undergoing a purely medical evaluation may be triaged to a multidisciplinary work-up following medical evaluation; they may need more diagnostic evaluation or they may go to medical treatment on either an out-patient or in-patient basis. In some cases, it may be felt that the pain clinic cannot help the person and he is sent back to the referring physician.

Step 2b. Those patients undergoing a multidisciplinary evaluation are seen separately by the physician and psychiatric/psychology teams and a family member or friend interviewed by the psychiatrist/psychologist. If return to work is a concern, a vocational rehabilitation counsellor may be part of the triage team. At this point, preferably the same day, the evaluation team meets to discuss the patient, their impressions and treatment suggestions. These are then communicated by the team directly to the patient and family members. The decision may be for in-patient or out-patient psychological, medical/surgical or multidisciplinary treatment, or for return to the referring physician for management. Further medical or psychological evaluation may be indicated before these decisions can be made and a further team meeting is then necessary with the patient to finalize treatment decisions.

At the completion of any stage of these procedures, communication back to the referring physician by the evaluators is made by letter. The initial evaluating physician and/or psychiatrist/psychologist becomes the patient's 'manager' and is responsible for the patient negotiating the route through evaluation and treatment. Should the manager not be part of the ultimate treatment team, that team takes over the responsibility for follow-up and communication to the referring physician.

Treatment options on an out-patient or in-patient basis vary. They may include pharmacological, anaesthetic (nerve block), rehabilitative (reactivation, vocational), surgical (very rare in our experience), psychological, behavioural modification, psychiatric or a combination. Most multidisciplinary in-patient or out-patient programmes centre around behaviour modification and physical reactivation, with lesser parts of treatment by other approaches mentioned. Withdrawal from narcotic and sedative/hypnotic medications is inevitably a part of most treatment decisions.

RESULTS

At the outset, it is necessary to be critical of the information to be presented so that these data can be seen in perspective. Outcome data continue to be presented and, in the best of all worlds, provide strong information for the clinic to which they apply, but may be less important in other contexts. The reason for this is that no two clinics function alike. Their structure and personnel are often quite different as is their focus of treatment, despite being 'multidisciplinary'. Pools of patients also are different from one clinic to another. Outcome studies show wide variance in admission criteria (if reported), treatment methods, outcome measures and length of follow-up. The majority of reported studies are anecdotal with little information and too few numbers to provide reliable data about outcome. The presence of control or comparison information is woefully lacking. Despite these drawbacks, the information available is encouraging in terms of long-term gains, which include increased activity, less pain reported, return to work, consumption of fewer medications and fewer hospitalizations.

Another concern in reviewing the data is knowing which type of intervention has been the most effective. The true multidisciplinary program is multidisciplinary both in evaluation and treatment and one treatment modality blends into another (Murphy and Anderson, 1984).

From a medical point of view, treatments are as follows:

(1) *Active physiotherapy*, which includes general conditioning with increasing strength, stretch and aerobic capacity but with emphasis on the previously injured part, e.g., back, neck, shoulder.

(2) *Passive physiotherapy*, which is part of a few programs and includes such modalities as transcutaneous electrical stimulation, traction, massage, heat, ultrasound, etc.

(3) *Medication withdrawal*. Of concern is the variability of this treatment from rigid withdrawal of all narcotics, sedatives, hypnotics and tranquilizers at a fixed rate to a laissez-faire encouragement to reduce.

(4) *Nerve blocks*, under which one can include specific procedures such as sympathetic blockade, epidural steroid injections as well as less specific procedures such as trigger point injections and acupuncture.

From a psychological viewpoint, treatments, or interventions are as follows:

(1) *Physiological*, where attempts are made through such methods as biofeedback, relaxation training, and/or exercise programs to control muscle tension, blood vessel tone and visceral responses, which may play a role in the genesis of the pain.

(2) *Operant conditioning*, which asserts that pain is represented by overt responses – complaining, guarding, taking medication and controlled by contingent reinforcers. Negative reinforcement (or no reinforcement) of these activities and positive reinforcement of well-behaviours such as increasing activity are the treatment (Fordyce, 1976; Fordyce et al., 1973).

(3) *Cognitive-behavioural therapies*, which rely on re-education of pain patients who are felt to behave according to their interpretation of physiological events using past experiences that have formed attitudes, beliefs and assumptions shaping affect and behaviour. Patients are taught basic physiology and psychology of chronic pain and using a changed understanding of their body processes are taught to identify negative habitual thoughts related to pain. They are also taught to recognize the relationship between these thoughts and consequent feelings and pain, and to substitute more adaptive thoughts. Based on this information, they are instructed in the use of coping strategies to reduce suffering.

From this melange of treatments, identification of the most important modality seems to depend to a great extent on the bent of the reviewer. This may be because one tends to rely on one's own expertise for treatment, and the emphasis from one multidisciplinary program to another will depend on the skill(s) of the personnel. However, few studies attempt to compare treatment strategies across a constant patient population.

The majority of the reviews look at psychological treatments and psychological outcomes (Linton, 1982; Linton, 1986; Maruta et al., 1976; Sturgis et al., 1984; Turner and Chapman, 1982; Turner and Romano, 1984). This is particularly true for those studies dealing with headache and temporo-mandibular joint problems. Those studies looking at low back pain or varied pain problems tend to have a broader range of treatment outcomes or focus on pain and function. The reviews mentioned above cover 25 studies with follow-up from 1 month to 8 years and patient populations of 5–200 (studies looking at results at the end of treatment without follow-up are not included here).

Looking at the outcome shows a varied response to treatment. In terms of the pain report where the variation in outcome is greatest, patients show 0–86% reduction at follow-up. When assessed (8 of the 25 studies), the percentage of patients working, looking for work or in retraining varies from 20 to 80%. Continued increase in mobility, exercise and activity is reported in all studies and in a few is quantified as being improved by 16% (early follow-up) to 69%. Medication intake was reduced in all at follow-up, in one group to zero, and varies greatly in degree because different philosophies on medication are espoused from clinic to clinic. Only two of the studies address health care utilization and indicate a decrease.

One of the most in-depth surveys bears review. This comes from the University of Minnesota (Roberts and Rheinhardt, 1980) and compares three groups of patients, one accepted and treated, one accepted but who refused treatment and a third who were rejected. Follow-up was 2–8 years. Seventy-seven percent of treated patients were leading normal productive lives without pain medication following treatment, whereas only 3% of the others had a similar outcome. There is a detailed description of the program, patient selection, outcome evaluation and statistics which deserves study by those concerned about treatment outcome of multidisciplinary approaches to relief of chronic pain.

A subsequent study using the format of treatment and evaluation from Roberts and Rheinhardt was performed at the University of Nebraska (Guck et al., 1985). This outcome study showed similar results, but in addition, showed a significant decrease in pain-related hospitalizations and surgeries during follow-up in the treated versus non-treated groups.

More detailed analysis of outcome studies was performed by Aronoff et al. (1983) with the emphasis on identifying methodological abnormalities. This is worth reviewing. An international look at pain relief clinic outcomes is also present in an article by Hallett and Pilowsky (1982), which identifies more clearly differences between patient populations and treatment strategies in selected studies. Of interest is the fact that this review shows that treatments for such diverse problems as cancer-related pain, orofacial pain, and a mixed bag of chronic non-malignant pains give similar outcomes. The treatments vary from surgical, pharmacological and nerve blockade to behavioural and psychiatric.

In conclusion, the need for accurate short- and long-term outcome information relating specific treatments to specific problems is obvious. National and international collaboration will be necessary to correlate information in a statistically meaningful way. The IASP, its component societies and the International Pain Foundation are attempting this task, but the process is embryonic. One is left to glean appropriate information from available studies in a piecemeal fashion until appropriate standardization allows more than the trends and impressions present in current studies.

REFERENCES

Aronoff, G.M., Evans, W.D. and Enders, P.L. (1983) A Review of Follow up Studies of Multidisciplinary Pain Units. *Pain*, 16, 1–11.

Bonica, J.J. (1953) *The Management of Pain*. Lea and Feibiger, Philadelphia.

Carron, H., Black, R.G., Bonica, J.J. et al. (1979) Pain Center/Clinic Directories. (ASA Publication not available).

Commission on Accreditation of Rehabilitation Facilities. 2500 North Pantano Road, Tucson, Arizona 85715 (602) 886–6575.

Fordyce, W.E. (1976) *Behavioral Methods for Chronic Pain and Illness*. C.V. Mosby, St. Louis.

Fordyce, W.E., Fowler, R.S., Lehman, S.F., Delateur, B.J., Sand, P.L. and Treischmann, R.B. (1973) Operant Conditioning in the Treatment of Chronic Pain. *Arch. Phys. Med. Rehab.*, 54, 399.

Guck, T.P., Skultety, F.M., Meilman, P.W. and Dowd, E.T. (1985) Multidisciplinary Pain Center Follow-Up Study: Evaluation with a No-Treatment Control Group. *Pain*, 21, 295.

Hallett, E.C. and Pilowsky, I. (1982) The Response to Treatment in a Multidisciplinary Pain Clinic. *Pain*, 12, 365–374.

Linton, S.J. (1986) Behavioral Remediation of Chronic Pain: A Status Report. *Pain*, 24, 125–141.

Linton, S.J. (1982) A Critical Review of Behavioural Treatments for Chronic Benign Pain Other than Headache. *B.J. Clin. Psychol.*, 21, 321–337.

Maruta, T., Swanson, D.W. and Swanson, W.M. (1976) Chronic Pain: Which Pains May a Pain Management Program Help? *Pain*, 7, 321–329.

Melzack, R. and Wall, P.D. (1965) Pain Mechanism. A New Theory. *Science*, 150, 971–979.

Murphy, T.M. and Anderson, S.A. (1984) Multidisciplinary Approach to Managing Pain. *Adv. Pain. Res. Ther.*, 7, 359–368, Raven Press, New York.

Roberts, A.H. and Rheinhardt, L. (1980) The Behavioral Management of Chronic Pain: Long-Term Follow-up With Comparison Group. *Pain*, 8, 151.

Sternback, R.A. (1974) *Pain Patients: Traits and Treatments*. Academic Press, New York.

Sturgis, E.T., Schafter, A.A. and Sikora, T.L. (1984) Pain Center Follow-up Study of Treated and Untreated Patients. *Arch. Phys. Med. Rehab.*, 65, 301.

Swerdlow, M. (1986) A Preliminary History of Pain Relief Clinics in Europe. *The Pain Clinic*, 1, 77–82.

Turner, J.A. and Chapman, C.R. (1982) Psychological Interventions for Chronic Pain – A Critical Review. *Pain*, 12, 1–22.

Turner, J.A. and Romano, J.N. (1984) *Evaluating Psychological Interventions for Chronic Pain: Issues and Recent Developments* Editors: C. Benedetti, C.R. Chapman and G. Morrica. *Advances in Pain Research and Therapy*, Raven Press, New York, 7, 257.

M. Swerdlow and J.E. Charlton (eds.) Relief of Intractable Pain
© 1989, Elsevier Science Publishers B.V. (Biomedical Division)

4

Assessment of the patient with chronic pain

Samson Lipton

INTRODUCTION

Some of the patients arriving at a pain clinic have had unsuccessful treatment for their pain. They hope for any method of pain relief which does not have unacceptable side effects or consequences. The cause of their pain may be diagnosed but the normal treatment does not work; or it may be that the pain is iatrogenic due to previous treatment; perhaps they are undiagnosed or have a condition such as cancer which is untreatable; they may have psychological pain which needs psychological methods to produce relief. In the final analysis, with or without a diagnosis, the patient wants relief.

The algologist deals with this problem in the same way that any physician approaches a medical problem. He makes enquiries about what is troubling the patient – in this case a pain or pains. He then goes into details of where the pain is, when it comes on, how it affects the patient, what type of pain it is and so on. Enquiry is made of personal and family history, previous illnesses, both physical and mental. A picture is gradually built up. In known pain syndromes, the diagnosis can be made from the history; in others, the physical examination, or the psychological profile help.

Finally, there are investigations, which confirm or refute the suspicions of the algologist. Further investigations are carried out. At some stage, either a diagnosis is made which suggests treatment, or no diagnosis is made and a treatment regime is drawn up in order to find out whether there is a treatment which will relieve the pain. As with any other physician, the algologist draws on his experience, knowledge and skill.

Normally, when a patient has a consultation, the physician does not obtain a neat chronological history with all his queries satisfied by tabulated answers.

Thus, although this chapter is divided into sections, it must be understood that answers to different sections come irregularly and are placed into proper order by the physician, and this takes training and knowledge.

Initially, in assessing chronic pain, a decision has to be reached, whether the patient has pathophysiologically developed pain or psychopathological pain. Thus, a decision is made as to whether the pain is physical, physical with psychological overlays, mainly psychological or frankly psychotic (Pilowsky and Spence, 1975; Chapman et al., 1979; Devine and Merskey, 1965). These divisions are arbitrary, as most patients with chronic pain suffer from psychological effects. Patients with minor psychological effects are best treated by physical means. Those psychologically affected by pain can be divided into four groups for treatment.

(1) With a known physical cause: this should be treated if results are expected in the short term.

(2) For pain previously treated unsuccessfully or when no cure is available, or where psychological overlay is marked, both physical and psychological treatment proceed together.

(3) Where major psychological or psychotic reactions are present, initial treatment is on psychological or psychiatric lines.

(4) When abnormal pain behaviour is exhibited and people and situations are manipulated, psychological methods are used.

These few remarks are simplistic and the reader is urged to read Chapter 2 in conjunction with this one.

A patient's assessment follows the standard methods used in all medical disciplines and begins with the history. This will be discussed shortly, but the initial contact has benefits apart from obtaining facts, e.g.,

(1) Empathy with the patient.

(2) Finding out what is important to the patient. This may have no relation to the illness, but is essential information.

(3) New facts or correlations may appear due to the algologist's specialised knowledge and structuring of the consultation.

(4) The patient is observed – attitude, appearance, speech, gait, movements and general demeanour.

PATIENT REFERRAL

The patient arrives by one of two routes, either:

(1) By referral from a primary or secondary clinic, or:

(2) Direct from the general practitioner.

The patient brings notes, often from more than one physician. With a long pain history, there may be many documents. There will be details, investigations and diagnoses by previous physicians but this does not mean that the algologist can accept them without confirmation. The difficult cases are those where the patient has a huge dossier of papers. The algologist must read these, but he must take his own history, make his own examination, and carry out his own investigations. Recent investigations may be accepted, repeated or extended. Nothing is taken for granted during these stages of history and examination, followed by investigation; then another review is carried out with further examination and enquiry, and detailed notes must be made and kept. Often a patient does not realise that there are associated defects present with his pain. These must be documented before treatment or the algologist will be blamed for their appearance after the treatment. It is best to demonstrate these deficits to the patient and his relatives beforehand. Making notes of what is found and done is of great importance, and full documentation is urged throughout all stages of consultation and treatment.

History

This gives, chronologically, the patient's previous illnesses; the present problem, its development and relation to previous illness; the family history and the patient's personal history and life-style.

In the history, the physician puts questions to the patient, the answer to one suggesting the following. In almost all cases the first question will be 'What is it that brought you to see me?' or a variation of it. It is designed to elicit what the patient is most worried about and where the pain is. Probably, it will not be the most important medical feature, but will be the one most important to the patient. In a chronic pain patient the answer should involve pain directly or indirectly: 'I can't walk. "Why?" Because of the pain', rather than 'I can't walk. "Why?" My legs won't move properly. "Since when?" Since the operation on my big toe. "How did you get up the stairs?" I got help', and so on. When a patient visits a 'pain' doctor and does not talk about pain, suspicions of a psychological problem are raised. This can be decided when the consultation is completed.

An overview

A quick survey of the situation is needed next to obtain an overall view of the problem. Some of the information elicited will be followed up in more detail later. Particular importance must be devoted to the type of pain; the areas of pain; if more than one, do they differ in these areas, or from time to time? Does it affect the patient's business, housework, appetite, sleep, activity and/or strength?

The questions 'where, when, how, why and how effective?' are used to get a rapid overview in relation to:

(1) This pain.
(2) Other pains.
(3) Other illness.
(4) Previous treatment.
(5) Previous medication.
(6) Time relations.

The enquiries of 'what, how much, how little, how frequently?' are used for the patient's activity. It is important to know what can't be done now that used to be possible. 'How did it come on? Slow, fast, or very suddenly? What is the result of rest, activity, graded exercise, analgesics?' Finally, 'What helps it; what worsens it; what makes no difference?' The answers to some of these questions enable further valuable judgements to be made (see below).

Note the relation between the patient's descriptions and his behaviour. Are these compatible? For instance, the patient may say the pain is so severe that he cannot sit on a chair for more than a few minutes, yet he sits still without wriggling for the whole of the consultation. He may smile while complaining of agony, or move when he says he cannot move. Is what he says reasonable? Is it possible that his pain never varies, or that he gets no sleep? Is his appearance compatible with an appetite so poor that 'food hardly passes his lips'. Does he look unhappy, discontented, depressed, anxious or agitated?

Does the history fit any of the known pain syndromes? Did the sciatic pain come on immediately or soon after lifting a heavy, awkwardly shaped article? Is the pain in the calves on walking of the severity of arterial claudication or is it the vague ache of a venous partial occlusion? Is the description of waking in pain at night, taking an analgesic and eventually getting off to sleep again due to a carcinoma, or is there a simpler explanation?

There are as many scenarios for the history as there are pain syndromes. It is up to the algologist to know these, to have read widely and to recognise their features. The initial complaint of pain will focus the attention on one or other part of the body. For instance, a complaint of pain in the leg coming on suddenly may signify disc disease, muscle trauma, sciatica or facet joint involvement. If it comes on slowly over some weeks it can be muscular, neoplastic, or again from a disc or facet joint. The type of pain and other features of its presentation are important. Some of these combinations form pain syndromes which are readily recognised. Some of the different pains and a few syndromes are given at the end of the next section in note form as examples. They are not meant to be comprehensive.

The initial history is of great importance and cannot be skimped. In a large number of patients, corroborative evidence will be required. The other elements of the consultation, the examination and the investigations provide this.

Type of pain

It is difficult to understand *exactly* what type of pain the patient has, and *exactly* where it is. Pain is a subjective sensation, so it is difficult for you and the patient to be on the same 'wavelength'. It is worthwhile taking time over this. It is also helpful in getting an idea of the patient's tolerance to pain. This is possible from the personal history – a previous toothache, cut, or broken limb (Chapman et al., 1985).

Not all patients can express themselves easily, so it may be necessary to present adjectives for the patient's consideration, such as hot, cold, burning, unpleasant, sharp, stabbing, like lightning, pins and needles, knife-like, stops you dead in your tracks. The words used in the McGill pain questionnaire are fairly comprehensive and easily understood (Melzack, 1975). They serve as a model and have the advantage of translation into different languages. The whole of the McGill pain questionnaire can be filled in by most patients at home on their own and assessed before the patient's consultation. It will provide a base line on the pain and gives some idea of the patient's psychological state. In many clinics, it is a standard pre-consultation procedure, usually organised and assessed by psychologists. The results are available at the initial consultation. Many clinics insist that the patient fills in the psychological assessment or McGill pain questionnaire under supervision at the clinic before the consultation. At home, if the patient has difficulty filling it in, a relative or spouse may help. It is not unusual for a spouse to be quite indignant that they are not allowed to 'help' the patient to fill in the questionnaire. 'It might not be filled in correctly' is not an unusual statement – and a very revealing one.

Visual analogue scale

The simplest method of quantifying a patient's severity of pain is by using the visual analogue scale (VAS). This is a 10 cm line; at one end is written 'no pain at all' and at the other end, 'the worst pain I could ever imagine'.

There are certain difficulties when using the VAS. In particular, it does not provide an accurate measurement between one patient's pain and that of another. The details are available (Murrin and Rosen, 1981).

Pain descriptions

The following descriptions have been used.
– Deafferentation pain... is burning, tingling, numb, uncomfortable, unbearable (Tasker, 1984).

- Nerve compression... severe constant ache, paraesthesiae, shoots.
- Nerve damage... burning, hyperpathia.
- Postherpetic neuralgia... shoots, constant ache, superficial burning, stabbing, dysaesthesia, hyperaesthesia. May last for years. Usually history of acute attack of shingles (Hope-Simpson, 1965).
- Fibrositis... widespread muscular aching.
- Trigger point... as fibrositis but more localised. Certain movements are limited, cause exacerbations, may refer some distance from trigger point (Travell and Rinzler, 1952; Travell and Simons, 1983; Lewitt, 1979; Glyn, 1971).
- Trigeminal neuralgia... intermittent bouts of lightning-like lancinating pain, uni-lateral, lasts a few seconds, in acute exacerbations bouts come every few min-utes. Quite incapacitating, patient may not wash or eat on one side of mouth (Loeser, 1984).
- Atypical facial pain... continuous uni- or bilateral pain in either or both sides of the face (Loeser, 1984).
- Intermittent claudication... increasingly severe pain in the muscles used during activity, usually in the calves during walking. Improves and disappears on cessa-tion of activity (Cousins et al., 1979; Mills, 1982).
- Rest pain... occurs usually at night in feet, may be improved by getting up and walking about, may occur in claudication, is due to arterial occlusion (Cousins et al., 1979).
- Bone pain... a deep ache, if inflammatory, throbs. In cancer often responds to non-specific anti-inflammatory drugs (NSAIDs), as prostaglandins are pro-duced by bony secondaries (Twycross and Lack, 1983; Galasco, 1980).
- Nerve entrapment... pain and paraesthesiae in distribution of trapped nerve, common in carpal tunnel in the median nerve distribution (Applegate, 1972).
- Meralgia paraesthetica... burning dysaesthesia in anterolateral thigh.
- Causalgia... hyperpathia, or hyperaesthesia in distribution of damaged nerve, extremely sensitive to touch, temperature, trophic changes in skin (Boas, 1983).
- Cancer pain... slowly increases in intensity, pain may be iatrogenic from pre-vious treatment. Remember, pain in a patient with cancer may not be related to the cancer at all (Twycross and Lack, 1983).

Mixtures of the types of pain mentioned are not uncommon (Wyant, 1979).

Position of pain

Details of where and how long the pain has been present are needed. Separation of the position of the pain in relation to time is not easy. Questions to ask are: 'Was it always in its present position? Did it start in one place and spread from there? Did it start in one place and then spread to several places? Dit it start in several places simultaneously? Are these places equally painful; do they vary and how; which is worse and when? How does it affect your way of life now? Can you go to work, or does it limit you?'

This question 'where is the pain?' requires persistence, as patients are not always sure of the answer. Answers such as 'all my arm' require supplementary questions, such as 'which arm?' and 'do you mean from the shoulder to the finger tips?' If a more limited area, then 'from where to where?' – ask the patient to show you what he means. Ask whether this includes the front and the back, the inside, or the outside? Put the patient's arm in the neutral position so the affected dermatomes can be easily seen. A chart of the whole body should be available so the patient can draw in the pain areas. It is best to use a blank chart without the dermatome lines drawn in, otherwise the patient follows these lines and the algologist tends to interpret pains dermatomally when such an interpretation may not be correct. When different types of pain are present, these can be shown by different types of cross hatching, or coloured pencils can be used.

Time scale of pain

It is necessary for some idea of the time scale and periodicity of the pain to be obtained. In any one patient, the pain suffered varies from time to time, and this will have diagnostic importance. To take an example from a well understood acute pain: the onset, type and frequency of indigestion depends, say, on whether it is caused by a gastric or a duodenal ulcer. These two will also be different from abdominal shingles, which will be different from the chronic condition of postherpetic neuralgia. All of them will differ from an acute gastritis. It is not only the time scale which distinguishes the conditions causing these pains. The type of pain, the course of exacerbations and improvements, the time scale of medication and its effects all help. Pains which do not vary over long periods of time may be psychological, but not necessarily. Steadily increasing pains which are unremitting, relieved in part by analgesics and wake the patient at night might suggest cancer, and that condition would need excluding.

Some of the questions to ask are: 'When did you first notice the pain; was the pain the same then as it is now; how did it vary? Was it as severe as it is now; how long before it became bad enough to need analgesic tablets? What did you use; for how long did they help; when did you go on to something else; how long did that help; what are you taking now and is it enough? Is there more than one pain; when do they come; how long does each last; do you have them all together, or in different places together? Can you remember what brings them on; how soon does it bring them on? What helps; how soon does it help; how long does it last?'

The time scale of the pain or pains is dealt with in detail. This information may appear also during the earlier history in a haphazard fashion. It needs arranging in chronological order. The same or similar questions are used in the different sections.

Personal history

The standard information of age, sex and previous illnesses combined with earlier details of the condition complained of may suggest one painful condition, for instance, rheumatoid arthritis is more common in women while ankylosing spondylitis is mostly a disease of men. A previous history of mental or psychological illness is important, but hypochondriacs can develop trigeminal neuralgia, cluster headache or a masticatory dysfunction syndrome, so such a patient complaining of pain in the head must be investigated properly. All patients should have a history taken and a careful examination made. First impressions are important and it is during the initial part of the history that an assessment is made of the accuracy, exaggeration, general attitude and truthfulness of the patient. Certain involuntary patient attitudes must be remembered. The patient may be worried about cancer and be scared; there may be litigation pending (Dworkin et al., 1985); the patient may be malingering, though this is rare; there may be pain behaviour and manipulation – of both the algologist and the patient's family (Sternbach, 1974; Fordyce, 1978; Pilowsky and Spence, 1975). This part of the history is no formality.

Enquiry is made into the sleep pattern and any alterations; the energy the patient has now compared to previously; his work in industry or in the house and how it has changed with time. Patients who have had chronic pain for some time give a good indication of activity by their 'up-time'. This is often used in psychological assessments, but is generally useful (Sternbach, 1979). The patient is asked to keep a 'pain diary' before the consultation. Comments are kept short or the diary becomes a book. Essential details are: up-time; variation of pain throughout the 24 h; the intensity of pain during this period. The relation to appetite, meals, analgesics, tobacco, excretion and total drug intake can be seen.

Use of 'street drugs' may be suspected. Appetite, weight loss and attitude are useful indicators, but illnesses producing similar effects, such as cancer or active rheumatic disease, need excluding.

Family history

The standard format is used, but the algologist is particularly interested in familial diseases such as the rheumatic conditions, chronic low back pain in the male patients, cardiac conditions, angina, high blood pressure and claudication. Gastric or duodenal ulcers, depression or other psychiatric conditions are all pointers to problems in the patient.

At this point in the consultation – before the physical examination – the algologist will have some ideas on the cause or the possible cause of the patient's pain and pays attention to these aspects. When a definite cause is found, the routine examination is not skimped. It is tempting to go no further, but the consultation should be completed as patients can have more than one condition and may have additional complications.

Physical examination

The physical examination is designed to check the normal functions and to find abnormalities and the cause of the present condition. It may not be possible to do this, but the examination is complete enough to determine whether there is no reason to explain the pain. In that case, the methods available in Chapter 2 are used. It is necessary to note which physical movements the patient is able to perform, as well as those he cannot perform, e.g., in a tennis elbow, which is an inflammatory response following trauma at the common tendinous origin of the extensors of the wrist at the lateral epicondyl of the humerus, movements which use the extensors of the wrist are sometimes impossible to perform, while movements at the uninvolved elbow are quite normal (Littler, 1980). Another example is that a stiff back, sciatica or prolapsed intervertebral lumbar disc prevents bending to touch the toes, but in lumbar facet joint disease, the pain occurs on straightening up again, not on going down – or at least it is worse on straightening.

Yet another example is the patient with long-standing diabetes and a stocking type of burning intractable leg pain; it may be concluded that the patient has a peripheral neuritis, but it would best be checked by diagnostic lumbar sympathetic block, as all or some of this pain may be due to a sympathetic dystrophy and not a diabetic neuropathy at all. If the patient has a stocking type of intractable pain with no other signs or symptoms, it is possible that the pain is of psychological origin.

If the patient has diabetes and migraine, it would be unwise to conclude that one causes the other. If the patient has long-standing diabetes, has lost a lower limb through vascular disease and has phantom limb pain, the explanation is different again – the patient has lost the limb probably due to the diabetes, but the phantom limb pain follows the amputation. The diabetic condition may make an already present circulatory problem worse, but it might not be causal. If the patient is young, it probably is causal. If the patient has brothers, some of whom have high blood pressure and vascular problems without diabetes, the causal relation of the patient's diabetes diminishes, particularly if the patient also has raised blood pressure (Arcangeli et al., 1976).

Sometimes, cause and effect are obvious, but with litigation spreading throughout the world, the algologist should not make uncorroborated statements or diagnoses.

THE CENTRAL NERVOUS SYSTEM

A complete examination should be made and complete notes of the findings should be placed in the case file. This examination should be repeated after any major diagnostic procedure or treatment, and the clinical effects and any side effects of the procedure should be documented.

Many patients are unaware that they have, say, a small area of analgesia or anaesthesia on their leg. However, if any procedure is carried out and the patient notices the defect afterwards, they will be convinced (with their relatives) that it is a new, recent feature and is the fault of the algologist. Thus, it is imperative that the documentation mentions the abnormality before the procedure. It is best to draw the patient's and also the relatives' attention to it before any procedure.

The examination of the central nervous system will cover movement, power, position sense and coordination; touch, pinprick, hot and cold sensation; vibration sense and reflexes. These apply to the cranial and spinal nerves alike. Thus, ocular movements, accommodation, nystagmus and papilloedema, visual acuity, smell, hearing and taste, balance and gait should be covered. Analgesic, dysaesthetic and hyperaesthetic areas are mapped out. This system is the key to our understanding of the pain process (Kellgren, 1977). The history, in conjunction with examination of this system, usually enables the algologist to arrive at a correct diagnosis, or exclude pathology in it. Naturally, pain in a particular part of the body will tend to expand the examination, e.g., pain or paraesthesia from neck to finger tips will direct attention to the possibilities of cervical disc (Nurick, 1975); facet joint disease (Mooney and Robertson, 1975); thoracic outlet syndrome (Lascelles et al., 1977) or tendinitis (Littler, 1980). If in addition there is a background of unremitting pain gradually getting worse over weeks or months, primary or secondary cancer is considered (Twycross and Lack, 1983). If the paraesthesia is worsened by elevating the arms, or the blood pressure varies with the arms in this position, then a cervical rib can be investigated. It is not proposed to go through all the possible combinations of pains, physical signs and history here as these are immense, but these must be understood by the algologist – and in considerable detail. A list of reading material is suggested at the end of this chapter.

OTHER BODY SYSTEMS

The patient must be fully examined, which means that the normal general examination is carried out. This will include the cardiovascular, respiratory, alimentary, dermatomal, endocrinal and reproductive systems. The presence of adenopathy, tenderness and trigger points is included (Travell and Simons, 1983). Particular attention is paid to painful areas and the muscles, skin and bones of those areas, and the possibility of referred pain.

INVESTIGATIONS

The physical examination and history should be enough to suggest the initial investigations. These fall broadly into two varieties; non-interventionist and interventionist.

Non-interventionist

This includes urine and faeces examinations, and probably the blood biochemistry can be included here, though strictly speaking the taking of blood is an intervention. Thermography can be used to show alteration of skin temperature in areas where the patient complains of pain. Skin thermometers can help, but they will not give such wide cover as thermography. Straightforward radiology and ultrasound e.g., of chest, heart or bone, is in this group. The algologist must know exactly what is needed in a particular investigation and ask for it. For instance, if a patient has previously had a lumbar spine fusion and reports a sudden return of pain on movement, an x-ray in the upright position is not enough. Films in normal position and obliques, in flexion and extension and in both lateral flexions will be necessary to exclude movement at the previous fusion site. It is best to consult the radiologist in advance for advice on which x-ray views would be best. If this is impossible, full notes must be sent to the radiologist in time to decide whether further radiological investigation will be needed. Computerised tomography (CT scan) is available to most hospitals now. Nuclear magnetic resonance (NMR) may be available and applicable.

In general terms, a CT scan will show soft tissue in, say, a lumbar spine. It can show a disc protrusion, but no further details. The pancreas is difficult to visualise by any method, but the best is ultrasound, provided there is not much bowel gas present. The NMR scan is not universally available, but it does not necessarily add more detail than the CT scan. Its great advantage is that the tomographic 'cuts' can be made in any desired direction, and information can be obtained from these special planes which is not available from the CT scan.

Interventionist

These investigations are of two types:

(1) Those such as myelograms, pyelograms, computer tomography with enhancement, bronchoscopy, oesophagoscopy and similar investigations are carried out by specialists of other disciplines. Nerve damage or compression may be corroborated by nerve conduction studies.

(2) Those carried out by the algologist. This latter type would include techniques such as nerve blocks to localise a pain pathway and sympathetic block, say,

when a sympathetic dystrophy is suspected. The intravenous lignocaine test seems
to be gaining adherents again. Here, 1.5 mg lignocaine per kg body weight is injected slowly intravenously. Pain due to a central process is improved or disappears, but not that due to a peripheral pain. In this way, pathophysiological pain
can be distinguished from psychopathological pain (Boas, 1983).

It must be remembered that all the tests and investigations mentioned have false
positive and false negative results. Thus, while they may be used to help with a
diagnosis, no single investigation should be allowed to decide the diagnosis without much careful thought regarding confirmation by some other method, or if this
is not possible, there should be a repeat investigation. The single most useful test
the author has found and used is the ESR. A raised ESR shows inflammatory
or neoplastic disease is present and therefore warrants persistent investigation.
The ESR is not raised in mechanical causes of pain.

REFERENCES

Applegate, W.V. (1972) Abdominal cutaneous nerve entrapment syndrome. *Surgery*, 71, 118–124.

Arcangeli, P., Digiesi, V., Rochi, O., Dorigo, B. and Bartoli, V. (1976) Mechanisms of ischemic pain
in peripheral arterial disease. In: *Advances in Pain Research and Therapy, Vol. 1*. Editors: J.J. Bonica
and D. Albe-Fessard. Raven Press, New York pp. 965–973.

Boas, R.A. (1983) The sympathetic nervous system and pain relief. In: *Relief of Intractable Pain, 3rd
Edn.*, Editor: M. Swerdlow. Elsevier, Amsterdam.

Chapman, C.R., Sola, A.E. and Bonica, J.J. (1979) Illness behaviour and depression compared in pain
center and private practice patients. *Pain*, 6. 1–7.

Chapman, C.R., Casey, K.L., Dubner, R., Foley, K.M., Gracely, R.H. and Reading, A.F. (1985) Pain
measurement: an overview. *Pain*, 22, 1–31.

Cousins, M.J., Reeve, T.S., Glynn, C.J., Walsh, J.A. and Cherry, D.A. (1979) Neurolytic lumbar sympathetic blockade; Duration of denervation and relief of rest pain. *Anaesth. Intensive Care*, 7,
122–135.

Devine, R. and Merskey, H. (1965) The description of pain in psychiatric and general medical patients.
J. Psychosom. Res., 9, 311–316.

Dworkin, R.H., Handlin, D.S., Richlin, D.M., Brand, L. and Vannuci, C. (1985) Unravelling the effects of compensation, litigation and employment on treatment response in chronic pain. *Pain*, 23,
49–59.

Galasco, C.S.B. (1980) The management of skeletal metastases. *J. R. Coll. Surg. Edinburgh*, 3,
148–151.

Glyn, J.H. (1971) Rheumatic pains: some concepts and hypotheses. *Proc. R. Soc. Med.* 64, 354–360.

Hope-Simpson, R.E. (1976) The nature of herpes zoster. A long-term study and a new hypothesis.
Proc. R. Soc. Med. 58, 9–20.

Kellgren, J.H. (1977) The anatomical source of back pain. *Rheumatol. Rehabil.*, XVI(1), 7–12.

Lascelles, R.G., Mohr, P.D., Neary, D. and Bloor, K. (1977) The thoracic outlet syndrome. *Brain*,
100, 601–612.

Lewitt, K. (1979) The needle effect in relief of myofascial pain. *Pain*, 6, 83–90.

Littler, T.R. (1980) Pain in rheumatic conditions. In: *Persistent Pain, Vol. 2*, Chapter 3, pp. 59–81.
Editor: S. Lipton. Academic Press, London.

Loeser, J.D. (1984) Tic douloureux and atypical facial pain. In: *Textbook of Pain, 1st Edn.*, Chapter 2.C.4, pp. 426–434. Editors: P.D. Wall and R. Melzack. Churchill Livingstone, Edinburgh.

Melzack, R. (1975) The Mcgill Pain Questionnaire; major properties and scoring methods. *Pain*, 1, 277–299.

Mills, K.R., Newham, D.J. and Edwards, R.H.T. (1982) Force, contraction frequency, and energy metabolism as determinants of ischemic pain. *Pain*, 14, 149–154.

Mooney, V.T. and Robertson, J. (1975) The facet syndrome. *Clin. Orthop. Relat. Res.*, 115, 149–156.

Murrin, K.R. and Rosen, M. (1981) Measurement of Pain. In: *Persistent Pain, Vol. 3*, Chapter 2, pp. 26–27. Editors: S. Lipton and J. Miles. Academic Press, London.

Nurick, S. (1975) Cervical spondylosis and the spinal cord. *Br. J. Hosp. Med.*, 13, 668–674.

Pilowsky, I. and Spence, N.D. (1975) Patterns of illness behaviour in patients with intractable pain. *J. Psychosom. Res.*, 19, 279–287.

Sternbach, R.A. (1974) *Pain Patients: Traits and Treatment.* Academic Press, New York.

Sternbach, R.A. (1979) Clinical aspects of pain. In: *The Psychology of Pain.* pp. 241–264. Editor: R.A. Sternbach. Raven Press, New York.

Tasker, R.R. (1984) Deafferentation. In: *Textbook of Pain, 1st. Edn.*, Chapter 1.9, pp. 119–132. Editors: P.D. Wall and R. Melzack. Churchill Livingstone, Edinburgh.

Travell, J.G. and Rinzler, S.H. (1952) The myofascial genesis of pain. *Postgrad. Med.*, 11, 425–434.

Travell, J.G. and Simons, D.G. (1983) *Myofascial pain and dysfunction. The trigger point manual.* Williams and Wilkins, Baltimore.

Twycross, R.G. and Lack, S.A. (1983) *Symptom Control in Advanced Cancer: Pain Relief.* Pitman, London.

Wyant, G.M. (1979) Chronic pain syndromes and their treatment. *Can. Anesth. Soc. J.*, 26, 216.

Additional reading

Bogduk, N., Tynan, W. and Wilson, A.S. (1981) The nerve supply to the human intervertebral discs. *J. Anat.*, 132(1), 39–56.

Foley, K.M. (1979) Pain syndromes in patients with cancer. In: *Advances in Pain Research and Therapy, Vol. 2*, pp. 59–77. Editors: J.J. Bonica and V. Ventafridda. Raven Press, New York.

Fordyce, W.E. (1976) *Behavioural Methods for Chronic Pain and Illness.* pp. 11–25. C.V. Mosby, St. Louis.

Fordyce, W.E. (1978) Learning processes in pain. In: *The psychology of pain.* pp. 49–72. Editor: R.A. Sternbach. Raven Press, New York.

Jeffrys, R.V. (1980) Cervical Spondylosis. In: *Persistent Pain, Vol. 3.* Chapter 5, pp. 115–141. Editor: S. Lipton. Academic Press, London.

Lance, J.W. and Anthony, M. (1966) Some clinical aspects of migraine. *Arch. Neurol.*, 15, 356–361.

Loh, L. and Nathan, P.W. (1978) Painful peripheral states and sympathetic blocks. *J. Neurol. Neurosurg. Psychiatry*, 41, 664–671.

Persistent Pain. Vols. 1–5 inclusive. Editors: S. Lipton and J. Miles. Academic Press, London.

Reid, W., Watt, J.K. and Gray, J.G. (1970) Phenol injection of the sympathetic chain. *Br. J. Surg.*, 57, 45–50.

Wall, P.D. and Melzack, R. (1984) *Textbook of Pain.* Churchill Livingstone, Edinburgh.

M. Swerdlow and J.E. Charlton (eds.) Relief of Intractable Pain
© 1989, Elsevier Science Publishers B.V. (Biomedical Division)

5

Drug treatment of chronic pain

J.Edmond Charlton

INTRODUCTION

It is a primary aim of medicine to reduce suffering. Any patient complaining of pain must be taken seriously and should not be allowed to remain in pain whilst a diagnosis, or lack of it, is established. In almost all cases this means that drug therapy will be introduced, or, if the patient is already on medicine, this may be changed. Thus, it is important that anyone caring for patients with chronic pain should have a good working knowledge of the drugs used.

This chapter will review commonly used groups of drugs such as opioids, non-steroidal anti-inflammatory drugs (NSAIDs), antidepressives and anticonvulsants. In addition, it will consider the claims of other groups of drugs to have a role in the management of chronic pain. Inevitably, there will be some omissions. Some drugs used in the treatment of acute pain have been omitted, except where it is useful to illustrate the management of chronic pain by a study performed on patients with acute pain.

As pain is usually multifactorial in its aetiology, no single treatment can expect to yield perfect pain relief. Thus, drug therapy must be considered as only part of the treatment that may be necessary. In addition, different parts of the pain problem may respond to different drugs, or even be caused by them. However, in many cases, drug therapy will be the chief component of treatment.

PHARMACOKINETICS AND PHARMACODYNAMICS

These terms are taken to mean the dynamics of drug absorption, distribution and elimination, the mechanisms of drug action and the relationship between drug

concentration and effect. For discussion of the basic principles of pharmacokinetics, see Benet and Sheiner (1985), and of pharmacodynamics, see Ross and Gilman (1985). Mather (1985) noted that those concerned with the relief of pain have
a tradition of ignoring kinetics when employing analgesic drugs. Kinetic differences between analgesic drugs are revealed by tests performed at different times
after administration. The concept of the 'total analgesia' to a given stimulus is represented as the area under the curve of effect plotted against time. This is appropriate unless the drugs have marked differences in rate of onset, intensity of
effect or duration of action. A more satisfactory method involves multiple comparisons between drugs given at different doses and observations being made over
a prolonged time (Janssen, 1982). From this sort of data, doses to produce equivalent effects can be calculated on a continuous basis, and this will yield information
about potency as well as the time-course of effects.

Problems arise from many sources, not the least being the individual variation
of patients. Among others of significance are acute and chronic pathophysiology,
which may alter drug response through changes in rates of absorption, distribution and/or elimination (Benet et al., 1984).

The majority of pharmacokinetic and pharmacodynamic studies have been
done on patients with acute pain. These studies have been important in establishing the action of opioid drugs given by non-traditional methods, such as epidural
administration. (Throughout this chapter the term opioid is used to designate a
group of drugs that are, to varying degrees, morphine-like in their properties.) The
studies of opioids have verified the bioavailability of such drugs given buccally
or rectally and have outlined the effects of pathology on drug elimination. However, there are vast differences between acute and chronic pain, and in addition,
the variability in pharmacokinetic parameters between patients is large and generally unpredictable.

STRATEGY OF OPIOID USE (MEAN EFFECTIVE ANALGESIC CONCENTRATION)

The individual patient is the correct person to judge the severity of pain and the
adequacy of pain relief. This is demonstrated by the effective analgesia that can
be achieved with patient-controlled analgesia systems. This method of drug delivery will allow, not only for individual differences in pharmacokinetics (i.e., rates of
distribution and clearance), but also for pharmacodynamics, which will consist of
many complex biochemical, psychological and physiological variables. Because of
the complexity of these variables, it may appear that the traditional subservience
to following pharmacokinetic principles is probably of limited use in the chronic
pain patient. Indeed, it is arguable that titrating to response, which would be ap-

propriate for acute pain management, is the wrong thing to do when dealing with chronic pain. Is this necessarily true? Using opioids as an example, patients may appear to be refractory to their effects due to tolerance from previous treatments, pathophysiology affecting pharmacokinetics, or myriad factors affecting pharmacodynamics. There may be a reluctance to increase dosage to obtain adequate clinical effect because of worries about side effects. Thus, pharmacokinetics may appear to be of limited value. However, it has been shown that patients have a reproducible minimum effective analgesic concentration (MEAC) for each individual drug, which is independent of the route of administration (Glynn and Mather, 1982; Mather and Glynn, 1982). The MEAC for the individual can also be of use when formulating treatment plans. For example, patients with very large values of MEAC, or who require heroic blood concentrations to provide pain relief, are probably candidates for alternative therapy, such as an analgesic with a different mode of action, or an appropriate destructive procedure. Alternatively, determination of pharmacokinetic parameters can identify those cases where blood concentrations, and therefore, doses, are inadequate to provide analgesia.

Oral medication remains the best way of treating most chronic pain patients. To be effective, an analgesic drug must have a high oral bioavailability and a low MEAC. Both these parameters can be determined easily and appropriate dosage schedules can be worked out. However, there remains a need to perform more long-term pharmacokinetic and pharmacodynamic studies in patients with chronic pain conditions. Those that are available are not usually related to patient treatment, but are biopharmaceutical. Recent textbooks of therapeutics do include pharmacokinetic and pharmacodynamic data where this is available, but it is clear that further studies are necessary (Avery 1980; Gilman et al., 1980). Patients who fail to achieve analgesia from any cause are more likely to become intractable because of therapeutic failure, and possible reasons for failure may go undetected without this knowledge.

It can be seen that the success of a dosing regimen is dependent upon many variables. Therapeutic monitoring is one way of making allowance for individual variations in response. However, merely checking a blood concentration does not substitute for clinical judgement, and any interpretation placed on a blood result must always be in the context of clinical data. The optimum therapeutic levels of the drug must be known, and these must be relevant to the group of patients or the individual being treated. About 25% of patients receive doses below or above the therapeutic range in a multiple dose regimen.

OPIOID PEPTIDES

The discovery of the endogenous opioid peptides and the identification of receptors for these substances have tended to obscure the fact that we need more data about the use of the drugs we possess at present. The impetus that these discoveries has given may yield new classes of analgesics, but that is still in the future.

Classification

There are at least five groups of naturally occurring opioid peptides (Hughes and Kosterlitz, 1983). Those that have attracted most interest comprise three families; the encephalins, the dynorphins and the endorphins. These opioid peptides may function as short-acting neurotransmitters or as long-acting neurohormones, and may show overlapping activity in their receptor-mediated actions. For a review of the significance of the various opioid systems and pain, see Millan (1986). The anatomical distribution of opioid peptides has been reviewed by Akil and her colleagues (1984). There are three main types of opioid receptor – mu, kappa and delta (Paterson et al., 1983), which have overlapping activity. The opioid peptides are widely distributed throughout the body and are found in the sensory and autonomic systems, limbic structures and neuroendocrine systems (Atweh and Kuhar, 1983), where they operate as part of a widespread inhibitory system. The system is inactive under normal conditions and only becomes active when an abnormal pathophysiological state supervenes. Thus, opioid peptides will not provide analgesia until a noxious stimulus occurs. This, to some extent, explains their role in transcutaneous nerve stimulation and acupuncture.

Clinical applications

The clinical use of endogenous opioids has been disappointing. This is unsurprising considering their widespread distribution and the likelihood that they carry out many different functions. Whilst it has been possible to achieve analgesia using opioid peptides, this has frequently been at the cost of marked side effects. Nonetheless, their discovery has opened the way for the spinal and epidural use of opioid drugs and it has concentrated research efforts towards finding drugs that are receptor-specific.

Morphine is taken as the typical agonist at the mu receptor. Drugs such as methadone, pethidine and codeine are clearly agonists at the mu receptor by their pharmacology and ability to substitute for morphine. Of the mixed agonist-antagonist drugs currently available, only buprenorphine appears to have partial mu agonist activity. The other mixed agonist-antagonists, of which pentazocine, nalbuphine and butorphanol are examples, show mu antagonist properties with kappa agonist activity, and all of them are analgesics.

Knowledge of the location of specific opioid receptor types may make it possible to utilize, for example, a selective kappa agonist to produce analgesia with a reduced incidence of respiratory depression. However, this might be at the cost of increased euphoria or sedation. To this end, several kappa agonists are already undergoing preliminary trials, and looking further into the future, it may be possible to achieve more selective analgesia with fewer side effects by employing partial kappa agonists. This sort of research may yield benefit to the clinician in time, but for the moment we must learn the effective use of the drugs we have.

ANALGESIC DRUGS

Opioid analgesics

Most studies of opioid analgesics have been carried out in volunteer subjects, acute pain patients or patients with cancer. There are few, if any, studies carried out on chronic pain patients. Much of the pharmacokinetic and pharmacodynamic data available relates to the spinal and epidural use of strong opioids and this will be considered separately (see p. 110). The prolonged use of strong opioids also carries problems with side effects, drug interactions, tolerance, dependence and abuse potential.

Chronic use

The prolonged use of strong opioids is still a matter of the finest judgement. Differences in law, politics, ethics and philosophy have led to wide variation in clinical practice throughout the world. It is true to say that there are many patients who are able to lead reasonable, productive lives, only because they are taking strong opioid analgesics on a regular basis. Conversely, there are many patients with cancer pain who continue to suffer severe pain because physicians or governments have reservations about the use of these drugs (Swerdlow and Stjernsward, 1982). The World Health Organization addressed this problem in a booklet entitled 'Cancer Pain Relief' (1986), which outlines basic strategies for the management of pain arising from cancer.

An analgesic ladder consisting of three steps is suggested. Firstly, a non-narcotic such as aspirin or paracetamol. Secondly, a weak opioid such as codeine, and thirdly, a strong opioid such as morphine. A fundamental principle is that if a drug is ineffective in controlling pain, another one that is clearly stronger should be prescribed. It is stated that the use of strong opioid analgesics should be instituted if the severity of the pain warrants it and, furthermore, that no account should be taken of expected survival time when the decision to introduce these drugs is taken. In addition, adjuvant drugs are administered as necessary. This analgesic protocol has been field-tested and found to be effective (Takeda, 1986).

There can be no justification for witholding adequate doses of strong opioids from patients with pain arising from malignant disease. The controversy is whether they should be used in patients with severe chronic pain that is *not* associated with malignancy. Many pain treatment programmes utilize drug withdrawal as part of their management strategy (Buckley et al., 1986). Others take the view that the use of strong opioids is permissable if the results justify it (Portenoy and Foley, 1986; Urban et al., 1986). Clearly, there is justification for both points of view. Experience with cancer patients suggests that tolerance and abuse are unlikely, and this view is supported by other studies which consider opioid use in non-cancer patients (Medina and Diamond, 1977; Porter and Jick, 1980). More important is the critical assessment of the patient's condition to determine whether treatment with opioids is indicated. Recent studies from Adelaide (Cherry et al., 1985) and Arner and Meyerson in Sweden (1988) have argued most cogently for the diagnostic use of opioids before long-term treatment is undertaken, as many pains commonly encountered in the pain clinic may not be opioid-sensitive. Only exceptionally is a strong opioid drug the best way to treat a patient with chronic non-cancer pain.

Therapeutic use of strong opioids

Equivalent dosages for representative opioids are shown in Table 5.1. Pratical experience would suggest variations from the dosages shown in this table, but as a general guide to relative analgesic activity it remains reasonable and has been used successfully as the basis of a drug management programme. Methadone is used as the standard in this table as this is the drug for opioid withdrawal in this protocol (Buckley et al., 1986).

Morphine

Pharmacology

This drug remains the gold standard by which all other opioids are judged. It is available as the sulphate or the hydrochloride, and there is no difference in the clinical effect between the two forms. In the blood, about one-third is bound to plasma proteins, which is less than other opioids (Olsen, 1975). Unbound morphine is predominantly ionised at physiological pH and it is very hydrophilic. It is rapidly distributed, primarily to muscle rather than fat (Paalzow, 1982), which would be the case for the majority of opiods which are more lipid-soluble (Mather, 1983). In the acute circumstance, this would suggest that patients with poor muscle blood flow might show a diminished response to i.m. morphine and an exaggerated one to i.v. injection. However, although morphine crosses the blood-brain barrier relatively poorly, clinical analgesia is achieved within a few

TABLE 5.1

Dosage equivalents for strong opioids

Drug	Dose (mg) equivalent to 10 mg of oral methadone	
	oral	i.m.
Agonists		
Codeine	200.0	130.0
Diamorphine (Heroin)	30.0	3.0
Fentanyl (Sublimaze)		0.1
Hydromorphone (Dilaudid)[a]	7.5	1.5
Levorphanol (Dromoran)		2.5
Methadone		8.0
Morphine	60.0	10.0
Oxycodone (Percodan)[a]	30.0	15.0
Oxymorphone (Numorphan)[a]		1.5
Papaveretum (Omnopon)		16.5
Pethidine/Meperidine (Demerol)	400.0	100.0
Partial agonists, agonist/antagonists		
Buprenorphine (Temgesic)		0.3
Butorphanol (Stadol)[a]		2.0
Nalbuphine (Nubain)		12.0
Pentazocine (Fortral/Talwin)	180.0	60.0

[a] Drug not available in United Kingdom.

Table modified from Buckley et al. (1986).

minutes of an i.v. injection.

Morphine is metabolized by glucuronidation in the liver and is then excreted by the kidney. The majority of work on the pharmacokinetics of morphine has been done as single-dose studies, which are of doubtful relevance to long-term chronic usage in patients with multisystem disease. However, Sawe and her colleagues (1983) have shown that the conjugation of morphine with glucuronic acid is proportional to the dose during long-term treatment with increasing doses. This study showed that the metabolic pathway for morphine does not become saturated even after very long periods of continuous treatment with increasing doses. This is illustrated by the demonstration of a linear relationship between the dose and the plasma levels of morphine, as well as its 3- and 6-glucuronidated metabolites, both of which are highly active and long-acting (Shelly et al., 1986; Osborne et al., 1986, 1988). They were also able to show that neither endogenous or exogenous factors, nor disease progression seemed to interfere with the metabolism of morphine. Other workers (Patwardhan et al., 1981) have shown that morphine is metabolized normally in patients with impaired liver function, although earlier studies suggested otherwise (Laidlaw et al., 1961). It would seem reasonable to exercise care when using morphine in patients with liver failure. Caution should also be exercised in patients with impaired ventilation, asthma and increased intracranial pressure (Inturrisi, 1982). These cautions extend to every other morphine-like drug.

Clinical use of morphine

Oral morphine

The metabolism of morphine, the 'first pass effect', means that higher doses of oral morphine are required to produce the same effect as a parenteral dose. Table 5.1 suggests an oral i.m. ratio of 6:1 (Inturrisi, 1984), but others have suggested that the ratio is about 3:1 (Twycross, 1984). Practical experience suggests that both are correct and that there is a widespread individual variation in response. Confirmation of this impression was obtained from an elegant study of the efficacy and pharmacokinetics of oral morphine in patients with cancer (Gourlay et al., 1986). This showed pronounced differences in the oral bioavailability of morphine. The values of the oral/parenteral ratio found in this study ranged from 2.5 to 10. Thus, variability in oral morphine bioavailability may be a major reason for apparent differences in response to oral morphine regimens. In addition, it is probably the main reason that oral regimens are thought to be less effective than the same drug administered intramuscularly or intravenously (Gourlay and Cousins, 1984).

Despite these problems, oral morphine remains the most widely used strong analgesic. It is chemically stable in water and its shelf life is determined by microbial contamination. The addition of chloroform water (0.25%, v/v) will prevent contamination for up to 3 weeks (Regnard and Davies, 1986). There is some evidence that sodium metabisulphite may be more effective (Regnard et al, 1984). The practical use of oral morphine solutions has been well reviewed by Walsh (1984a). This article emphasizes that treatment must be tailored to the needs of the individual, and recent pharmacokinetic data support this premise (Sawe et al., 1981a, 1983; Neumann et al., 1982; Gourlay et al., 1986). Morphine is given on a regular, time contingent basis. The use of time contingent, rather than pain contingent analgesic schedules, enables continuity of analgesia to be established and maintained.

Initial dosage of oral morphine is usually dependent upon the patient's previous analgesic requirements. There is no correlation with weight, height or surface area (Regnard and Davies, 1986). Elderly patients may require smaller doses than younger patients (Neumann et al., 1982). Obviously, doses should be titrated to relief of the patient's pain. Effective doses are of the order of 10 – 30 mg 4-hourly, with a range of 5 mg or less, up to 500 mg 4-hourly. It should be emphasized that if morphine dosages are reaching the higher levels mentioned, a critical appraisal of whether the pain is opioid-sensitive should be undertaken. Too frequently, there is a blind adherence to the use of these drugs, and the response to every change in the patient's symptoms is a reflex increase in the amount of opioid prescribed.

It may be necessary to prescribe oral morphine solutions more frequently than 4-hourly. In these circumstances, repeated dosing may mean disturbed or poor sleep patterns, with the possibility of loss of pain control if the patient is allowed to sleep too long. One solution may be to give an increased dosage at night. There is no evidence that this practice leads to an increased mortality (Regnard and Davies, 1986). Another solution would be to switch to a different formulation, such as slow-release morphine, or to switch to another strong opioid. Houde (1974) has shown that, in patients with pain due to cancer, cross-tolerance tends to be incomplete and that there may be some advantage in switching from one drug to another when dose escalation or unacceptable frequency of dosing becomes a problem.

Slow-release morphine

Sustained-release morphine preparations are now widely available. There are studies purporting to show advantages for this preparation over conventional oral morphine, but other clinical studies are less supportive (Twycross and Dewhurst, 1981; Walsh, 1984b). In particular, there are no extensive studies of the bioavailability and pharmacokinetic profiles of these formulations. It seems likely that there is little difference in bioavailability and that such advantage as there is rests purely with the convenience of the reduced dosing frequency (Walsh, 1984b; Hanks and Trueman, 1984; Hoskin et al., 1987). However, compliance may be improved and there may be fewer side effects related to high plasma levels. It should be remembered that controlled-release tablets may contain a large dose of drug, and if the drug is rapidly released, a systemic toxic reaction may occur. Nor can these formulations lengthen the dosage interval reliably. The usual transit time through the major site of drug absorption, the small bowel, is about 6 h, and a tablet taken on an empty stomach may well deliver most of its contents to the large bowel, where almost no drug absorption takes place. Thus, on theoretical grounds, the effectiveness of a strict 12-hourly dosing regime seems unlikely, and more frequent dosing schedules appear to have more likelihood of success.

Conversion from oral morphine solutions to controlled-release morphine, and vice versa, can be achieved by taking the total daily dose in mg and starting the same daily dose of the drug at an appropriate frequency. For example, 120 mg of morphine solution (i.e., 20 mg 4-hourly) is equivalent to 120 mg of controlled-release morphine (i.e., 60 mg 12-hourly).

Alternative routes

Morphine can also be given buccally, rectally or vaginally, although other agents may be more appropriate when these routes are used. Delivery by spread across a mucous membrane may be useful when the oral route is denied, for example, by disease progression or because of vomiting or dysphagia. There are no long-term studies of the bioavailability of morphine by these routes. Bioavailability from buccal administration appears to be the same as that from oral intake (Hoskin et al., 1987). Buccal morphine has been shown to be as effective as intramuscular morphine in a study of postoperative pain (Bell et al., 1985). Such data as are available suggest that absorption may be very variable in the case of the rectal and vaginal routes, and a dose increase of about one-third is usually necessary.

Continuous infusions

These can be intravenous (Holmes, 1987; Miser et al., 1980; Adams et al., 1984) or subcutaneous (Campbell et al., 1983; Miser et al., 1983; Ventafridda et al., 1986). The obvious advantage of these methods of delivery is that the dose delivered is unaffected by metabolic change, as is the case with the oral route. Most kinetic studies have been carried out on patients with postoperative pain. However, such data as there are relating to the use of these methods in the long-term relief of cancer pain (Miser et al., 1980, 1983; Nahata et al., 1984) supports a dose of 0.05 mg/kg per h (range 0.025–2.6 mg/kg per h) for both intravenous and subcutaneous routes. Both methods have been used most successfully for pain relief in patients receiving high dose chemotherapy with concomitant damage to mucous membranes, and who are unable to take drugs orally. They work particularly well in children.

   Although there are relatively few indications for parenteral analgesia in cancer patients, the subcutaneous route may be useful in some circumstances. Examples are, where vomiting is difficult to control and antiemetic treatment is taking effect; where there is acute pain and rapid effect is required; in patients with dysphagia and in patients in the last few days or hours of life. There are obvious advantages over intermittent intramuscular or subcutaneous injections. The equipment required is reasonably simple, and this method is not as intimidating to patients and staff as the use of the epidural or spinal route. In an anecdotal study, Ventafridda and his associates (1986), have reported the successful use of morphine infusions in adults over periods of time ranging from 4 to 17 weeks.

Diamorphine

Diamorphine (diacetylmorphine/heroin) is a pro-drug for morphine. Following absorption, it is rapidly deacetylated to 6-acetylmorphine and morphine and can be used in an identical fashion to morphine (see Table 5.1 for dosage). The oral solution has a short shelf life once it has been prepared (Evans, 1983). Controlled studies conducted in patients with advanced cancer receiving maintenance oral morphine or diamorphine and in cancer patients postoperatively have shown no difference between the two drugs (Twycross, 1977; Kaiko et al., 1981). More recent pharmacokinetic and opioid receptor binding studies have shown that diamorphine's actions are mediated through its metabolites and that this represents a relatively inefficient way of delivering morphine (Inturrisi et al., 1983; Inturrisi et al., 1984). It seems that the only possible advantage of diamorphine over morphine is the fact that diamorphine is eight times more soluble than morphine (100 mg will dissolve in 0.2 ml). However, the development of techniques such as subcutaneous infusion has rendered this advantage illusory. In addition, hydromorphone is almost as soluble as diamorphine and is at least eight times as potent (Beaver, 1980).

Brompton cocktail

There have been many variations on this traditional mixture of a strong analgesic (morphine or diamorphine), cocaine, a phenothiazine, alcohol, syrup and chloroform water. It was assumed uncritically that all the constituent parts were necessary for effective use (Mount et al., 1976; Melzack et al., 1976). However, in a later study, the same group of workers have shown that there is no difference in clinical effects or side effects between the Brompton cocktail and an oral morphine solution (Melzack et al., 1979). A recent, controlled study has clearly demonstrated that cocaine, in the doses normally employed in Brompton cocktail (10 mg by mouth), has no positive virtues in the management of chronic malignant pain. If anything, the effects upon the mood of the patients with chronic malignant pain were negative (Kaiko et al., 1987).

Methadone

This drug has a high oral bioavailability of about 80% (range 60–95%) as reported by Nilsson et al. (1982) and Gourlay et al. (1986). This compares with an oral bioavailability for morphine reported as varying between 38% (Sawe et al., 1981) and 26% (range 10–43%) reported by Gourlay and his colleagues (1986). Methadone has the longest half-life of any of the commonly available strong opioids. The terminal half-life is of the order of 30–40 h, and the clearance is much slower than that of other opioids. However, there is a fairly large variation in the half-life, and this necessitates care in adjusting the dosing interval in individual patients (Gourlay et al., 1986). However, this same study also showed that the bioavailability for morphine was even more variable.

Recently, efforts have been made to estimate methadone clearance and use this as a method of estimating analgesic requirement (Plummer et al., 1988). This study showed that in the elderly and in patients with malignant disease, the measurement of methadone clearance does not predict accurately the patient's analgesic needs.

It has been suggested that methadone is cumulative (Twycross, 1984). This is certainly true when the drug is introduced, and would be a problem if the 4-hourly dosing regimens necessary with morphine were employed. The implication is that methadone continues to accumulate whatever happens, as though none of it is ever metabolized or excreted. However, as we shall see, when used in an appropriate fashion, methadone is probably the drug of choice for long-term pain relief. It has also been stated that there is no straightforward relationship between plasma levels and degree of analgesia (Twycross, 1984). However, there is clear evidence that there is an excellent relationship between plasma levels and analgesia as shown by studies on postoperative pain (Gourlay et al., 1982a, 1982b, 1984) and in chronic pain (Paalzow et al., 1982; Gourlay et al., 1986).

Because of its unusual pharmacokinetic profile, methadone medication is best started slowly. This can either be done using an initial intravenous injection followed by once or twice daily dosing (Gourlay et al., 1986) or a patient-controlled dosing regimen (Sawe et al., 1981b). The latter method uses a fixed dose (determined by the patients pre-existing opioid intake) taken at time intervals chosen by the patient. Sawe et al. found that there was a decrease in the amount of drug taken and an increase in the dosing interval over the first 2 weeks; thereafter it became stable, with excellent pain relief. Gourlay et al. report that effective pain control was maintained with a dosing regime of one or two doses every 24 h, whereas for comparable effectiveness oral morphine solution required doses to be given 4–8 times or more per 24 h. It appears that daily fluctuations in blood concentrations will be much less with methadone than with morphine. Therefore, the potential for side effects associated with repeated peaks of blood opioid concentration immediately following a dose, and later with sub-therapeutic concentrations, is likely to be more pronounced with morphine. It is worthwhile repeating, however, that the dose and dosing interval for methadone must be carefully determined, as the potential for prolonged side effects exists if doses are too large and the dosing interval too short.

Pethidine/Meperidine

It is difficult to understand why this drug is given to any patient with chronic pain. There is a large first-pass effect, resulting in moderate to poor oral potency.

The young and the elderly are known to be sensitive to the effects of all opioids, but are particularly sensitive to pethidine, perhaps because of changes in plasma protein levels affecting binding. In addition, it is known that liver disease may increase bioavailability and prolong clearance and half life (Neal et al., 1979).

The major metabolite is norpethidine, which has a very long half-life of over 14 h, and thus accumulation may be a problem in the early stages of use. This problem may be greater in patients with renal impairment because the renal clearance of norpethidine exceeds the glomerular filtration rate. It has been incriminated in the production of a central nervous system irritability syndrome, but this has been debated (Austin et al., 1980). The use of this drug is contraindicated in patients taking monoamine oxidase inhibitors. Despite these problems, pethidine is being used in the treatment of patients with intractable pain (Glynn and Mather, 1982). However, its short length of action may lead to ineffective analgesia at night, although this could be overcome by the use of suppositories (Mather and Denson, 1986).

OTHER STRONG AGONISTS

The drugs mentioned in this section are alternatives to methadone or morphine in the management of severe intractable pain. Pharmacokinetic and pharmacodynamic data and controlled clinical trials are not available for the majority of these agents.

Dipipanone (Diconal)

This drug is available in Britain as a 10 mg tablet combined with 30 mg cyclizine, a phenothiazine antiemetic. Dipipanone has a longer length of action than morphine (up to 5 h), and has been suggested as a good intermediate drug, with potency between the weak and strong opioids (Twycross, 1978). It is claimed to produce good analgesia when taken regularly (Evans, 1981), but the present author believes that this combination should never be used on a long-term basis because of the presence of the phenothiazine.

Dextromoramide

This drug is a diphenylpropylamine, as is dipipanone. It is of limited use in the management of long-term pain because of its short duration of clinical effect (2–4 h). This is at variance with such pharmacokinetic data as are available, which indicate a long plasma half-life (Caddy and Idowu, 1979; quoted by Twycross, 1984). It is claimed to be less constipating than other similar drugs, but it is also quite sedative. 5 mg is alleged to be equivalent to 15 mg of morphine. A 10 mg suppository form is available.

Phenazocine

This is a benzmorphan derivative little used in chronic pain relief and of which even less is written. It is available as a 5 mg tablet, which has a length of action of up to 6 h. Claimed to be less sedating than morphine, its main virtue is that it is active when used sublingually and when used in this fashion, is not as irritant as many other drugs.

Levorphanol

Levorphanol is related to phenazocine and is alleged to have a duration of action of 6–8 h orally or by intramuscular injection. This drug has a long half-life and is like methadone in its characteristics (Dixon et al., 1983). Available as a tablet or injection, it is five times more potent than morphine. It is claimed to produce less nausea and vomiting than morphine and to be less sedative.

Oxycodone

This drug is only available as a suppository in the United Kingdom in the form of oxycodone pectinate. In this form, it can produce useful analgesia at night for up to 8 h. Oxycodone is available in the USA as a 5 mg tablet, a solution, and in various combinations with aspirin, paracetamol and caffeine. It is equipotent with morphine but has greater oral activity. It is well known in most pain clinics as a drug which produces modest, short-acting pain relief and long-acting behavioural problems when withdrawal is contemplated (Maruta and Swanson, 1981). The combinations with paracetamol and aspirin will limit dose escalation.

Oxymorphone

Not available in the United Kingdom, it is available in the United States as an injection and a suppository. It is very similar to morphine and the normal dose of 1 mg is reported to be equivalent to 10 mg of subcutaneous morphine and to have a similar duration of action (Twycross, 1984).

Hydromorphone

Hydromorphone is not available in the United Kingdom. Elsewhere, it is marketed in a variety of strengths as a tablet and an injection containing 2 mg per ml, and a new high potency formulation containing 10 mg per ml intended for chronic pain relief in the tolerant patient. It is extremely soluble and even stronger solutions are theoretically possible. A suppository is also available. Only limited clinical data are available, usually in the form of open trials, where it appears that, although more potent than morphine, the analgesia offered by hydromorphone is somewhat shorter in duration.

SIDE EFFECTS OF STRONG OPIOIDS

All strong opioids have major effects upon the central nervous system (CNS). Many of these limit the clinical usefulness of these agents and, on occasion, may

TABLE 5.2

Plasma half-lives of strong opioids

Drug	Plasma half-life (h)
Morphine	2–3
Pethidine	3–4
(Norpethidine)	14–21
Methadone	15–30
Levorphanol	12–16
Diamorphine[a]	0.05
Hydromorphone	2–3

[a] Biotransformed to morphine.

For references, see text.

necessitate their withdrawal because of persistent problems. The most obvious CNS effect is analgesia. This may be accompanied by changes in mood that may be pleasant to some patients and intensely upsetting to others. Mental impairment, as with most side effects, settles down with long-term use, but appears to be dose-related and may prove a problem as high dosages are introduced. Sedation, too, is frequent during the initial introductory period. This may be prolonged for up to 2 weeks in the case of methadone but will disappear with time. Forrest and his colleagues (1977) have studied the use of CNS stimulants to overcome the problem of sedation. The results were surprising in that 10 mg of dextroamphetamine not only reversed the sedating effects of morphine but also potentiated the analgesia. This method of treatment may be suitable for short-term use but is unlikely to be of long-term benefit.

Respiratory depression is a well known and consistent side effect with this group of drugs. Again, it may be a cause of concern when the drug is being introduced, but it is not usually a problem except in those with pre-existing respiratory compromise. Nausea and vomiting is the most common acute side effect, and most distressing to the patient. In general, this will settle down within 3–4 days, and if it does not, a further cause should be sought. Metoclopramide (10 mg i.m.) has been suggested as the most suitable antiemetic for opioid-induced vomiting, and if this is unsuccessful, either droperidol (2.5 mg i.m.) or haloperidol (0.5 mg i.m.) may be useful.

This group of drugs also have peripheral actions, and those upon the gastrointestinal tract are most prominent. Gut motility is slowed and sphincter tone is increased, primarily due to a direct neuronal effect. Thus, all opioids produce constipation, and this is the one side effect of opioids that never goes away. The constipation is dose related and requires prophylactic treatment whenever opioid medication is introduced. If it passes clinical trials successfully, the new drug Cisapride, which increases gastrointestinal motility in the face of opioids may solve this problem. It is not yet known what effect this drug has upon sphincters and thus, the problem of increase in biliary tract tone may remain.

TOLERANCE, DEPENDENCE AND ADDICTION

Tolerance

The cessation of side effects is an example of tolerance. Tolerance to analgesic effects of strong opioids is unpredictable in its onset, but it can be said to have occurred when increasing doses of drug are required to produce the same clinical effect. Clinically, tolerance is usually noted first as a decrease in the duration of analgesia. When the pharmacological basis for this decrease in duration is not understood by the medical and nursing staff, the patient is accused of being a clock watcher or an addict. The confusion associated with this phenomenon stems from the fact that the rate at which tolerance to analgesics develops may vary enormously. The reason for this is not understood. In general, the need to increase doses or change the frequency of dosing in patients with pain arising from cancer may be of pharmacological interest, but it is of little importance clinically because the drug continues to be effective. In addition, there are data to show that the vast majority of patients treated with strong opioids do not require heroic dosages (Twycross, 1984).

Dependence

Dependence is when the characteristic signs of a withdrawal syndrome occur. The severity of this will depend on the drug being taken and the dose and the duration for which it has been taken. Drug-seeking behaviour by the patient is more likely to occur when inadequate doses are being prescribed, and is due to tolerance and not dependence.

Addiction

There are advantages to the prescribing of strong opioids in the form of a 'pain cocktail', as this places control of the contents in the hands of the prescribing physician and makes withdrawal more straightforward (see Buckley et al., (1986) for details of withdrawal protocols). This is undoubtedly the best approach to adopt if it is felt that the intake of strong opioid medication is for social or recreational purposes rather than for pain relief. The recognition of addiction and abuse of drugs may be difficult. However, there is little evidence to support the view that this happens as a result of medical prescription. Sensible guidelines for the long-term use of strong opioids have been issued by the California Medical Association and are reprinted by Fields in his excellent monograph (1987).

SPINAL AND EPIDURAL OPIOIDS

Spinal and epidural opioids have been the growth industry of pain relief in the last decade, following the initial report of analgesia mediated through the direct spinal action of opioids (Yaksh and Rudy, 1976). This was followed by reports of the clinical use of intrathecal (Wang et al., 1979) and epidural (Behar et al., 1979) opioids in man. Recognition of the usefulness of subarachnoid and epidural opioids in the relief of acute and chronic pain is an advance, and hundreds of reports of the use of a number of different agents have appeared in the literature. Most of these reports concern acute pain relief, and are open and uncontrolled. Experience is available with the use of certain strong opioids in the control of chronic pain associated with cancer. The most significant achievement of the introduction of spinal and epidural opioids is the reawakening of interest in the kinetics of cerebrospinal fluid (CSF) and the drugs used. A discussion of the mechanisms of action of spinal and epidural opioids is beyond the scope of this chapter. Extensive reviews have been published (Yaksh, 1981; Jacobson, 1984; Cousins and Mather, 1984; Cousins, 1988a, b).

Opioids injected directly into the CSF become diluted and then passively diffuse into the spinal cord, producing profound segmental analgesia by an effect upon opioid receptors found predominantly near the substantia gelatinosa. A proportion of the drug will be bound by protein and lipid tissues, and a proportion will be removed by vascular absorption. The analgesic contribution from systemic uptake will depend on the physical characteristics of the drug used. In general, subarachnoid injections of opioids will produce cord concentrations which are far in excess of those seen after normal parenteral use.

Epidural opioids produce their effect by a combination of systemic absorption (Weddel and Ritter, 1981), dural penetration and uptake by epidural fat. Systemic absorption begins immediately and may result in plasma levels of drug similar to those achieved by intramuscular injection. For a review of the factors involved in the subarachnoid and epidural use of opioids see Bullingham et al. (1984) and Cousins (1988a, b).

The vast majority of studies concerning spinal and epidural opioids deal only with clinical effects. However, there have been pharmacokinetic studies of morphine in plasma and CSF following spinal and epidural use (Gustafsson et al., 1982a, 1984; Nordberg, 1984; Nordberg et al., 1984; Watson et al., 1984; Sjostrom et al., 1987a, b). The problems with studies of this nature have been reviewed by Cousins (1987).

Subarachnoid opioids

Most physicians have opted to use the epidural route, although there is no reason to believe that this offers any advantage or disadvantage, other than the fact that it offers a more suitable route for long-term use and for continuous delivery systems. Virtually all experience with subarachnoid opioids has been gained with morphine, although most strong opioid analgesics have been tried (Jacobson,

1984). Morphine is probably the most suitable agent for the relief of chronic pain as it is the best-documented drug. Its long length of action means bolus doses need be given only once or twice daily. However, there is no reason why other drugs cannot be used.

Clinical experience

Wang has reviewed his experience with the use of subarachnoid morphine since his original paper in 1979 (Wang, 1985). This experience is illustrative of some of the pitfalls that accompany this method. During the initial testing with a dose range of 0.5–2.0 mg, 74% of his patients experienced reasonable pain relief. 26% failed to obtain satisfactory pain relief, or developed intolerable side effects. Six of 28 patients with an intrathecal catheter developed a persistent CSF leak. 43% of those with catheters and 50% of those with implanted pumps developed either tolerance or severe complications.

Dosage for chronic use

In a retrospective, multiphysician survey, Yaksh and Onofrio (1987) have considered the doses of intrathecal morphine given via chronic infusion. Infusions were given for a mean of 13 weeks. As might be expected, there was a time-dependent increase in the infusion dose from the initial level of approximately 4 mg/day. The magnitude of the increase was 3-fold at 3 months, and 5-fold at 6 months. This corresponds to previously reported levels, although there is a wide range (Auld et al., 1985; Krames et al., 1985; Shetter et al., 1986). The incidence of complications was low.

   Although experience is still sparse and there are no prospective controlled studies, it appears that the subarachnoid route offers an effective way of controlling the pain of malignant disease. The drug of choice is probably morphine, which will produce profound, prolonged analgesia and is suitable for both intermittent and continuous use. The optimal starting dose for the relief of acute pain is 0.5–2 mg, but it is probably necessary to use higher doses in the relief of chronic pain as parenteral opioids will invariably be used. It is suggested that 2–4 mg is used initially. The site of injection is probably not critical when morphine is used, and changes in dose and volume of injectate can be made where other drugs are employed. It has been claimed that the duration of analgesia can be increased, and the incidence of side effects reduced by using a hyperbaric solution (Caute et al., 1988).

Side effects

The major side effects are drug-related or system-related. There is little experience with any drug other than morphine. Side effects vary from the irritating to the downright dangerous. These have been summarized by Jacobson (1984) and vary from acute and delayed respiratory depression, nausea and vomiting, to pruritus and urinary retention. Technical side effects associated with catheters and implantable systems include blockage and kinking of the catheters, haemorrhage, infection and CSF leakage.

Up to 45% of patients given subarachnoid opioids develop pruritus. This may be less frequent with preservative-free morphine, but is not related to histamine release. The pruritus can be either segmental or widespread and particularly affects the head and neck; it can be abolished by small doses of naloxone (0.2 mg) that are insufficient to abolish analgesia. This topic is reviewed by Ballantyne and her colleagues (1988). Nausea and vomiting are common to the use of opioids by any route and affect up to 25% of patients given subarachnoid morphine. Urinary retention will occur in about 20% of males and is less common in females. The mechanism is not known but may be related to the loss of sensation in the bladder, and an associated increase in sphincter tone (Bromage et al., 1982a).

Respiratory depression is the most serious side effect and will occur in up to 5% of patients treated with subarachnoid morphine. This is ten times greater than the incidence following epidural morphine. Both early and late respiratory depression are seen. The former results from vascular uptake, and the latter from slow rostral spread of the hydrophilic morphine in the CSF. Kafer and her colleagues (1983) in a study of epidural morphine showed a biphasic depression of ventilatory response to carbon dioxide, the first at 1–2 h from vascular uptake and the second at 8 h from the cephalad movement of the morphine in the CSF. It has been suggested from a study of 9300 patients that respiratory depression is more likely in patients aged 70 or over, in those with impaired respiratory function, where the thoracic epidural route has been employed, and where there is concomitant use of other opioids (Gustafsson et al., 1982b).

Epidural opioids

Epidural opioids work partly by diffusion across the dura, and thus the clinical effect will be determined, to some extent, by the physical characteristics of the dura and the drug employed. Moore and his colleagues (1982) have suggested that transfer of opioids across the dura is proportional to their molecular weight. Their studies indicate that when the concentration gradient to the spinal cord is high, for example, immediately after an epidural injection, the primary determinant of the permeability constant is the molecular weight of the drug injected. Thus, drugs with similar molecular weights, such as morphine and methadone, will cross the dura at the same rate. Although diamorphine is more lipid-soluble, and thus might be expected to work quickly, the increased molecular weight means that it will diffuse at the same rate as the other two drugs. Highly lipid-soluble, bulky drugs such as buprenorphine will have negligible transfer to the CSF. The exception to this is fentanyl, which is a sausage-shaped molecule and seems to be able to diffuse faster because of this. Further variation will occur with the site of injection, as the dura is thicker at the top and thinner at the bottom. The role of epidural fat is unclear, but it seems likely the more lipophyllic drugs will be taken up to a greater degree by this fat and this may serve as a depot for drugs and act as a sustained-release mechanism which may have significance when chronic dosage is employed.

The rate of systemic absorption competes with the rate of dural penetration by reducing the concentration of drug available to penetrate the dura. Other factors are important in the clinical effect. For example, the volume of the injectate will increase the amount of dura in contact with the drug; height and posture will have similar effects; age may be a factor, as evidenced by the increased number of complications in the elderly, and the addition of adrenaline may inhibit transport across the dura, as shown by lowered plasma levels of drug (Bromage et al., 1983).

Clinical experience

Epidural morphine is recognized as a highly effective long-term treatment for cancer pain (Magora et al., 1980; Howard et al., 1981; Zenz et al., 1981; Coombs et al., 1982; Gustafsson et al., 1982b; Crawford et al., 1983). Patients can be managed on a domiciliary basis and maintain full activity (Christensen, 1982). Systems employed range from percutaneous catheters (Zenz et al., 1981) to totally implanted systems with rechargeable, programmable infusion pumps (Coombs et al., 1982). The type of system employed depends on the resources available and the needs of the patient, but most clinical circumstances can be served by an implanted reservoir into which the drug can be delivered by intermittent injections, or via an external syringe driver as required. It seems likely that the use of epidural opioid infusions at a constant slow rate poses a lower risk of tolerance developing (Cousins and Mather, 1984).

Other drugs used epidurally to treat pain caused by malignant disease are pethidine (Glynn et al., 1981; Gustafsson et al., 1982b) and buprenorphine (Crawford et al., 1983; Pasqualucci et al., 1987). However, systematic studies are lacking and there are few comparative studies to indicate the relative efficacy and safety of the various opioid drugs when used epidurally for cancer pain. There is scope for further studies to delineate the optimum volume, site of injection and delivery system. There is some evidence that the site of epidural injection is important and that this should be reasonably close to the site of pain. If this cannot be achieved for anatomical reasons, it may be possible to counteract this with manipulations in choice of drug, volume of injectate and dosage.

There are isolated anecdotal reports of the use of epidural opioids in non-malignant pain (Chayen et al., 1980; Crawford et al., 1983; Gorski et al., 1982). No conclusions whatsoever can be drawn from these reports. Indeed, the veracity of some of them must be cast into doubt by conclusions drawn from a systematic and specific analysis of pain likely to respond to epidural morphine.

Arner and Arner (1985) have analysed the analgesic response to epidural morphine of various types of pain associated with cancer. Their conclusion was that the best response was obtained when the pain was continuous and arising from deep somatic structures. Pain was less reliably relieved when associated with a neurogenic or cutaneous origin. Incident pain, such as that arising from a pathological fracture or an obstructed bowel, was not helped. They stress that careful analysis of the type and pattern of pain is mandatory before embarking upon invasive therapy.

The use of diagnostic epidural opioids has been suggested by the Adelaide group as a way of differentiating between organic and functional pain (Cherry et al., 1985). Possible pitfalls in this approach have been discussed by Arner and Meyerson (1988), who found opioids to be relatively ineffective by any route for idiopathic and neuropathic pain.

Dosage for chronic use of epidural opioids

In the absence of systematic studies, it is difficult to be certain about optimum dosage of any strong opioid used epidurally. Certainly it is unwise to give excessive amounts in the hope of achieving a greater clinical effect (Knill et al., 1981). Data from dose-response studies performed in patients with acute pain indicate that the optimum starting dose of morphine is 2–6 mg (Martin et al., 1982; Kafer et al., 1983). Higher doses may give a longer duration of action, but this may be at the cost of increased side effects (Bromage et al., 1982b). Systemic uptake is at a rate similar to that seen after intramuscular injection. The study of epidural morphine requirements in patients with chronic cancer pain by Samuelsson and his colleagues (1987) suggests that higher doses of the order of 18 mg per day were needed to obtain pain relief. With continuing use up to 3 months, dose requirement increased 4- to 5-fold. Interestingly, no correlation was found between pain relief and CSF morphine concentrations in this study. It would appear that morphine requirements may show considerable variation between patients as well as in the individual patient.

Similar variation in dose requirement has been demonstrated in acute pain studies for pethidine (Sjostrom et al., 1987a, b), diamorphine (Watson et al., 1984) and buprenorphine (Pasqualucci et al., 1987). As tolerance develops with continued use, dosage requirements will rise. Various solutions to this problem have been suggested, among them injections of local anaesthetic which, it is alleged, 'rests' the opioid receptors (Chayen et al., 1980; McCoy and Miller, 1982), using the delta agonist D-Ala-D-Leu-encephalin (Krames et al., 1985), switching drug and using the alpha-adrenergic agonist clonidine (Coombs et al., 1985; Glynn et al., 1987).

Side effects

Side effects present with the use of subarachnoid opioids occur less with epidural opioids. For example, itching occurs in 8.5% of cases with epidural opioids and in 46% when the drug is administered by the subarachnoid route (Ballantyne et al., 1988). Other problems that have been reported include pain on injection, a seizure (Landow 1985), euphoria, anxiety and hallucinations (Gustafsson et al., 1982b) and metastatic carcinoma following prolonged use of a catheter (Pedersen and Madsen, 1985).

Methods of delivery

Many different systems are now being marketed for the delivery of opioids either intrathecally or epidurally. For techniques and descriptions, see Mather and Raj (1986).

WEAK OPIOIDS

Drugs of this type are prescribed frequently by primary care physicians for a wide variety of painful disorders and it is not unusual to encounter patients attending the pain clinic who have taken them for many years. There are three major drugs in this group: codeine, dihydrocodeine and dextropropoxyphene. These are prescribed frequently in combination with other analgesics. They are recommended by the World Health Organization for cancer pain that is not responsive to non-opioid analgesics. Despite this recommendation, there are almost no modern data concerning the use of these drugs in chronic pain. All drugs in this group have an equal potential for addiction, but this is lower than with the strong opioids.

116

Codeine

Codeine is suggested as the first choice drug in this group. It is structurally similar to morphine and is approximately two-thirds as effective orally as when given parenterally. This is due to less first-pass metabolism in the liver. About 10% of the codeine is demethylated to form morphine, and it is possible that the analgesic effect may be due to this. However, it should be noted that it has distinct actions of its own and is a powerful cough suppressant and is very constipating. The plasma half-life is 2–3 h (Jaffe and Martin, 1985). Normal clinical dosage is 30–60 mg orally every 4 h to a maximum of 360 mg. In combination with aspirin-like drugs, the analgesic effects are usually additive, but the variability in response is considerable (Cooper and Beaver, 1976).

Dihydrocodeine

Dihydrocodeine is only available in a few countries and is chemically related to codeine. It has properties similar to codeine when used at the same dosage, and is slightly more potent. It has a shorter length of action than codeine and this makes its value in the management of chronic pain extremely limited. It is contraindicated in pain of dental origin, as a dose-related hyperalgesic effect has been reported (Seymour et al., 1982). This caveat may apply to the use of all opioids in dental pain.

Dextropropoxyphene

Dextropropoxyphene is an amazingly popular drug and is prescribed in vast amounts, either alone, or in combination with other analgesics such as aspirin and paracetamol. The pharmacokinetic data for this drug are incomplete, but suggest

TABLE 5.3

Dosage equivalents – weak opioids

Drug	Dosage (mg)
Codeine	30
Dihydrocodeine	30
Dextropropoxyphene (hydrochloride)	65
Dextropropoxyphene (napsylate)	100

a bioavailability of about 50%, with a long half-life, plus metabolism to an active metabolite (norpropoxyphene), which also has a long half-life (Mather and Raj, 1986). Thus, this drug has the potential for steadily developing toxicity. Patients with hepatic dysfunction and poor renal function are particularly at risk.

Dextropropoxyphene is associated with problems in overdosage (Editorial, 1977), notably a non-naloxone reversible depression of the cardiac conducting system, and this may be associated with its local anaesthetic activity. Furthermore, Miller and his colleagues (1970) reviewed 243 reports of the use of this drug and concluded that there were few hard data on its therapeutic value. Using similar data, Smith (1971) concluded that the analgesic efficacy of this drug is less than that of aspirin and barely more than that of placebo. Despite these facts, this drug still has some notable supporters (Twycross, 1984; World Health Organization, 1986). Dextropropoxyphene studies fail to show any analgesic superiority over codeine, and thus it is difficult to see any reason for the popularity of this drug, either alone or in combination. Codeine is much cheaper and is known to be effective, thus the role of dextropropoxyphene as a modern analgesic is in serious doubt.

AGONIST-ANTAGONISTS AND PARTIAL AGONISTS

Most of the drugs in this section are either competitive antagonists at the mu receptor (i.e., they can bind to this site, but exert no action) or they exert only limited actions (i.e., they are partial agonists). Those that are antagonists at the mu receptor can provoke withdrawal in patients receiving conventional agonist opioids.

Pentazocine

Pentazocine is a benzomorphan derivative which is a very weak antagonist at the mu receptor. It has less abuse potential than the conventional agonists such as morphine. It produces an analgesia which is clearly different from morphine and is probably due to agonist actions at the kappa receptor. There are no detailed studies of its use in chronic pain, but basically it is a high clearance drug with a low oral bioavailability of about 20% and a half-life of 2–3 h (Ehrnebo et al., 1977). Normal analgesic dosages are 30–60 mg of pentazocine by injection, which is alleged to be equivalent to 10 mg of morphine. An oral dose of 50 mg will yield analgesia equivalent to that produced by 60 mg of codeine. Side effects are common, with sedation, sweating and dizziness the most common. Nausea is less common than with morphine. At doses slightly higher than those normally used clinically, pentazocine produces psychotomimetic side effects. This problem, and its short length of action, make it an unsuitable drug for use in chronic pain. The pharmacology of pentazocine has been reviewed by Brogden and associates (1973).

Nalbuphine

This drug is structurally related to the pure mu agonist oxymorphone and the pure mu antagonist naloxone. It is a prominent antagonist at the mu receptor and is probably unique in being a partial agonist at the kappa receptor. Nalbuphine has a half-life in plasma of about 5 h. Given orally, it has about a 20% bioavailability (Beaver et al., 1981). Ten mg of nalbuphine intramuscularly is equivalent to 10 mg of intramuscular morphine, with a slightly longer duration of action. Nalbuphine causes respiratory depression similar to morphine in the useful clinical dose range of up to 30 mg. After this, there is a 'ceiling effect' in that no further respiratory depression occurs, but neither does any more analgesia; indeed, both respiratory depression and analgesia tend to reverse with further increase in dosage. Nalbuphine has virtually no effect whatsoever on the cardiovascular system (Lake et al., 1982), and it may also have an advantage in that it may not raise biliary tract pressure. It is difficult to envisage any major role for this drug in the relief of chronic pain.

Butorphanol

Butorphanol is a morphinan congener with a clinical profile similar to that of pentazocine. Butorphanol is a high-clearance drug with a half-life of 3 h. It would

TABLE 5.4

Plasma half lives of agonist/antagonists and partial agonist

Drug	Plasma half-life (h)
Pentazocine	2–3
Nalbuphine	5
Butorphanol	3
Meptazinol	2–3
Buprenorphine[a]	3

[a]Partial agonist. High receptor affinity prolongs clinical effect.

be expected to undergo extensive first-pass metabolism which would markedly limit its use in chronic administration. Parenterally, 2–3 mg of butorphanol produces analgesia and respiratory depression equivalent to 10 mg of morphine, with a similar length of action. Its side effects are very similar to those of pentazocine, including the potential for psychotomimetic problems at the upper levels of dosage. It is no longer marketed in the United Kingdom and will be of little or no use in the management of chronic pain.

Buprenorphine

This drug is a semi-synthetic, highly lipophilic opioid derived from thebaine. Like butorphanol, it is a high-clearance drug with a half-life of about 3 h. It undergoes extensive metabolism when taken orally, and to avoid this effect it is given sublingually. Pharmacokinetic analysis indicates that the bioavailability is variable after both intravenous and sublingual administration and can be in excess of 90%. Buprenorphine (0.4 mg) is equivalent to 10 mg of morphine given intramuscularly with a duration of action of 6 h. Thus, the short half-life bears little relationship to the duration of its clinical effects and this may be accounted for by its extremely high receptor affinity. For a review of the pharmacology of this agent, see Heel et al. (1979).

Side effects are similar to those produced by morphine, but the incidence of nausea and vomiting appears to be substantially higher. However, respiratory depression and constipation are somewhat less. The long duration of action and high bioavailability would suggest a role for this drug in the management of chronic pain. However, it is difficult to find any controlled studies in the literature, and the high incidence of side effects seems the likely reason (Evans, 1983). Those patients who can tolerate this drug appear to get long-lasting effective analgesia. Andriaensen and Van de Waale (1976), quoted by Evans (1983), reported good analgesia with dosages ranging from 0.15 to 0.8 mg, but with a 50% incidence of side effects. A comparative study of intramuscular morphine and buprenorphine in the treatment of chronic pain of malignant origin showed a similar result (Kjaer et al., 1982). For epidural use, see Pasqualucci et al. (1987).

Meptazinol

This drug belongs to a chemical series known as hexahydroazepines. It is known to act as a mixed agonist-antagonist at opioid receptors, but differs from all conventional drugs of this type by having an analgesic action that is independent of this. It has been suggested from animal studies that this is due to an effect at central cholinergic synapses. The pharmacokinetic data are not clear about this drug, and there may be a marked variation in bioavailability. Dosage is 75–100 mg intramuscularly, and duration of effect is similar to that of pethidine (Charlton, 1985). It may be more effective intramuscularly than by intravenous infusion (Harmer et al., 1983), and less effective orally; doses of 200 mg orally will give analgesia equivalent to 60 mg of codeine. Side effects are similar to those reported for buprenorphine. This drug has little to commend it for use in chronic pain.

Naloxone

Naloxone is a competitive antagonist at all the opioid receptors. Given on its own, it produces no discernible subjective effects in dosages up to 12 mg. Thus, any opioid-induced effect, either endogenous or exogenous, can be reversed by naloxone. It has been demonstrated that it will decrease the pain tolerance of individuals with high pain thresholds, reverse the effects of placebo and antagonize the analgesia produced by low frequency acupuncture and low frequency electrical stimulation. The presumption is that all these effects are mediated through endogenous opioids (Jaffe and Martin, 1985).

It has also been suggested that naloxone has a role in reversing some of the troublesome side effects of subarachnoid and epidural opioids. Small doses (0.4 mg) given intramuscularly will reverse respiratory depression without antagonizing the analgesia (Korbon et al., 1985). However, the length of action of naloxone may be as little as 1 h, so that subsequent doses may be required. The potential for reversing the analgesia always accompanies the use of this drug in this fashion.

Budd (1985) has reported the use of naloxone in large doses to treat the pain of thalamic syndrome. Anecdotal reports have suggested that doses ranging from 4 to 12 mg may yield analgesia ranging from a few days to several years. The drug can either be given as a single infusion, or as a series of infusions utilizing gradual increases in dosage (Ray and Tai, 1988). As cardiac arrest has been reported following reversal of opioids with naloxone, full cardiovascular monitoring should be employed during naloxone infusions (Cuss et al., 1984). There is no obvious mechanism for this analgesic effect, and controlled studies are needed.

Nefopam

Nefopam is a centrally acting drug that is chemically related to orphenadrine and diphenhydramine. It is not an opioid, nor is it a non-steroidal anti-inflammatory drug, nor is it an antihistamine. The mechanism of analgesic action is unknown. As a non-opioid, it is free from problems of habituation and respiratory depression. Normal dosage is 30–90 mg 8-hourly by mouth, or 20 mg 6-hourly by intramuscular injection. This drug has a high side effects profile and the side effects include dry mouth, insomnia, sickness, dizziness and headache. Side effects appear to be dose-related and may be linked in some way to the sympathomimetic actions of the drug. The pharmacological properties and its efficacy have been reviewed by Heel et al. (1980). McQuay and his colleagues have reported the use of nefopam in chronic back pain (1986). They were able to demonstrate a dose-response curve for analgesic effect in the single-dose part of this trial. With long-term usage, the doses required to produce analgesia caused frequent side effects, and two-thirds of the patients withdrew from the study because of side effects or lack of clinical effect.

NON-OPIOID ANALGESICS

This large group of drugs includes the non-steroidal anti-inflammatory drugs (NSAIDs) and paracetamol. These drugs are prescribed commonly, and frequently are effective in the relief of mild to moderate acute pain arising from the musculoskeletal system, toothache, headache, dysmenorrhoea and other minor pains. They may have a smaller role to play in the management of long-term pain because of the high number of side effects associated with their use.

This section cannot be comprehensive by virtue of the sheer volume of literature available. In addition, many of these papers are sponsored by manufacturers and tend to compare inappropriate drugs, or inappropriate doses of appropriate drugs. Scientific methods are often absent, and many of the papers presented at sponsored symposia fall into the 'modern impressionist' school of investigation.

Mode of action

Until recently, the relief of pain and inflammation provided by NSAIDs was thought to be due to inhibition of the enzyme cyclooxygenase (Vane, 1972). Vane suggested that membrane disruption allowed lipid components to be acted upon by phospholipases to produce arachidonic acid. End-products in the cascade of arachidonic acid breakdown include endoperoxides and prostaglandins, but how these substances mediate information remains incompletely understood. Various problems have been encountered with the so-called Vane hypothesis, and these have been summarized by Kantor (1988).

Metabolism of NSAIDs

All NSAIDs are metabolized to inactive compounds by conjugation in the liver. The conjugated compounds, most of which are glucuronides, are then excreted by the kidney. Thus, it follows that the effect of hepatic or renal pathology must be considered when prescribing NSAIDs. Some NSAIDs undergo such extensive metabolism that they may be safe even when there is extensive renal impairment. This property has been claimed for ketoprofen (Kantor, 1986). However, it is worth remembering that the elderly have a markedly reduced number of functioning nephrons, and they may have decreased liver function as well. In addition, the elderly show differences in the distribution and protein binding of these drugs that may make the dose-activity relationship greater. This effect is more of a problem with those drugs that have long half-lives. However, this property is generally regarded as being an advantage in both chronic pain patients and the elderly, where simple dosing regimens offer the advantage of higher compliance. It is wise to warn patients of the possibility of increased biological effect when prescribing the longer-acting drugs, such as naproxen, piroxicam or those agents with shorter half-lives presented in sustained-release form. It should be noted that plasma half-life does not always correlate with duration of action, nor do pharmacokinetic data explain the widespread individual variation in response to these drugs (Huskisson, 1984). Age-associated changes in response to aspirin and similar compounds have been reviewed by Baskin and his colleagues (1981).

Side effects

As the clinical use of this group of agents is limited frequently by side effects, it is reasonable to consider this topic next. There is no doubt that NSAIDs are highly effective in relieving the symptoms of arthritis and of conditions where the inflammatory component to the disease process is causing pain. However, there does not appear to be any drug of choice, and frequently the limiting factor in the choice of NSAID has been the incidence of side effects. Several members of this group of drugs have been withdrawn in recent years because of serious adverse reactions.

There seems little doubt that inhibition of cyclooxygenase is an explanation for the adverse effects of NSAIDs. Prostaglandins are physiological substances with a variety of roles in the body. The presence of PGE_2 and prostacyclin in the gastric mucosa will affect gastric physiology and the cytoprotection of the gastric mucosa. The same substances will modulate the effects of pressor substances on the renal blood supply. Other serious side effects, less clearly linked with prostaglandin inhibition, involve the skin, and, rarely, the liver and bone marrow. NSAIDs can also provoke acute asthma in susceptible individuals.

Gastric problems

Gastric irritation, erosion and peptic ulceration all become more likely when there is inhibition of prostaglandin synthesis. This will lead to loss of the mucous barrier and reduce mucosal blood supply. The dosage and duration of treatment are the most important determinants of mucosal damage (Weber and Griffin, 1986). Although problems are more common in the elderly, this probably reflects prescribing practice (Langman, 1986; Walt et al., 1986). However, adverse reactions in the elderly are more likely to be serious, or even fatal (Pickles, 1986; Henry et al., 1987). There appears to be little correlation between the symptoms produced and gastroscopic findings. There is about 30% incidence of gastrointestinal side effects, but only a 1–2% incidence of peptic ulcer (Jick and Porter, 1978). Worryingly, there may be large asymptomatic ulcers (Roth and Boost, 1975). There do not appear to be any differences between drugs (Rossi et al., 1987).

Uncoated aspirin damages gastric mucosa by cyclooxygenase inhibition and also breaks the mucosal barrier by a direct effect. However, enteric-coated aspirin is on a par with other NSAIDs as far as the production of gastrointestinal side effects is concerned.

Management of gastric problems

There are several possibilities for management of gastrointestinal problems. Firstly, it may be possible to switch from one NSAID to another, as there are differences between the agents. However, it would require immense fortitude to do this in the face of active gastrointestinal toxicity and without further therapeutic measures being taken, especially when one considers that as many as 4000 people die each year in the United Kingdom from gastrointestinal complications of NSAIDs, a mortality similar to that associated with self-poisoning (Cockel et al., 1987).

Antacid therapy does provide some protection, but this is at the cost of reduced absorption and increased renal excretion. The histamine-2 receptor blockers have proved disappointing. Perhaps the most promising research concerns the use of sucralphate to protect the gastric mucosa. This has led to a reduction in symptomatology in 75% of patients. In another approach, trials of synthetic prostaglandins are showing positive protective results (Charlet et al., 1985). However, this latter group of drugs might cause uterine contractions, which may complicate their clinical use.

Renal problems

The mechanisms of renal toxicity have been reviewed by Orme (1986) and Kantor (1988). In general, the end-products of the cyclooxygenase pathway are vasodilators and protect the kidney against pressor effects. If this effect is lost, as in NSAID therapy, unopposed pressor influences cause salt and water retention, which in turn can lead to congestive heart failure. In addition, the effect of all diuretics may be blunted, and NSAIDs may counteract the response to all antihypertensive drugs and thus the blood pressure may rise. A few patients develop a severe interstitial nephritis, which may lead to renal failure.

Management of renal problems

Regular monitoring of renal function is advisable, especially where this is likely to be reduced. In patients with reduced renal function, there are theoretical grounds for the use of pro-drugs such as Sulindac. Although renal problems are still possible, there appears to be a reduced renal toxicity, probably because the inactive parent drug is preferentially excreted (Ciabattoni et al., 1987).

Clinical use of NSAIDs

When prescribing NSAIDs, the following general principles should be borne in mind (Anonymous, 1983).

(1) All NSAIDs act symptomatically, and there is no evidence that they alter the underlying disease process.

(2) There is nothing to be gained from prescribing more than one NSAID at a time, as they all have the same mode of action.

(3) In general, all drugs within a group have the same clinical effect.

(4) Dosage should be started at the lowest level and titrated against symptom relief. However, they should be tried to full dosage (side effects permitting) before being rejected as ineffective. All NSAIDs appear to have a ceiling dose, that is to say, a dose beyond which increments fail to yield additional analgesia. This ceiling dose will vary from patient to patient.

(5) Warn the patient that perfect pain relief is not possible. Explain the risks and ask that any adverse effects be reported. There is a widespread variation in response on the part of the patients, and their preferences may be an important guide. Thus, there is no 'drug of choice' for all patients, and equally, there is little point in persevering with a drug when there is no clinical benefit to the patient. This can usually be seen in 1–2 weeks.

A logical basis for the selection of NSAIDs would be on the basis of efficacy, safety and cost, in that order (Anonymous, 1987). Thus, the propionic acid derivatives would probably be first, followed by the acetic acid derivatives, aspirin and related compounds and then indomethacin and related compounds.

Propionic acid derivatives

This drugs in this large group (Table 5.5) are equally effective as anti-inflammatory drugs providing that they can be tolerated. It may be necessary to give quite

TABLE 5.5

Non-steroidal anti-inflammatory drugs

Salicylates	Pyrazoles	Propionic acid derivatives
Aspirin	Phenylbutazone	Fenoprofen
Sodium salicylate	Azapropazone	Flurbiprofen
Diflunisal		Ibuprofen
Choline magnesium		Ketoprofen
trisalicylate		Naproxen
		Fenbufen[a]
		Tiaprofenic acid
Indole derivatives	Fenamates	Acetic acid derivatives
Indomethacin	Mefenamic acid	Diclofenac
Sulindac		Fenclofenac
Tolmetin		Fenbufen[a]
Oxicams	Pyranocarboxylates	Alkanones
Piroxicam	Etodolac	Nabumetone

[a] Fenbufen is a pro-drug with two active metabolites in different groups.

large doses for a clinical effect; up to 2.4 g with ibuprofen. Although better tolerated than most other groups of NSAIDs, they will still cause gastrointestinal upsets in 30% of patients. Despite frequent claims to the contrary, there is no evidence that one drug or another causes fewer gastrointestinal side effects. Many have a long length of action, and this may offer an advantage in dosing or in improving compliance, but if there is a beneficial clinical effect, there is rarely a problem with compliance. Several drugs in this group are two to three times as expensive as ibuprofen.

Recent work has shown that drugs in this group may exist in different forms, called enantiomers. These are designated the *R* and *S* forms. Naproxen only exists in the *S* form, and in the case of flurbiprofen, most of the analgesic activity occurs in the *S* form (Sunshine et al., 1987). This work raises the possibility of enhanced clinical effect, or of reduced toxicity. There are many reasons why this discovery may not yield clinical benefits, but it has provoked much activity on the part of the pharmaceutical houses, and the future holds promise.

Acetic acid derivatives

Drugs in this group have been implicated with a high incidence of rashes, but otherwise seem well tolerated. Diclofenac seems to be less likely to give rise to problems, and should be first choice in this group. Fenbufen is a pro-drug for two active metabolites, one of which is a member of this group.

Salicylates

Aspirin is a very effective anti-inflammatory drug at doses of 2.4–8 g. However, at these dose levels there may be problems with dyspepsia, tinnitus and gastrointestinal bleeding. To combat this, a number of pro-drugs have been developed. These agents and enteric-coated formulations cause fewer side effects than aspirin alone. In addition, these can be minimised further by taking the drug after food. There appears to be little difference between the various formulations.

Benorylate is an aspirin-paracetamol complex that is metabolized to the active drugs. Salsalate, choline magnesium trisalicylate and diflunisal all give rise to active drug after ingestion.

Indole derivatives

Indomethacin is a well established anti-inflammatory drug, with an equally well established incidence of adverse effects. These include all the 'normal' side effects of NSAIDs, with the addition of severe headache and dizziness, which are particularly common in the elderly. Improvement may occur if the dosage is lowered, or sometimes, if a slow-release form is used. It has been suggested that indomethacin is more effective in the control of bone pain than other NSAIDs (Brodie, 1974).

Sulindac is a pro-drug and a derivative of indomethacin. It has a long half-life and also causes headache and dizziness, but to a lesser extent than indomethacin. Constipation is an unusual side effect which is reported by about 10% of patients taking this drug. Tolmetin is closely related to the withdrawn drug zomepirac and appears to have little to distinguish it from other members of this group.

Pyrazoles

Phenylbutazone is only available in the United Kingdom for the treatment of ankylosing spondylitis. It is the most toxic NSAID, and is second only to chloramphenicol as a causative factor in fatal aplastic anaemia. In addition, it causes all NSAID side effects to a greater degree than other drugs, and has been implicated in fatal gastrointestinal haemorrhage, water retention that has led to congestive heart failure, a high incidence of skin rashes and nephrotoxicity.

Fenamates

Mefenamic acid is an analgesic with only minor anti-inflammatory activity. Thus, it is used more frequently as an analgesic. Adverse reactions may be severe and include diarrhoea and occasional blood dyscrasias.

Other NSAIDs

Piroxicam is a drug with a long half-life of about 2 days. This may lead to problems with accumulation when first starting the drug and this may be pronounced in the elderly patient. It is alleged to give rise to more gastrointestinal side effects than other NSAIDs, but a large retrospective survey has failed to confirm this, despite piroxicam being the top ranked drug.

Etodolac and nabumetone are two newer agents and there are insufficient published data to comment on their relative value compared to other NSAIDs.

PARACETAMOL (ACETAMINOPHEN)

Paracetamol cannot be included with aspirin and the other NSAIDs as it has no demonstrable anti-inflammatory activity. The peripheral prostaglandin synthetase inhibition seen with aspirin is not found with paracetamol, and this is an important point to consider when prescribing for patients with conditions that have an inflammatory basis. The dose-response relationship for paracetamol has not been established unequivocally. For example, although 650 mg doses are more effective than 300 mg doses, an increase to 1000 mg may not provide any more analgesia, and a ceiling dose for maximum analgesia has not yet been determined (Mather and Denson, 1986).

Paracetamol is rapidly absorbed when taken orally and peak concentrations are reached in about an hour. Unlike aspirin, it is not absorbed through gastric mucosa and absorption is dependent upon gastric-emptying time. It has relatively few side effects and does not produce gastric irritation, or interfere with platelet function. It has no effect upon oral anticoagulants and shows no cross-sensitivity with aspirin. Hypersensitivity is most uncommon. It is metabolized in the liver by conjugation reactions and the hepatotoxicity seen in overdose is caused by minor metabolites. Glutathione exerts a protective effect in these circumstances (Mitchell et al., 1974).

CAFFEINE

This drug is a weak stimulant which is often included in small doses in analgesic preparations. The British National Formulary (1988a) states that it does not contribute to the analgesic or anti-inflammatory effect of the preparation and may possibly aggravate the gastric irritation caused by aspirin. The authors also suggest that in excessive dosage, or on withdrawal, caffeine may itself induce headache. All pain clinic physicians are probably aware of one or two cases where painful conditions have remitted following withdrawal from a large daily intake of coffee or cola drinks.

However, evidence has been presented that suggests that caffeine does have a useful role to play when used as part of a combination analgesic tablet (Laska et al., 1984). 40% more analgesic drug was required to provide the same amount of analgesia as a caffeine/analgesic combination. See also the accompanying Editorial by Beaver (1984b).

COMBINATION DRUGS

The fact that different classes of drugs act by different mechanisms has encouraged manufacturers to combine drugs in the hope of increasing the beneficial effect. This has led to a natural concern about using these drugs, as the combinations may be inappropriate or the dosages unrealistic. However, there is reasonable evidence to suggest that relatively low doses of two drugs can yield analgesia that is superior to that of either drug at a higher dose, and with fewer side effects (Beaver, 1984a). However, there is no virtue in combining two drugs with the same mechanism of action. The main problems with fixed combination tablets stem from the difficulty in making dose adjustments when these prove necessary. Against this is the fact that when a dose is established, combination tablets may make the patient's life simpler and improve compliance.

CORTICOSTEROIDS

Despite vast amounts of research, the mechanism of action of the corticosteroids remains largely unknown. They are known to suppress both humoral and cellular responses. Corticosteroids are pure anti-inflammatory drugs and have no analgesic action. Thus, they relieve pain only by their local anti-inflammatory action. They have a low therapeutic ratio and should be prescribed only after careful consideration of the diagnosis and alternative therapies. The overriding principle must be to use the lowest dose possible for the shortest possible time.

Used carefully, corticosteroids are useful in the management of a number of rheumatic diseases. There is no argument about their use in polymyalgia rheumatica, polymyositis and sometimes in systemic lupus erythematosus. There is debate about when and how to use them in rheumatoid arthritis. In general, they should be reserved for those cases where there is acute disease which is unresponsive to other therapy, where there is severe disease progression and where it is important to keep the patient mobile whilst waiting for another form of therapy to work, such as gold, penicillamine or an immunosuppressive. Steroids have also been used in the treatment of algodystrophy (see p. 149, 250).

OTHER DRUGS USED IN PAINFUL DEGENERATIVE DISEASE

Analgesics relieve pain, whatever the cause. Anti-inflammatory drugs relieve inflammation, whatever the cause. Other drugs may relieve pain in specific disease processes. This may be because their action is upon a specific part of the disease process and thus may take a prolonged time for the full effect to be seen. Examples are penicillamine, gold or immunosuppressive drugs for rheumatoid arthritis; allopurinol or uricosuric drugs for gout, and diphosphonates, calcitonin and mithramycin for Paget's disease. A detailed consideration of these agents is beyond the scope of this chapter and the reader is referred to an excellent specialized monograph on the clinical pharmacology of anti-inflammatory agents (Brooks et al., 1986).

ANTICONVULSANTS, ANTIDEPRESSIVES, NEUROLEPTICS AND ANXIOLYTICS

To be regarded as an analgesic, a drug must relieve pain in well-known animal models of pain and must give demonstrable and reliable pain relief in patients with a painful disease. Drugs such as the opioids and the NSAIDs clearly are analgesics. The evidence is much less clear for the drugs in this section, and although traditional methods would not classify these drugs as analgesics, they all appear to have indications for use in the treatment of various aspects of chronic pain.

Anticonvulsants

The usefulness of this group of drugs has only been established for the treatment of neuropathic pain with a paroxysmal component such as trigeminal neuralgia. Excellent reviews of the use of anticonvulsants in the treatment of neuralgic pain have been written by Swerdlow (1984, 1986).

Trigeminal neuralgia is the best known painful condition for which anticonvulsants are effective. Shortly after phenytoin was established to be an effective and relatively non-sedating anticonvulsant medication, it was found to be of value in the treatment of trigeminal neuralgia. Subsequently, carbamazepine was found to be even more effective for this condition, and as newer anticonvulsants are introduced, they, too, are tried in painful conditions of a similar nature.

Conditions which may respond to anticonvulsants include trigeminal neuralgia, glossopharyngeal neuralgia, tabetic lightning pains, various neuropathies, lancinating pains arising from conditions such as postherpetic neuralgia and multiple sclerosis, and similar pains that may follow amputation or back surgery. All of these conditions are characterized by a lancinating or paroxysmal component and all have nerve damage as a feature of the condition. The pathological basis for this sort of pain is yet to be established, and it is unlikely that we will understand how anticonvulsants work until this is known. Current thought suggests that anticonvulsants work in a similar fashion to local anaesthetic drugs and their effect is mediated through the sodium channels in the spinal cord. By this action, they suppress foci of abnormal impulse generation that develop in damaged nerve.

Carbamazepine

At present, carbamazepine remains the first-line drug for the treatment of lancinating neuropathic pain. Absorption of carbamazepine from the gut is slow and probably incomplete, as a parenteral form is not available; bioavailability, calculated to be 80–90% can only be an estimate. The drug is metabolized in the liver, partly to carbamazepine 10,11-epoxide, which also has anticonvulsant activity. It has a long half-life of about 48 h, but this becomes much less with prolonged administration. This is due to autoinduction of metabolism, and an increase in dosage may be required to maintain control after about a month of treatment. As with all anticonvulsants, a true 'therapeutic range' does not exist and there is debate as to the need to monitor plasma levels. It seems likely that maximum therapeutic benefit is in the range 6–12 mg/l (25–50 μmol/l). One justification for monitoring blood levels is that drug interactions are so common that it is dangerous practice not to do it. This observation applies to a large number of the drugs used in the management of chronic pain, and the author monitors drug levels wherever possible.

In trigeminal neuralgia, approximately 70% of patients will have significant pain relief (Loeser, 1984). However, up to one-third of these may have intolerable side effects. It is usual to start with a dose of 100 mg twice daily and then increase the dose every 2 days by 100 mg daily to a total daily dosage of 600 mg. If, after 2 weeks at this dose level, there is neither pain relief or side effects, the dosage can be increased by 200 mg to a maximum total daily dosage of 1200 mg.

Side effects are dose-related and include nausea, dizziness, slurred speech, ataxia, skin rashes and somnolence. Rarely, bone marrow depression may develop. This usually occurs within 3 months of exposure to the drug and a full blood count should be carried out regularly. A major fall in any component necessitates immediate cessation of the drug; prompt restoration of marrow function is the usual outcome.

Sillanpaa (1981) has reviewed the use of carbamazepine in numerous conditions with lancinating pain as a feature. With regard to trigeminal neuralgia and other facial pain, he summarizes 33 papers covering the treatment of over 1700 patients. Although the criteria of pain quality and pain relief varied considerably, carbamazepine yielded pain relief in 70–80% of cases. In those studies with an effective design the figure was still in excess of 60%, which by any standards is an impressive result. Carbamazepine appears to be just as effective in cases of facial pain that have a lancinating component, but who do not have typical trigeminal neuralgia. Most authorities regard carbamazepine as being ineffective in cases of atypical facial pain without a lancinating component.

The effect of carbamazepine appears to be extremely rapid in those cases who respond. In the study of Rasmussen and Riishede (1970), the paroxysms had disappeared within 24 h in 74% of cases, and within 96% of cases within 48 h. In addition, the long-term results are good, approximately two-thirds of patients remaining well controlled for at least 2 years.

Many painful conditions other than trigeminal neuralgia have been treated with carbamazepine, and these have been reviewed by Sillanpaa (1981). They include glossopharyngeal neuralgia, tabetic lightning pains, phantom limb and stump pain, paroxysmal pain associated with multiple sclerosis, metabolic and diabetic neuropathies. Although good results have been reported in all of these cases, controlled studies have been carried out only in patients with diabetic neuropathy. A representative study is that of Wilton (1974), who utilized a double-blind, within-patient crossover study of carbamazepine against placebo. Carbamazepine was definitely superior and about 80% of cases experienced pain relief. Other controlled studies showing similar results are reviewed by Swerdlow (1986). Good results are also claimed in the treatment of migraine and cluster headache (Friedman, 1968; Rompel and Baurermeister, 1970), but this view is contradicted by Fields and Raskin (1976).

Phenytoin

Swerdlow (1986) has emphasized that 1942 was a landmark in the history of the treatment of chronic pain when it was first demonstrated that phenytoin could relieve the pain of trigeminal neuralgia (Bergouignan, 1942). Like carbamazepine, the oral absorption is slow, variable and sometimes incomplete. Bioavailability is about 90%. The most important determinant of absorption is particle size, which is affected by the dosage form (salt or free acid) and the excipients used. Thus, marked changes in serum levels may be expected if the formulation is changed.

Phenytoin is one of a handful of drugs that exhibit zero-order kinetics in therapeutic dosage (Richens and Dunlop, 1975). As the circulating concentration rises, the liver enzyme system becomes saturated, and this has the important clinical implication that the relationship between dose and concentration is non-linear. A small increment in dose can lead to a substantial rise in plasma level, and conversely, the circulating concentration can fall by an unexpectedly large amount when the dose is cut back. Elimination half-life is in the order of 9–22 h following a single dose, but is considerably longer at high concentrations and it may take up to 3–4 weeks for steady-state to be reached in some patients. This has the implication that unexpected toxicity may occur up to a month after beginning or altering therapy.

The optimum plasma concentration for phenytoin has not been established when this drug is used to treat painful conditions. However, the plasma concentrations of carbamazepine required to control epilepsy and trigeminal neuralgia are the same, and it would appear reasonable to believe that the same would apply to other anticonvulsants. Thus, the target range for plasma concentration would be 10–20 mg/l (40–80 μmol/l). However, this can only be regarded as a guide to therapeutic decision making.

The long half-life of phenytoin permits single daily dosing, although paradoxically, either sedation or insomnia may require divided dosage. Most patients require about 300 mg/day (5 mg/kg), but some exhibit saturation of metabolism at doses as low as 100–150 mg. Others may require doses in excess of 600 mg/day for effective pain control. Therapy should begin with 200 mg daily. If symptoms of toxicity occur, the serum concentration should be measured and the dose reduced appropriately. If pain relief has not been obtained, dosage increments of 100 mg are appropriate. Therapy should be maintained within the therapeutic range for 6 weeks before it can be said to be unsuccessful. It should be noted that the dose range suggested here is much less than that quoted by others (Loeser, 1984; Fields, 1987). There is no evidence to suggest that doses up to 1000 mg are more effective; indeed, they may lead to substantial toxicity.

Cosmetic side effects such as gingival hyperplasia, acne and hirsutism make this a drug to be used with reluctance in the young. Severe reactions may include erythroderma, hepatotoxicity, blood dyscrasias, systemic lupus, sensory neuropathy, intellectual deterioration and irreversible cerebellar degeneration. Signs of concentration-dependent toxicity include nausea, vomiting, drowsiness, dysarthria, tremor and ataxia. Nystagmus is often the earliest sign.

There are few controlled studies of the use of phenytoin in chronic pain. Such studies as there are suggest that phenytoin is not as effective as carbamazepine in similar conditions (Chinitz et al., 1966; Lockman et al., 1973; Chadda and Mathur, 1978).

Clonazepam

Clonazepam is a benzodiazepine developed for its anticonvulsant activity. Swerdlow (1986) states that this drug, and other benzodiazepines, enhance polysynaptic GABA-ergic inhibition at all levels of the CNS. It has also been suggested that clonazepam acts by mimicking the effects of glycine at its receptor sites.

It is rapidly and completely absorbed, and dosage is 0.5–2 mg per day in divided doses. The clinical usefulness of this drug is likely to be limited by prominent sedative side effects. Other side effects are ataxia, hypotonia, slurred speech and behavioural problems. Clinical experience with this drug in the treatment of lancinating pain is extremely limited and there have been no large well-controlled trials. In an open study, Swerdlow and Cundill (1981) reported less problems with this agent when compared to other anticonvulsant drugs in the treatment of lancinating pain. In addition, they felt it was the most effective. Maciewicz et al. (1985), reviewing the drug treatment of neuropathic pain, cite 11 reports of the use of clonazepam as a treatment for chronic pain, chiefly for cranial neuralgias.

Sodium valproate

There is disagreement about how this drug works, but the likely mechanism of action almost certainly involves GABA. It is rapidly and completely absorbed. Once more, no well-controlled trials have been carried out, but there is an increasing body of anecdotal evidence that suggests that this drug may be most useful in the management of lancinating pain (Raftery, 1979; Peiris et al., 1980; Swerdlow and Cundill, 1981).

Dosage is 400–800 mg/day in divided doses. Plasma concentrations are not as useful a guide to therapy as with other anticonvulsants. This drug has widespread metabolic side effects, which may be dose-related, and these may include gastric irritation, nausea and thrombocytopenia. There has been recent concern over severe hepatic or pancreatic toxicity. Liver function should be kept under review during therapy with this drug, and any case of acute abdominal pain should have an immediate estimation of the plasma amylase.

Other anticonvulsants

Mephenesin and chlormephenesin have been reported as being of some value when other therapy fails (King, 1958). However, use of these agents must be regarded as speculative at best, as these are elderly drugs with a short action, widespread toxicity and without any body of literature to support their use. Swerdlow (1986) has reported the use of nitrazepam in doses of 2.5 mg 2–4 times daily: 6 out of 11 patients who received the drug obtained improvement. No other studies have been reported. Tizanidine is a clonidine derivative that is undergoing trial for the treatment of trigeminal neuralgia. Preliminary results indicate that it offers no advantages over carbamazepine (Vilming et al., 1986).

ANTIDEPRESSIVES

Persistent chronic pain is frequently accompanied by depression. Indeed, it would be surprising if it were not, and thus the use of antidepressives and other psychoactive drugs has become part of standard practice. However, there is evidence that at least some of these drugs have analgesic properties that are independent of their psychological effects. In this context, the term antidepressive is preferred to antidepressant because these drugs do not antagonise depressants, that is to say, drugs depressing the nervous system, but are active in depressive illness.

Tricyclic antidepressives

The tricyclic antidepressives (TCAs) are those most frequently used for the treatment of chronic pain conditions. The term tricyclic is misleading as there are now one-, two- and four-ring structured drugs with broadly similar properties. For the purposes of this chapter, all are termed tricyclic. An early, frequently quoted article by Paoli et al. (1960) describes the use of imipramine for treatment of chronic pain. Saunders (1963) discussed TCAs for pain associated with cancer. Since these early papers, a substantial body of literature has grown. Unfortunately, the vast majority of this is uncontrolled anecdote, and there are few scientific data on mechanisms of action, dosage, inter-drug variability, or long-term efficacy. Many reports illustrate the use of TCAs in combination with other agents without adequate comparisons against these drugs separately or in combination.

Neurophysiology and neuropharmacology

The biochemical activity of the TCAs suggests that their main effect will be in the bulbospinal system, where serotonin acts as a neurotransmitter. There is a substantial body of evidence to support the role of the bulbospinal system as a prime modulator of pain transmission. Much of the evidence comes from work on stimulation-produced analgesia and from the neuropharmacology of the endogenous and exogenous peptides. The reader is referred to reviews by Basbaum and Fields (1978) and Butler (1984). There is also some evidence of a spinal site of action (Hwang and Wilcox, 1987).

The TCAs inhibit the reuptake of serotonin and/or noradrenaline by the nerve-terminal that releases them, thereby increasing the concentration of the neurotransmitter at the synapse and thus increasing activity in the neural pathways where these substances act as neurotransmitters. However, it is difficult to accept this action of TCAs as the sole explanation for their clinical effect. This is chiefly because of the timing of the response. Acute administration of the agents leads to uptake inhibition of the neurotransmitter within minutes (Ross and Reny,

1975). However, the clinical effect in chronic pain is not usually seen for 2–4 weeks, although some authors claim that the analgesic effect appears in 3–7 days (Davis et al., 1977; Monks and Merskey, 1984). Other possible mechanisms of action are a straightforward antidepressive action, or by modulating the activity of other biologically active amines such as the endogenous opioids. Evidence for these differing modes of action in depressed and non-depressed patients has been reviewed by Feinmann (1985). The neurophysiological evidence is considered by Fields (1987). Further supporting evidence for the use of TCAs is supplied by Rosenblatt et al. (1984).

Fields (1987) points out that both serotonergic and noradrenergic neurones on the brainstem project to, and inhibit, nociceptive transmission cells in the spinal cord. The presence of these biogenic amine links in the pain-modulating systems suggests that TCAs can produce analgesia by enhancing the inhibitory action of serotonin and noradrenaline upon spinal cord transmission neurones. There is experimental evidence that supports this hypothesis, as TCAs administered systemically (Lee et al., 1983; Rigal et al., 1983) or intrathecally (Botney and Fields, 1983; Taiwo et al., 1985) will enhance the antinociceptive action of morphine given systemically. This enhancement can be blocked by the appropriate antagonists.

Levine and his colleagues studied the effect of amitriptyline (a relatively selective serotonin uptake inhibitor) or desipramine (a relatively selective noradrenaline uptake inhibitor) or placebo on the effect of a single dose of morphine given for postoperative dental pain (Levine et al., 1986). Desipramine, but not amitriptyline increased and prolonged the morphine analgesia. Thus, it may be that the noradrenergic component contributes to endogenous opioid-mediated analgesia. Interestingly, Watson and Evans (1985), in a study of postherpetic neuralgia, reported that amitriptyline was superior to the withdrawn drug, zimelidine, a very highly serotonergic antidepressive. This effect was independent of an effect upon depression.

Clinical experience

There is a wealth of clinical data on the use of TCAs, but much of it is inconclusive and difficult to organize. It would appear reasonable to suggest that any clinical trial should be double-blind and controlled, and that any study of a psychotropic medicine should include a placebo. It seems likely that patients who are depressed are likely to do best (Pilowsky et al., 1982). There is reasonable evidence of an analgesic effect for TCAs in headache, facial pain, low back pain, arthritis, denervation pain, and, to a lesser degree, cancer. They do not appear to have an effect on sympathetically maintained pain, phantom pain or neuroma. The data available have been reviewed by Butler (1984) and Monks and Merskey (1984). Only studies that are controlled are included unless a statement to the contrary is made.

Headache

There are several studies of the use of TCAs in headache of differing aetiologies. There are two studies using low dose amitriptyline for the treatment of migraine, and they showed 55 and 80% improvement, respectively. Couch et al. (1976) found the non-depressed patient to be most benefitted. Gomersall and Stuart (1973) found those patients with headaches of short duration to respond best.

There are three studies of TCAs in tension headache. Diamond and Baltes (1971) showed low dose amitriptyline to be slightly superior to high dose amitriptyline and both to be superior to placebo. Lance and Curran (1964) found low dose amitriptyline to be superior to placebo in a crossover design trial. Carrasso (1979) compared amitriptyline and clomipramine and found clomipramine to be more effective. The amitriptyline dosage in this trial was higher than in the other trials mentioned in the text, and this may represent the phenomenon of the 'therapeutic window' to be discussed later. In a more recent study, maprotiline was found to be superior to placebo in a well-designed study (Fogelholm and Murros, 1984). Patients who were only slightly or not at all depressed responded better than those with more severe depression.

There are other studies of headache with depression or psychogenic overlay, and in these, both amitriptyline and doxepin have been shown to be effective. Anxiety and depression were good predictors of benefit (Okasha et al., 1973; Ward et al., 1979).

Facial pain

There are few reports on the efficacy of TCAs in the management of chronic facial pain. Feinmann et al. (1984) have shown an analgesic effect for TCAs, as have Sharav and co-workers (1987). The latter paper demonstrated an analgesic effect for amitriptyline that was independent of any effect on depression.

Low back pain

There are few well-conducted studies of the use of TCAs in low back pain, despite the frequent use of this group of drugs on an empirical basis. Two studies of imipramine versus placebo showed conflicting results. A study by Jenkins et al. (1976) demonstrated no difference between placebo and imipramine. However, this study was for a 4 week period only and used a lower dose of TCA than that of a subsequent study by Alcoff et al. (1982), which did show improvement with imipramine after 8 weeks of treatment.

Hameroff et al. (1982) examined the effects of doxepin in antidepressive doses against placebo in the treatment of low back pain and found doxepin to be superior. Interestingly, they found that the more active subjects and those with less sleep disturbance responded better. They also found that improvement was related to adequate serum levels of doxepin and that therapy had to be maintained for a minimum period of 4 weeks to be effective. None of this information helps in elucidating a mechanism of action, but it does suggest that further studies should be undertaken.

Arthritis

Very little work has been published on the effect of TCAs in arthritis. The first study reported was an open study of patients having a condition referred to as 'non-articular rheumatism' but included patients with rheumatoid arthritis as well. Over 60% reported an improvement with imipramine (Kuipers, 1962). This anecdotal paper was followed by a double-blind crossover study of patients with rheumatoid arthritis and no history of psychiatric disorder. Patients were prescribed imipramine or placebo and the drug was clearly superior, both on patient's preference and by improvement in grip strength (McDonald Scott, 1969). This study was repeated over a longer period, with similar results in a larger number of patients (Gingras, 1976).

There have been two studies utilizing low dose clomipramine. The first was an open study of patients with 'arthralgia', and indicated improvement, as measured by a decrease in analgesic intake, a decrease in stiffness and an increase in activity. Improvement was observed in about 60% of participants (Regalado, 1977). A larger study of low dose clomipramine versus placebo was double-blind without crossover and failed to show any difference between the active drug and placebo (Ganvir et al., 1980).

It is difficult to reconcile these findings with the role of TCAs in the arthritic diseases. Clearly, depression, anti-inflammatory effects and central serotonin metabolism play a part, but the exact contribution of each to the clinical response remains to be delineated.

Denervation states

Postherpetic neuralgia is the condition that is reported most frequently to respond to TCAs. The vast majority are anecdotal case studies of dubious value. Various TCAs have been utilized (amitriptyline, clomipramine and nortriptyline) with or without phenothiazines and anticonvulsants. The drug doses have varied considerably, but most are low, of the order of 25–100 mg/day. Few of these studies consider the problems of accompanying depression, serum drug levels or inter-drug comparisons when two drugs are used at the same time.

In contrast to this, the double-blind crossover study of amitriptyline and placebo in postherpetic neuralgia by Watson and his colleagues (1982) considers the problems of age, symptom duration, depression and serum levels in relation to clinical effect. These authors reported that the age of the patient and duration of symptoms did not relate to clinical effect, and that depressed patients responded better than non-depressed patients, although no change in their depression was documented. Drug dose and serum level of amitriptyline were shown to be of significance. In three of the subjects in this study, the effect of the 'therapeutic window' was observed, in that as doses increased, the pain-relieving effect was diminished, only to increase again as doses were lowered.

Turkington (1980) conducted a well-controlled study of patients with diabetic neuropathy. All patients were initially challenged with phenytoin therapy for 2 weeks, followed by carbamazepine therapy for a week, before being entered into a double-blind study with imipramine, amitriptyline or diazepam. At the end of the 10 week study period, there was a 100% success rate for abolishing pain in the imipramine and amitriptyline groups. The diazepam group showed no change in pain symptoms, but had 100% relief of pain on antidepressive doses of imipramine. Studies of depression before and after treatment indicate that the primary problem was depression and that relief of pain was associated with the reversal of depression occasioned by the TCAs. In a small study of patients with painful diabetic neuropathy, Knivesdal and her colleagues (1984) showed clear evidence of benefit from low dose imipramine in a placebo-controlled trial over a 10 week period. There was no evidence of depression in any of the patients studied.

Davidoff et al. (1987) report upon the use of trazodone in the treatment of dysaesthetic pain in traumatic myelopathy. No benefit was noted, and a fairly high incidence of side effects was seen. However, this trial has been criticized, as the numbers of patients were probably too small to draw valid conclusions (Tyrer and Matthews, 1988).

Once more, it is difficult to make any sense out of the published work. On one hand, it is possible that low dose TCAs may be successful in the management of postherpetic neuralgia, and that this may be more successful if the patient is depressed. Equally, it may be that pain relief is associated only with the decline of depression. One would like to see many more careful trials carried out to assess these points and to differentiate between relief of pain and relief of depression.

Cancer pain

Although used frequently in cancer pain, the majority of reports on antidepressives are anecdotal – for example, recent surveys of their use in Germany (Kocher, 1979) and Italy (Magni et al., 1987). The lack of controlled trials is assumed to be due to the ethical problems of conducting long-term double-blind trials, and the large number of different sources for pain which may be present in cancer patients. There is only one adequately controlled trial, which reports a mildly positive result to the use of imipramine in cancer pain (Fiorentino, 1967, quoted by Monks and Merskey, 1984).

In summary, TCAs have been tried in a wide variety of painful conditions. It has been suggested that this use stems from the belief that many pain syndromes represent a form of depression. However, the role played by depression is unclear, and without clinical or biological markers to predict drug response, it is difficult to see a method of overcoming this problem. It is possible that TCAs produce a major part of their clinical effect through an action upon depression, but there is enough evidence to suggest that they may exercise an analgesic effect of their own. Although it has been argued that the case for an analgesic effect for TCAs has yet to be made (Pilowsky et al., 1982), there is enough evidence from animal and human studies to continue treating patients with certain conditions with every expectation of success.

Clinical use of TCAs

In general, TCAs possess long half-lives, which makes steady-state plasma concentrations difficult to assess in less than 3–4 weeks. In addition, there is a widespread individual variation in metabolism and the monitoring of serum levels should be encouraged (Editorial, 1978). A complicating factor is that the principal metabolites of the parent drugs are themselves potent TCAs. For example, amitriptyline is metabolized to nortriptyline and imipramine to desipramine. Thus, at least initially, the effects may be additive. In addition, nortriptyline is an example of a drug that has a 'therapeutic window', where there is a strong correlation between the clinical response and plasma concentrations below 200 μg/l and above 50 μg/l (Editorial, 1978). This drug is ineffective above or below these levels.

TCAs are powerful drugs with a wide range of side effects. Introduction of these agents at therapeutic dose levels may cause a marked reduction in compliance because of adverse effects. Thus, it is reasonable to introduce these agents slowly. Using amitriptyline as an example, it is normal to introduce this as a single dose of 25 mg orally about an hour before bedtime. This can be increased by 25 mg after 2–3 days if tolerated by the patient. It is the author's practice to maintain the dose at 50–75 mg at night for 3–4 weeks. If there is no therapeutic effect by that time, the dosage is again increased by 25 mg aliquots until a total daily dosage of 150 mg is reached. This level is maintained for a further 3–4 weeks and if there is no therapeutic result, the drug is withdrawn in 25 mg/day decrements. Gradual withdrawal is recommended as withdrawal syndromes can occur with TCAs, although these are rare. The serum levels of the drug should be checked at intervals during therapy for absorption and compliance.

If a response occurs, therapy can be maintained for 3–6 months. After this peri-

TABLE 5.6

Pharmacological properties of antidepressive drugs

Drug	Type	Anticholinergic effect	Sedative effect
Tricyclic compounds			
Amitriptyline	tertiary amine	+ + +	+ +
Clomipramine	tertiary amine	+ +	+ +
Nortriptyline	secondary amine	+ +	0
Doxepin	tertiary amine	+ + +	+ +
Dothiepin	tertiary amine	+	+ +
Related compounds			
Maprotiline	secondary amine	+	+
Mianserin	tertiary amine	0	+ +
Unrelated compounds			
Trazodone		0	+ +

	Noradrenaline uptake/inhibition	Serotonin uptake/inhibition
Amitriptyline	+	+ + +
Clomipramine	+	+ + +
Nortriptyline	+ + +	+
Doxepin	+	+
Dothiepin	+ +	+
Maprotiline	+ + +	+
Mianserin	0	0
Trazodone	0	+ +

od, slow withdrawal of the drug can be tried, but the patient should be closely monitored for return of symptoms or depression. Where there is no response to therapy, this may be due to non-compliance or to inadequate dosage and monitoring of the serum levels may be helpful and allow adjustment of dosage to the correct level. If there is no response to an adequate trial of one TCA, another with different properties may be tried. For example, if amitriptyline yields no therapeutic result, clomipramine [serotonergic] and then maprotiline [catecholaminergic] could be tried.

Choice of TCA

TCAs can be roughly divided into those with markedly sedative properties, and those without. The newer antidepressives have not been studied as rigorously in clinical trials as the earlier TCAs such as amitriptyline and imipramine. The studies of the newer agents have failed to show any advantages in terms of clinical effect. However, the newer agents may be more selective in terms of pharmacological specificity and less likely to produce side effects. Despite this, pharmacologically specific responses have not been seen. Thus, there is little evidence that allows the clinician to choose a specific drug for a specific condition, except for clomipramine, which seems to be more effective for patients with depression associated with obsessional illness (Thoren et al., 1980).

The available antidepressives appear to have much the same efficacy whether prescribed for depression or for pain relief, and there is no way of predicting who will respond to what drug. Thus, choice will be determined by differences in safety, adverse effects, length of clinical experience and cost. Dosage frequency is not a factor, as almost all can be given once or twice a day, and sustained release compounds are expensive and unnecessary. Sedative TCAs given at night can help to promote sleep, but at the cost of daytime sedation. There is no reason to believe claims that some of the newer agents have an earlier onset of clinical effect.

Safety

This is an important factor in selecting an antidepressive agent, as depressed patients are at risk of suicide and the TCAs are a common cause of death from poisoning. Some of the newer agents should be safer than the TCAs because of their different pharmacological actions, but this cannot be confirmed until they have been used more widely. The fatal toxicity of antidepressive drugs has been studied by Cassidy and Henry (1987). They concluded that the toxicity of amitriptyline, desipramine and dothiepin was higher than other drugs, whilst that of clomipramine, imipramine, protriptyline and trimipramine was lower. Of drugs introduced since 1973, maprotiline had a toxicity similar to the older drugs, while other newly introduced drugs had lower toxicity, with mianserin, trazodone and viloxazine being significantly lower.

Side effects

Cardiovascular toxicity

The TCAs will cause conduction defects and arrhythmias in therapeutic dosage as well as in overdose. This problem may not be obvious on routine examination and care should be taken when prescribing these drugs for the elderly, or patients with heart disease. Newer drugs such as mianserin and trazodone are safer. The most common, and serious complication of TCAs is postural hypotension. This may occur at low doses and may occur in 20% of individuals (Glassman and Bigger, 1981).

Anticholinergic problems

These are often troublesome, especially with the older agents. Dry mouth, blurred vision, urinary retention and constipation are all unpleasant and may decrease compliance with treatment. Particular care must be exercised when prescribing for the elderly, who should be started on a lower dose. Paroxysmal sweating is not uncommon and the association with TCAs may go unrecognized.

Serious side effects

There have been reports of convulsions, and of haematological and hepatic reactions. These are much commoner with the newer agents, and maprotiline has caused convulsions, and mianserin has been associated with hepatic problems and blood dyscrasias.

5-HT ANALOGUES

The amino acid L-tryptophan is the precursor of 5-HT and is used as an antidepressant. There are no controlled trials of its use in the treatment of chronic pain. There are anecdotal reports that L-tryptophan loading reverses opioid tolerance (Hosobuchi et al., 1980) and reduces pain and increased sensory deficits in post-cordotomy or -rhizotomy cases where these had regressed (King, 1980).

MONOAMINOXIDASE INHIBITORS

These drugs are potent antidepressives but are used far less frequently than TCAs in the treatment of chronic pain because they are capable of producing dangerous adverse effects in combination with other drugs, and certain foods and drinks. Monoaminoxidase inhibitors (MAOIs) have been used successfully in a study of atypical facial pain where depression was a prominent feature (Lascelles, 1966). There has also been a trial of phenelzine in migraine. There was no correlation between serum levels of the drug and clinical response (Anthony and Lance, 1969). It is difficult to see a role for this group of drugs in the management of chronic pain.

LITHIUM

Lithium salts are used for their mood-regulating action in the treatment of manic illness and in the prevention of manic and depressive illness. Lithium has complex actions on central catecholamine and serotonin systems, and it has been used in several uncontrolled trials as a treatment for cluster headache, where high success rates were claimed (Kudrow, 1977; Mathew, 1978; Pearce, 1980). It has also been used for the treatment of painful shoulder (Tyber, 1974). Lithium salts have a very narrow therapeutic/toxic ratio and should not be prescribed unless monitoring of serum concentrations is possible. There are several different preparations of lithium and bioavailability may vary widely. A decrease in serum sodium can enhance lithium toxicity and careful patient selection is mandatory, as overdose may be fatal. In addition, there may be significant interactions with other drugs used in the management of chronic pain. However, levels of lithium required for the successful treatment of cluster headache may be lower than those required for the control of mania (Pearce, 1980); nonetheless, extreme caution must be exercised. For a review of the use of lithium in migraine and cluster headache, see Peatfield (1981).

NEUROLEPTICS AND ANXIOLYTICS

There are many drugs that fall into these categories, and as they may exert powerful central and peripheral effects, it was inevitable that they should be used for the relief of chronic pain. The phenothiazines have been given on many occasions, usually in conjunction with a TCA, but the evidence for associated analgesic activity is tenuous at best. The same may be said for the butyrophenones. The benzodiazepines are frequently prescribed for conditions that are painful, but again, there is no convincing evidence to support a pain-relieving action for these agents.

Phenothiazines

There are few data to support any analgesic activity for the majority of drugs in this group, despite their widespread use. In addition, any pain-relieving properties they may possess do not seem to be related to the relief of anxiety. For a review of possible mechanisms of action, see Oxman and Denson (1986). Most systematic studies of the use of phenothiazines in pain relief concern postoperative pain. The Belfast group studied nine different phenothiazines given parenterally, and of these, only methotrimeprazine was found to be an effective analgesic (Moore and Dundee, 1961; Dundee et al., 1963). In studies of acute pain, methotrimeprazine has been confirmed as an effective analgesic by itself, or in combination with other drugs (McGee and Alexander, 1979; Petts and Pleuvry, 1983). McGee and Alexander have reviewed several studies of the use of phenothiazines as analgesics or when they were used to potentiate opioid analgesia for acute pain relief. They concluded that the risk of side effects was greater than the possible benefit. Oxman and Denson (1986) suggest that the major effect of phenothiazines on chronic pain is derived from changes in sleep pattern or non-specific sedation rather than analgesia.

Monks and Merskey (1984) review the use of these drugs, either alone or in conjunction with TCAs, for the control of chronic pain. These authors accept the uncontrolled nature of all reported studies, and also note that the majority of trials lasted less than 3 months. Despite these problems, they still believe that these reports support the use of neuroleptics in patients with denervation pain, postherpetic neuralgia, cancer pain and thalamic pain. Phenothiazine/TCA combinations have also been used for the relief of pain associated with diabetic neuropathy (Turkington, 1980; Gomez-Perez et al., 1985). Although success was reported in both trials, the trial design did not allow for comparison of the effect of the individual drugs or the combination.

The use of phenothiazines carries attendant risks. They have a tendency to produce drowsiness and dysphoria. This mild dysphoria may progress to overt depression, and this was one of the reasons for the use of phenothiazine/TCA combinations. It is conceivable that the benefits ascribed to the phenothiazines were, in fact, in response to the TCA, which was being prescribed to treat a potential side effect of the phenothiazine. Other troublesome side effects of phenothiazines include the whole range of cholinergic side effects encountered with the TCAs and the rare, but more serious, problems of blood dyscrasias, neuroleptic syndrome, cholestatic jaundice and skin pigmentation. Patients who take phenothiazines for a long time may develop extrapyramidal symptoms and may progress to a tardive dyskinesia. The true incidence of this serious problem is not known, but Monks and Merskey (1984) quote a range of 1–45%.

Thus, the role of phenothiazines is far from clear. Fields (1987) believes they should be reserved for selected individuals when more established therapies have been unsuccessful. Methotrimeprazine is probably the first choice drug. This should be given in an initial dose of 10 mg at night, and the total daily dosage should not exceed 100 mg. Depressive reactions are reported to occur most frequently above 50 mg/day. The same pattern of use should be applied to other drugs in this group, such as chlorpromazine or pericyazine, with appropriate alterations in the daily dosage. Drugs in this group are more sedative and have fewer extrapyramidal side effects.

Where the patient is more likely to be troubled by cholinergic side effects, such as when these drugs are being used in combination with TCAs, fluphenazine (1–3 mg/day) or perphenazine (4–16 mg/day) may be helpful, but these agents have more pronounced extrapyramidal side effects. The greatest care must be taken with the use of these powerful agents, and potential benefits weighed against the undoubted risks. It is possible they may be of some value in cases where purely anti-anxiety and antidepressive drugs have failed to work. Therapy with phenothiazines should rarely be for a period greater than 3 months.

Butyrophenones

Drugs in this group tend to resemble the less sedative phenothiazines in their action. Haloperidol is the only drug with any reported effect in the management of chronic pain. Maltbie et al. (1979) have suggested that this drug may work by its effect on dopamine blockade and by a direct opioid receptor agonist activity. Support for this theory was provided by the work of Creese et al. (1976), who found that several butyrophenones and the closely related drug pimozide were nearly as potent opioid receptor binders as morphine. However, Clay and Brougham (1975) were unable to show this effect, and this contrast may reflect different experimental techniques.

Clinical reports of the use of haloperidol are confined to the work of Cavenar and Maltbie (1976a,b; Maltbie and Cavenar, 1977). These workers have published anecdotal reports of a tiny number of patients on several occasions. Controlled clinical trials are lacking and there is no reason to believe that this drug has any place in the management of chronic pain. The use of pimozide has also been reported, but without the support of adequate controls.

Benzodiazepines

This group of drugs may be used for the relief of pain in conditions associated with acute muscle spasm, and they are sometimes prescribed in an attempt to reduce the anxiety and muscle tension which are associated frequently with chronic pain complaints. However, except in specific conditions, most authorities believe their use in chronic pain is questionable. There is unequivocal evidence that benzodiazepines produce pharmacological dependence at a therapeutic dosage (Ashton, 1984; Tyrer, 1984).

Therapeutic benefit has been reported in pain of psychological origin (Okasha, 1973), diabetic neuropathy (Turkington, 1980) and chronic tension headache (Lance and Curran, 1964). In all cases, the benefit was less than that obtained by the TCA therapy to which it was being compared. However, clonazepam has been shown to be of value in the treatment of lancinating pain (Swerdlow and Cundill, 1981) and clobazam has been reported to relieve phantom limb pain (Rice-Oxley, 1986). In addition, there is still a place for the use of longer-acting drugs such as diazepam in the management of painful spasticity, due to acute injury or to spinal cord injury.

ANTIHISTAMINES

There has been a vast amount of animal work on the analgesic properties of the antihistamines. There is reasonable evidence supporting an analgesic action for chlorpheniramine, diphenhydramine, hydroxyzine, pyrilamine and promethazine (Rumore and Schlichting, 1985). The same review suggests that cinnarizine and cyproheptadine do not have analgesic activity. With regard to human studies, the same authors have concluded that diphenhydramine, hydroxyzine, orphenadrine and pyrilamine exhibit analgesic activity on their own (Rumore and Schlichting, 1986).

These agents were introduced into management of chronic pain because of their sedative and muscle relaxant properties. These actions are non-specific and there is nothing to suggest that the analgesia produced is related to sedation or muscle relaxation. It is not even clear whether the clinical effect is mediated centrally or peripherally. Although we know there are histamine-containing neurones within the CNS, it is not known whether they are concerned with pain transmission, although a peripheral nociceptive role is beyond doubt. In an important study, Krabbe and Olesen (1980) showed that infusions of histamine could provoke and maintain headache in patients with a history of migraine. This study also showed that injection of an antihistamine could relieve the pain.

Most clinical studies have been carried out with hydroxyzine, which has shown benefit in well-conducted studies of acute pain (Beaver and Feise, 1976; Bellville et al., 1979; Hupert et al., 1980), tension headache (Zaualeta, 1976), and cancer pain (Stambaugh and Lane, 1983). The usual oral dose is 25–100 mg every 6 h. A similar dosage can be given intramuscularly when the oral route is not available. There is some evidence that this drug is less effective by mouth (Kantor and Steinberg, 1976). Orphenadrine has been used primarily for the treatment of musculo-skeletal pain (Gold, 1978; Mok et al., 1979). Dosage is 50 mg orally four times daily. There is evidence that analgesic combinations of antihistamines and both NSAIDs and opioids may yield greater analgesia than that provided by each drug alone (Rumore and Schlichting, 1986).

SKELETAL MUSCLE RELAXANTS

Drugs described in this section are used for the relief of muscle spasm or spasticity. It is axiomatic that the underlying cause of the spasticity should be treated, and where possible, any aggravating factors (for example, pressure sores or infections) should be treated. Skeletal muscle relaxants usually help spasticity, but this may be at the cost of decreased muscle tone elsewhere, which may lead to a decrease in the mobility of the patient and thus make matters worse. An excellent review of the drug therapy of spasticity has been written by Young and Delwaide (1981).

The drug of first choice is probably dantrolene, which differs from other drugs in this section by having a peripheral site of action, working directly upon skeletal muscle. Dantrolene reduces contraction of skeletal muscle by a direct action on excitation-contraction coupling, apparently by decreasing the amount of calcium released from the sarcoplasmic reticulum (Van Winkle, 1976). Dantrolene does not affect neuromuscular transmission, nor does it change the electrical properties of skeletal muscle membranes (Davidoff, 1978). Absorption of dantrolene is slow and incomplete, but plasma levels can be used to monitor therapy. It has a half-life of about 9 h. The usual starting dose is 25 mg once a day. This can be increased by increments of 25 mg every week to a maximum of 400 mg given in four divided doses. This drug has the potential for severe hepatotoxicity, and if no benefit has accrued after 45 days of treatment, it is recommended that the drug is stopped. The most common side effect is weakness.

Baclofen is a derivative of the inhibitory neurotransmitter gamma-aminobutyric acid (GABA). It is believed to work by depressing monosynaptic and polysynaptic transmission in the spinal cord, and many of its effects are superficially similar to the actions of GABA. For a review of possible modes of action, see Bianchine (1985). Baclofen is rapidly absorbed after oral administration and has a half-life of 3–4 h. The normal starting dosage is 5 mg given twice daily; this can be increased by 5 mg every 3 days to a maximum of 80 mg daily in divided doses. The use of this drug may be limited by adverse effects which may include drowsiness, dizziness, weakness, ataxia and mental confusion. Gradual withdrawal is recommended after chronic administration. It is alleged that baclofen is most effective for the treatment of spasticity caused by multiple sclerosis or other diseases of the spinal cord, particularly traumatic lesions. It is not recommended for the spasticity caused by rheumatic disorders, stroke, cerebral palsy or the rigidity of Parkinsonism (Young and Delwaide, 1981). Baclofen has also been used successfully for the treatment of trigeminal neuralgia and a number of painful conditions including postherpetic neuralgia, tabetic pain and arachnoiditis (Steardo et al., 1984). There are no controlled trials of its use in these conditions.

It is presumed that benzodiazepines work by enhancing the efficiency of GABA-ergic transmission. At the spinal cord level, this may be manifest by enhancement of presynaptic inhibition of afferent neuronal terminals in the primary reflex arc (Bianchine, 1985). Although most benzodiazepines could be expected to help, diazepam is probably the most used drug in the treatment of spasticity. It is thought to be particularly useful in the treatment of patients with spinal cord lesions, although it is probably not as effective as baclofen in relieving intermittent flexion spasms (Young and Delwaide, 1981). The principle side effect is sedation, although this and its anxiolytic properties may be clinically useful (Lossius et al., 1980). Dosage should be titrated upward to maximal clinical effect, side effects permitting.

There are no controlled trials of any other drugs that show any clinical benefit for the management of acute or chronic muscle spasms.

Drugs acting on smooth muscle

The belladonna alkaloids and their synthetic substitutes have been employed for many years in the management of increased tone or 'spasm' of the gastrointestinal tract, or 'irritable bowel syndrome'. There is no convincing evidence that any of these agents have any effect on this condition (Ivey, 1975).

DRUG THERAPY OF MIGRAINE

There are several theories regarding the aetiology of migraine, but the two most widely held are that migraine is a manifestation of a CNS disorder of vasomotor regulation, or a systemic metabolic disorder. Probably the most important mechanism is the central and peripheral modulation of synaptic serotonin. For a fuller discussion of the pathophysiology of migraine, see Dalessio (1984). Most of the drugs currently used for the treatment and prophylaxis of migraine appear to have a role in altering the role of the neurotransmitter properties of serotonin, and this has been reviewed by Raskin (1981). When treating migraine, it is important to assess and correct, where possible, aggravating factors such as drugs, diet or emotional stress.

Ergotamine

This drug remains an important agent for the symptomatic relief of the pain of migraine, particularly in those patients who fail to gain relief from simple analgesics like aspirin and the NSAIDs. These latter drugs may act by lowering serotonin release from platelets. Ergotamine can be given orally or sublingually in a dose of 1–2 mg to a maximum dose of 6 mg per attack and no more than 12 mg per week. Ergotamine can also be given by inhalation or suppository if the oral route is not available, for example, as a result of vomiting. The smallest amount possible for the relief of headache should be employed. This drug is not useful in preventing attacks, but will relieve the majority of acute cases. Ergotamine is often prescribed in combination with caffeine, which has been shown to enhance its action.

Pizotifen

This drug is an antihistaminic and antiserotonergic drug that is structurally related to the TCAs. Its mechanism of action is not yet understood, but it offers good prophylaxis against classical migraine and a number of variants (Capildeo and Rose, 1982). Dosage is 0.5 mg initially, to a maximum of 3 mg. It may cause anticholinergic side effects including drowsiness and weight gain.

Beta blockers

This group of drugs have been used extensively in the prophylaxis of migraine, and have been reviewed by Weerasuriya et al. (1982). Propranolol has been demonstrated convincingly to be effective in a dosage of 80–160 mg/day (Diamond et al., 1982). The dosage should be titrated against clinical effect and should be discontinued after 6 weeks if satisfactory results have not been achieved. The decrease in dosage should be undertaken gradually over a 2 week period. In addition, metoprolol, atenolol, nadolol and timolol are all effective (Forssman et al., 1983; Ryan et al., 1983; Tfelt-Hansen et al., 1984). No significant effects have been found for pindolol, alprenolol, oxprenolol or acebutol (Peatfield, 1983).

Amitriptyline

Amitriptyline in doses of between 25 and 100 mg may be effective for migraine prophylaxis (Couch et al., 1976). The effect appears to be independent of any antidepressive action, since non-depressed patients with severe migraine have responded.

Calcium channel blockers

Several agents in this group have shown promise for the prophylactic treatment of migraine and cluster headache (Peroutka, 1983; Peroutka et al., 1984). Although older agents such as verapamil and nifedipine are effective, newer drugs such as flunarizine and nimodipine may be more useful (Amery, 1983; Diamond and Schenbaum, 1983; Gelmers, 1983). The mechanism of action proposed is that they act by causing changes in vascular tone in cerebral blood vessels.

Other drugs

Methysergide is a potent serotonin antagonist which is slightly less effective than propranolol (Saper, 1978). The usual clinical dosage is 4–8 mg/day. The major disadvantage of this drug is the danger of developing retroperitoneal fibrosis or fibrosis of the heart valves and pleura. It should only be used on cases that are resistant to treatment with other drugs and therapy should be discontinued for 1 month in every 6.

Cyproheptidine has antiserotonin, antihistamine and calcium channel blocking activity. It has been suggested for the treatment of refractory cases. The usual adult dose is 4 mg three or four times daily. Clonidine is a partial alpha-2 adrenergic agonist. It has been suggested for the prophylaxis of migraine where the attacks are triggered by foodstuffs containing tyramine (Williams, 1986). However, it is probably little better than placebo, and it may aggravate depression and cause insomnia (British National Formulary, 1988b).

DRUG TREATMENT OF ALGODYSTROPHY

The algodystrophies (causalgia, reflex sympathetic dystrophy) are painful conditions associated with overactivity of the sympathetic nervous system. Treatment is directed at blocking sympathetic overactivity, reducing pain and instituting aggressive physiotherapy to facilitate a return to normal function. Sympathetic blockade can be achieved by formal blockade of the nerves using local anaesthetic, or by the technique of intravenous regional sympathetic block (IRSB), described by Hannington-Kiff (1974; 1984). It is postulated that the guanethidine will first cause the release of noradrenaline, and second, prevent its reuptake, the result being a profound sympathetic block for up to 3 days. This technique has been accepted uncritically and has achieved widespread popularity, but large controlled studies are lacking. Bonelli and associates (1983), in a comparison with stellate ganglion block, showed that fewer IRSBs were required to achieve the same clinical result. The technique has also been applied to numerous other painful conditions (Loh et al. 1980). The adrenergic blocking agents reserpine and bretylium (Hannington-Kiff, 1984; Lief et al., 1987), the mixed alpha- and beta-adrenergic blocker labetalol (Parris et al., 1987), and the serotonin antagonist ketanserin (Lagas and Meijer, 1987) have been used successfully in a similar fashion to guanethidine. Oral beta-adrenergic blockers have been used successfully in a dose range of 120–240 mg/day in divided doses (Simson, 1974; Visitunthorn and Prete, 1981). There is a case report of the alpha-blocking agent prazocin (Abram and Lightfoot, 1981) and a series using phenoxybenzamine, another alpha-adrenergic blocker (Ghostine et al., 1984).

Other drugs that have been used successfully include corticosteroids. These are usually given as large doses of prednisone, 60–80 mg for 2–4 days and then tapered over a period of 6 weeks (Kozin et al., 1976; Schwartzman and McLelland, 1987). Methylprednisolone and dexamethasone have also been used. There are theoretical grounds for believing that calcium channel blocking drugs might be helpful in the management of the algodystrophies, and there are preliminary reports of the successful use of nifedipine, diltiazem and the angiotensin-converting enzyme captopril in the treatment of Raynaud's phenomenon, and nifedipine has been used in one study treating reflex sympathetic dystrophy. Tricyclic antidepressives, anticonvulsants, ketanserin and calcitonin have all been reported as effective, but, as with every other drug mentioned in this section, there are no controlled studies which indicate whether one drug or technique is superior.

MISCELLANEOUS DRUGS USED IN THE TREATMENT OF PAIN

Much of the work reported in this section is speculative at best, and has not been subjected to scientific trial. Some drugs are considered elsewhere and are mentioned in this section to note a report of an additional application.

Calcitonin

This agent is involved with parathyroid hormone in the regulation of bone turnover and hence in the homeostasis of calcium. It is used to lower the plasma calcium concentration in patients with hypercalcaemia, most notably in malignant disease. It is used in the treatment of the pain associated with severe Paget's disease of bone. Calcitonin has been used for the treatment of phantom pain (Kessel and Worz, 1987), reflex sympathetic dystrophy (Kleibel and Schmidt, 1984), and has been given intrathecally and epidurally for the management of pain associated with advanced malignancy (Chrubasik et al., 1987). The mechanism of analgesia is unknown.

Anticholinesterases

Schott and Loh (1984) reported a reduction in pain with the oral administration of anticholinesterase drugs. As yet unpublished studies suggest that all anticholinesterase drugs may have some analgesic activity, particularly where a central mechanism is involved. Distigmine, which only needs to be given once or twice daily, may be the most appropriate (Free, 1987).

D-Phenylalanine

There are conflicting reports about the value of this amino acid in the management of chronic pain (Budd, 1983; Walsh et al., 1986). It is alleged that this agent works by inhibiting carboxypeptidase A, an enzyme concerned in the breakdown of the endogenous opioids. However, a recent controlled study showed no evidence of significant analgesia compared with placebo (Walsh et al., 1986).

Adenosine monophosphate

There are recent reports of the value of this agent in the treatment and prevention of postherpetic neuralgia (Sklar et al., 1985). This work must be regarded as tentative as the number of patients involved was extremely small, and without substantial well-designed trials, the potential for toxicity as well as benefit cannot be assessed (Sherlock and Corey, 1985).

Aldose reductase inhibitors

It is possible that this group of drugs may be important in the treatment of symptomatic diabetic neuropathy. A small trial showed improvement in both symptomatology and function (Jaspan et al., 1983).

Local anaesthetics and their congeners

There are anecdotal reports of the value of local anaesthetic infusions. Benefit is reported for both esters (Schnapp et al., 1981; Phero et al., 1983) and amides (Boas et al., 1982; Edwards et al., 1985; Kastrup et al., 1987; Petersen and Kastrup, 1987). It is known that local anaesthetics will block high frequency neural activity by sodium channel inactivation. The clinical action is presumed to be one of membrane stabilization, and that benefit might be expected in conditions where anticonvulsants have been found to be beneficial. The clinical effect appears to be long-lasting and can be prolonged by the use of oral agents such as flecainide, mexiletine (Petersen and Kastrup, 1985) and the highly toxic tocainide (Lindstrom and Lindblom, 1987).

Beta blockers

Beta blockers have been reported as being of benefit in the algodystrophies (Simson, 1974), phantom limb pain (Ahmad, 1979; Marsland et al., 1982), and trigeminal neuralgia (Aparis et al., 1972). However, in the only controlled trial available, little benefit was seen (Scadding et al., 1982). It is suggested that this therapy should be reserved for cases where other therapeutic endeavours have failed.

Clonidine

There has been much interest in the alpha-adrenergic agonist clonidine, which has been shown to produce analgesia in both animal models and humans (Coombs et al., 1985; Glynn et al., 1987). There is evidence that both morphine and clonidine produce a dose-dependent inhibition of spinal nociceptive transmission, which is mediated through different receptors (Ness and Gebhart, 1988). This may explain why clonidine has also been shown to work synergistically with morphine when given intrathecally (Drasner and Fields, 1988). It is possible that epidural

clonidine has less potential for cardiovascular problems than intrathecal clonidine, and the results of controlled trials are awaited.

Somatostatin

Epidural somatostatin has been reported to be an effective analgesic (Chrubasik
et al., 1984, 1985). It is known to inhibit substance P and is said to have its analgesic effect through this action. These studies have been heavily criticised, as animal work has shown few analgesic effects and severe disturbances of neural function following intrathecal injection (Gaumann et al., 1988). Somatostatin has been
given by infusion for the treatment of cluster headache (Sicuteri et al., 1984). Extreme caution in the use of this agent is advised.

Capsaicin

Topically applied capsaicin (0.025% solution) has been used in the treatment of
postherpetic neuralgia. It is not possible to judge whether this will become a practical method of management. Although some patients improved, others did not
continue treatment because of intolerable burning sensations in the painful area
as the drug was applied. Clinical trials are proceeding (Watson et al., 1988).

REFERENCES

Abram, S.E. and Lightfoot, R.W. (1981) Treatment of long-standing causalgia with prazosin. *Reg. Anesth.*, 6, 79–81.

Adams, J.D., Diehl, L.F. and Wilson, J.P. (1984) Ambulatory use of high-dose intravenous morphine for severe pain. *Drug Intell. Clin. Pharm.*, 18, 138–140.

Ahmad, S. (1979) Phantom limb pain and propanolol. *Br. Med. J.*, 278, 415.

Akil, H., Watson, S.J., Young, E., Lewis, M.E., Katchaturian, H. and Walker, J.M. (1984) Endogen-ous opioids: biology and function. *Annu. Rev. Neurosci.*, 7, 223–255.

Alcoff, J., Jones, E., Rust, P. and Newman, R. (1982) Controlled trial of imipramine for chronic low back pain. *J. Fam. Pract.*, 14, 841–846.

Amery, W.K. (1983) Flunarizine, a calcium channel blocker: a new prophylactic drug in migraine. *Headache*, 23, 70–74.

Andriaensen, H. and Van de Waale, J. (1976) Clinical use of buprenorphine in chronic administration. *Acta Anaesth. Belgica*, 26, 187–189.

Anonymous (1983) Which anti-inflammatory drug? *Northern Regional Health Authority Drug Newslet-ter*, 18, 69–72.

Anonymous (1987) Which NSAID? *Drug and Therapeutics Bulletin*, 25, 81–84.

Anthony, M. and Lance, J.W. (1969) Monoamine oxidase inhibition in the treatment of migraine. *Arch. Neurol.*, 21, 263–268.

Aparis, O., Vidal, C. and Revol, J. (1972) Du traitement des neuralgies faciale par le propanolol. *Bordeaux Med.*, 7, 857–859.

Arner, S. and Arner, B. (1985) Differential effects of epidural morphine in the treatment of cancer-related pain. *Acta Anaesth. Scand.*, 29, 332–336.

Arner, S. and Meyerson, B.A. (1988) Lack of analgesic effect of opioids on neuropathic and idiopathic forms of pain. *Pain*, 33, 11–23.

Ashton, H. (1984) Benzodiazepine withdrawal: an unfinished story. *Br. Med. J.*, 288, 1135–1140.

Atweh, S.F. and Kuhar, M.J. (1983) Distribution and physiological significance of opioid receptors in the brain. *Br. Med. Bull.*, 39, 47–52.

Auld, A.W., Maki-Jokela, A. and Murdoch, D.M. (1985) Intraspinal narcotic analgesia in the treatment of chronic pain. *Spine*, 10, 777–781.

Austin, K.L., Stapleton, J.W. and Mather, L.E. (1980) Multiple intramuscular injections: a major source of variability in analgesic response to meperidine. *Pain*, 8, 47–62.

Avery, G.S. (1980) *Drug Treatment: Principles and Practice of Clinical Pharmacology and Therapeutics.* Adis Press, Sydney.

Ballantyne, J.C., Loach, A.B. and Carr, D.B. (1988) Itching after epidural and spinal opiates. *Pain*, 33, 149–160.

Basbaum, A.I. and Fields, H.L. (1978) Endogenous pain control mechanisms: Review and hypothesis. *Ann. Neurol.*, 4, 451–462.

Baskin, S.I., Smith, L., Hoey, L.A., Levy, P.I. and Goldfarb, A.H. (1981) Age-associated changes of responses to acetylsalicylic acid. *Pain*, 11, 1–8.

Beaver, W.T. (1980) Management of cancer pain with parenteral medication. *J. Am. Med. Assoc.*, 244, 2653–2657.

Beaver, W.T. (1984a) Combination analgesics. *Am. J. Med.*, 77 (Suppl. 3A), 38–53.

Beaver, W.T. (1984b) Caffeine revisited. *J. Am. Med. Assoc.*, 251, 1732–1733.

Beaver, W.T. and Feise, G.A. (1976) Comparison of the analgesic effect of morphine, hydroxyzine and their combination in patients with postoperative pain. In: *Advances in Pain Research and Therapy, Vol. 1.* pp. 553–557. Editors: J.J. Bonica and D. Albe-Fessard. Raven Press, New York.

Beaver, W.T., Feise, G.A. and Robb, D. (1981) Analgesic effect of intramuscular and oral nalbuphine on postoperative pain. *Clin. Pharmacol. Ther.*, 29, 174–180.

Behar, M., Olshwang, D., Magora, F. and Davidson, J.T. (1979) Epidural morphine in the treatment of pain. *Lancet*, i, 527–528.

Bell, M.D.D., Mishra, P., Weldon, B.D., Murray, G.R., Calvey, T.N. and Williams, N.E. (1985) Buccal morphine – a new route for analgesia? *Lancet*, i, 71–73.

Bellville, J.W., Dorey, F., Capparell, D., Knox, V. and Bauer, R.O. (1979) Analgesic effects of hydroxyzine compared to morphine in man. *J. Clin. Pharmacol.*, 19, 290–296.

Benet, L.Z., Massoud, N. and Gambertoglio, G. (1984) *Pharmacokinetic Basis for Drug Treatment.* Raven Press, New York.

Benet, L.Z. and Sheiner, L.B. (1985) Pharmacokinetics: the dynamics of drug absorption, distribution and elimination. In: *The Pharmacological Basis of Therapeutics, 7th Edition.* Chapter 1, pp. 3–34. Editors: A.G. Gilman, L.S. Goodman, T.W. Rall and F. Murad. Macmillan, New York.

Bergouignan, M. (1942) Cures heureuses de neuralgies faciales essentielles par le diphenylhydantoinate de soude. *Rev. de Laryngol. Otol. et Rhinol.*, 63, 34–41.

Bianchine, J.R. (1985) Drugs for Parkinson's disease, spasticity and acute muscle spasms. In: *The Pharmacological Basis of Therapeutics, 7th Edition.* Chapter 21, pp. 473–490. Editors: A.G. Gilman, L.S. Goodman, T.W. Rall and F. Murad. Macmillan, New York.

Boas, R.A., Covino, B.G. and Shahnarian, A. (1982) Analgesic responses to IV lignocaine. *Br. J. Anaesth.*, 54, 501–505.

Bonelli, S., Conoscente, F., Movilia, P.G., Restelli, L., Francucci, B. and Grossi, E. (1983) Regional intravenous guanethidine vs. stellate ganglion block in reflex sympathetic dystrophies: a randomized trial. *Pain*, 16, 297–307.

Botney, M. and Fields, H.L. (1983) Amitryptiline potentiates morphine analgesia by a direct action on the central nervous system. *Ann. Neurol.*, 13, 160–164.

British National Formulary (1988a) Number 15. Compound analgesic preparations. 4.7.1.1. p. 168.

British National Formulary (1988b) Number 15. Prophylaxis of migraine. 4.7.4.2. p. 177.

Brodie, G.N. (1974) Indomethacin and bone pain. *Lancet*, ii, 1160.

Brogden, R.N., Speight, T.M. and Avery, G.S. (1973) Pentazocine: a review of its pharmacological properties, therapeutic efficacy and dependence liability. *Drugs*, 5, 6–91.

Bromage, P.R., Camporesi, E.M., Durant, P.A.C. and Nielsen, C.H. (1982a) Non-respiratory side effects of epidural morphine. *Anesth. Analg.,* 61, 490–495.

Bromage, P.R., Camporesi, E.M., Durant, P.A.C. and Nielsen, C.H. (1982b) Rostral spread of epidural morphine. *Anesthesiology* 56, 431–436.

Bromage, P.R., Camporesi, E.M., Durant, P.A. and Nielsen, C.H. (1983) Influence of epinephrine as an adjuvant to epidural morphine. *Anesthesiology*, 58, 257–262.

Brooks, P.M., Kean, W.F. and Buchanan, W.W. (1986) *The Clinical Pharmacology of Anti-Inflammatory Agents.* Taylor and Francis, London.

Buckley, F.P., Sizemore, W.A. and Charlton, J.E. (1986) Medication management in patients with chronic non-malignant pain. A review of the use of a drug withdrawal protocol. *Pain*, 26, 153–165.

Budd, K. (1983) Use of D-phenylalanine, an enkephalinase inhibitor, in the treatment of intractable pain. In: *Advances in Pain Research and Therapy, Vol. 5.* pp. 305–308. Editors: J.J. Bonica, U. Lindblom and A. Iggo. Raven Press, New York.

Budd, K. (1985) The use of the opiate antagonist naloxone in the treatment of intractable pain. *Neuropeptides*, 5, 419–422.

Bullingham, R.E.S., McQuay, H.J. and Moore, R.A. (1984) Principles of use of extradural and intrathecal narcotics. In: *Anaesthesia Review 2.* Chapter 10, pp. 137–147. Editor: L. Kaufman. Churchill Livingstone, Edinburgh.

Butler, S.H. (1984) Present status of tricyclic antidepressants in chronic pain therapy. In: *Advances in Pain Research and Therapy. Vol. 7.* pp. 173–197. Editors C. Benedetti, C.R. Chapman and G. Morrica. Raven Press, New York.

Caddy, B. and Idowu, R. (1979) Oxidative determination of dextromoramide (Palfium) in body fluids. *Analyst*, 104, 328–333.

Campbell, C.F., Mason, J.B. and Weiler, J.M. (1983) Continuous subcutaneous infusion of morphine for the pain of terminal malignancy. *Ann. Int. Med.*, 98, 51–52.

Capildeo, R. and Rose, F.C. (1982) Single-dose pizotifen, 1.5 mg nocte: a new approach in the prophylaxis of migraine. *Headache*, 22, 272–275.

Carasso, J.L. (1979) Clomipramine and amitryptiline in the treatment of severe pain. *Internat. J. Neurosci.*, 9, 191–194.

Cassidy, S. and Henry, J. (1987) Fatal toxicity of antidepressant drugs in overdose. *Br. Med. J.*, 295, 1021–1024.

Caute, B., Monsarrat, B., Gouaderes, C., Verdie, J.C., Lazorthes, Y., Cros, J. and Bastide, R. (1988) CSF morphine levels after lumbar intrathecal administration of isobaric and hyperbaric solutions for cancer pain. *Pain*, 32, 141–146.

Cavenar, J.O. and Maltbie, A.A. (1976a) Another indication for haloperidol. *Psychosomatics*, 17, 128–130.

Cavenar, J.O. and Maltbie, A.A. (1976b) The analgesic properties of haloperidol. *U.S. Navy Medicine*. 67, 16–17.

Chadda, V.S. and Mathur, M.S. (1978) Double-blind study of the effects of diphenylhydantoin sodium on diabetic neuropathy. *J. Assoc. Physic. India*, 26, 403–406.

Charlet, N. Gallo-Torres, H.E. Bournameaux, Y. and Wills, R.J. (1985) Prostaglandins and the protection of the gastroduodenal mucosa: a critical review. *J. Clin. Pharmacol.* 25, 564–582.

Charlton, J.E. (1985) Newer analgesics in the control of postoperative pain. In: *Care of The Postoperative Surgical Patient.* Chapter 3. pp. 39–57. Editors. J.A.R. Smith and J. Watkins. Butterworths, London.

Chayen, M.S., Rudick, V. and Borvine, A. (1980) Pain control with epidural morphine in terminal care. *Anesthesiology*, 53, 338–339.

Cherry, D.A., Gourlay, G.K. McLachlan, M. and Cousins, M.J. (1985) Diagnostic epidural opioid blockade and chronic pain: preliminary report. *Pain*, 21, 143–152.

Chinitz, A., Seelinger, D.F. and Greenhouse, A.H. (1966) Anticonvulsant therapy in trigeminal neuralgia. *Am. J. Med. Sci.*, 252, 62–67.

Christensen, F.R. (1982) Epidural morphine at home in terminal patients. *Lancet*, i, 47.

Chrubasik, J., Meynadier, J., Blond, S., Scherpereel, P., Ackerman, E., Weinstock, M., Bonath, K., Cramer, H. and Wunsch, E. (1984) Somatostatin: a potent new analgesic substance. *Lancet*, ii, 1208–1209.

Chrubasik, J., Meynadier, J., Scherpereel, P. and Wunsch, E. (1985) The effect of epidural somatostatin on postoperative pain. *Anesth. Analg.*, 64, 1085–1088.

Chrubasik, J., Falke, K.J., Blond, S., Meynadier, J. and Zindler, M. (1987) Epidural salmon calcitonin-in-infusion in treatment of cancer pain. *Schmerz-Pain-Douleur*, 8, 23–27.

Ciabattoni, G., Boss, A.H., Patrignani, P., Catella, F., Simonetti, B.M., Pierucci, A., Pugliese, F., Filabozzi, P. and Patrono, C. (1987) Effects of sulindac on renal and extrarenal eicosanoid synthesis. *Clin. Pharmacol. Ther.*, 41, 380–383.

Clay, G.A. and Brougham, L.R. (1975) Haloperidol binding to an opiate receptor site. *Biochem. Pharmacol.*, 24, 1363–1367.

Cockel, R. (1987) NSAIDs – Should every prescription carry a government health warning? *Gut*, 28, 515–518.

Coombs, D.W., Saunders, R.L. and Pageau, M. (1982) Continuous intraspinal narcotic analgesia: technical aspects of an implantable infusion system. *Reg. Anesth.*, 7, 110–113.

Coombs, D.W., Saunders, R.L., Lachance, D., Savage, S., Ragnarsson, T.S. and Jensen, L.E. (1985) Intrathecal morphine tolerance: use of intrathecal clonidine, DADLE, and intraventricular morphine. *Anesthesiology*, 62, 358–363.

Cooper, S.A. and Beaver, W.T. (1976) A model to evaluate mild analgesics in oral surgery outpatients. *Clin. Pharmacol. Ther.*, 20, 241–250.

Couch, R.J., Ziegler, D.K. and Hassanein, R. (1976) Amitryptiline in the prophylaxis of migraine. Effectiveness and relationship of antimigraine and anti-depressant effects. *Neurology*, 26, 121–127.

Cousins, M.J. and Mather, L.E. (1984) Intrathecal and epidural administration of opioids. *Anesthesiology*, 61, 276–310.

Cousins, M.J. (1987) Comparative pharmacokinetics of spinal opioids in humans: a step towards determination of relative safety. *Anesthesiology*, 67, 875–876.

Cousins, M.J. (1988a) The spinal route of analgesia for acute and chronic pain. In: *Proceedings of the Vth World Congress on Pain. Pain Research and Clinical Management. Vol. 3.* Chapter 51. pp. 454–471. Editors: R. Dubner, G.F. Gebhart and M.R. Bond. Elsevier, Amsterdam.

Cousins, M.J. (1988b) New horizons. In: *Neural Blockade in Clinical Anesthesia and Management of Pain. 2nd Edition.* Chapter 32. pp. 1139–1145. Editors: M.J. Cousins and L.D. Bridenbaugh. Lippincott, Philadelphia.

Crawford, M.E., Andersen, H.B., Augustenborg, G., Bay, J., Beck, O., Benveniste, D., Larsen, L.B., Carl, P., Djernes, M., Eriksen, J., Grell, A.-M., Henriksen, H., Johansen, S.H., Jorgensen, H.O.K., Moller, I.W., Pedersen, J.E.P. and Ravlo, O. (1983) Pain treatment on outpatient basis utilizing extradural opiates. A Danish multicentre study comprising 105 patients. *Pain*, 16, 41–47.

Creese, I., Feinberg, A.P. and Snyder, S.H. (1976) Butyrophenone influences on the opiate receptor. *Eur. J. Pharmacol.*, 36, 231–235.

Cuss, F.M., Colaco, C.B. and Baron, J.H. (1984) Cardiac arrest after reversal of opiates with naloxone. *Br. Med. J.*, 288, 363–364.

Dalessio, D.J. (1989) Headache. In: *Textbook of Pain.* Chapter 26, pp. 386–401. Editors: P.D. Wall and R. Melzack. Churchill Livingstone, Edinburgh.

Davidoff, G., Guarracini, M., Roth, E., Sliwa, J. and Yarkony, G. (1987) Trazodone hydrochloride in the treatment of dysesthetic pain in traumatic myelopathy: a randomized, double-blind, placebo-controlled study. *Pain*, 29, 151–161.

Davidoff, R.A. (1978) Pharmacology of spasticity. *Neurology*, 28, 46–51.

Davis, J.L., Lewis, S.B., Gerich, J.E., Kaplan, R.A., Schultz, T.A. and Wallis, J.D. (1977) Peripheral diabetic neuropathy treated with carbamazepine and fluphenazine. *J. Am. Med. Assoc.*, 238, 2291–2292.

Diamond, S. and Baltes, B.J. (1971) Chronic tension headache – treatment with amitryptiline – a double blind study. *Headache*, 11, 110–116.

Diamond, S., Kudrow, L., Stevens, J. and Shapiro, D.B. (1982) Long-term study of propranolol in the treatment of migraine. *Headache*, 22, 268–271.

Diamond, S. and Schenbaum, H. (1983) Flunarizine, a calcium channel blocker, in the prophylactic treatment of migraine. *Headache*, 23, 39–42.

Dixon, R., Crews, T., Inturrisi, C.E. and Foley, K.M. (1983) Levorphanol: pharmacokinetics and steady state plasma concentrations in patients with pain. *Res. Commun. Chem. Pathol. Pharmacol.*, 41, 3–17.

Drasner, K. and Fields, H.L. (1988) Synergy between the antinociceptive effects of intrathecal clonidine and systemic morphine in the rat. *Pain*, 32, 309–312.

Dundee, J.W., Love, W.J. and Moore, J. (1963) Alterations in response to somatic pain associated with anaesthesia. Part XV: further studies with phenothiazine derivatives and similar drugs. *Br. J. Anaesth.*, 35, 597–609.

Editorial (1977) Dangers of dextropropoxyphene. *Br. Med. J.*, 274, 668.

Editorial (1978) Tricyclic antidepressant concentrations and clinical response. *Br. Med. J.*, 277, 783–784.

Edwards, W.T., Habib, F., Burney, R.G. and Begin, G. (1985) Intravenous lidocaine in the management of various chronic pain states. A review of 211 cases. *Reg. Anesth.*, 10, 1–6.

Ehrnebo, M., Boreus, L. and Lonroth, U. (1977) Bioavailability and first-pass metabolism of oral pentazocine in man. *Clin. Pharmacol. Ther.*, 7, 421–433.

Evans, P.J.D. (1981) Narcotic addiction in patients with chronic pain. *Anaesthesia*, 36, 597–602.

Evans, P.J.D. (1983) Opiates in the management of chronic pain. *Clin. Anaesth.* 1, 71–94.

Feinmann, C.P. (1985) Pain relief by antidepressants: possible modes of action. *Pain*, 23, 1–8.

Feinmann, C.P., Harris, M. and Cowley, R. (1984) Psychogenic facial pain: presentation and treatment. *Br. Med. J.*, 288, 436–438.

Fields, H.L. (1987) *Pain*. McGraw-Hill, New York.

Fields, H.L. and Raskin, N.H. (1976) Anticonvulsants and Pain. In: *Clinical Neuropharmacology, Vol. 1*. Chapter 15. pp. 173–184. Editor: H.L. Klawan. Raven Press, New York.

Fiorentino, M. (1967) Sperimentazione controllata dell'Imipramina come analgesico maggiore in oncologia. *Rivista Med. Trent.*, 5, 387–396.

Fogelholm, F. and Murros, K. (1984) Maprotiline in chronic tension headache: a double-blind cross-over study. *Headache*, 25, 273–275.

Forrest, W.H., Brown, B.W., Brown, C.R., Defalque, R., Gold, M., Gordon, H.E., James, K.E., Katz, J., Mahler, D.L., Schroff, P. and Teutsch, G. (1977) Dextroamphetamine with morphine for the treatment of postoperative pain. *N. Engl. J. Med.*, 296, 712–715.

Forssman, B., Lindblad, C.J. and Zbornikova, V. (1983) Atenolol for migraine prophylaxis. *Headache*, 23, 188–190.

Free, C.W. (1987) Anticholinesterase drugs in the treatment of chronic pain. *Pain* (Suppl.), 4, 71.

Friedman, A.P. (1968) The migraine syndrome. *Bull. NY Acad. Med.*, 44, 45–62.

Ganvir, P., Beaumont, G. and Seldrup, J. (1980) A comparative trial of clomipramine and placebo

158

as adjunctive therapy in arthralgia. *J. Internat. Med. Res.*, 8 (Suppl. 3), 60–66.

Gaumann, D., Yaksh, T., Rodriguez, M. and Post, C. (1988) Intrathecal somatostatin causes severe hindleg dysfunction in cats and is devoid of analgesic effects. *Reg. Anesth.*, 13. (Suppl.), 44.

Gelmers, H.J. (1983) Nimodipine, a new calcium antagonist, in the prophylactic treatment of migraine. *Headache*, 23, 106–109.

Ghostine, S.Y., Comair, Y.G., Turner, D.M., Kassell, N.F. and Azar, C.G. (1984) Phenoxybenzamine in the treatment of causalgia. *J. Neurosurg.*, 60, 1263–1268.

Gilman, A.G., Goodman, L.S., Rall, T.W. and Murad, F. (1985) *The Pharmacological Basis of Therapeutics, 7th Edition.* Macmillan, New York.

Gingras, M. (1976) A clinical trial of Tofranil in rheumatic pain in general practice. *J. Internat. Med. Res.*, 4 (Suppl. 2), 41–49.

Glassman, A.H. and Bigger, J. (1981) Cardiovascular effects of therapeutic doses of tricyclic antidepressants: a review. *Arch. Gen. Psychiatry*, 38, 815–820.

Glynn, C.J., Mather, L.E., Cousins, M.J., Graham, J.R. and Wilson, P.R. (1981) Peridural meperidine in humans: analgetic response, pharmacokinetics and transmission into CSF. *Anesthesiology*, 55, 520–526.

Glynn, C.J. and Mather, L.E. (1982) Clinical pharmacokinetics applied to patients with intractable pain: studies with pethidine. *Pain*, 13, 237–246.

Glynn, C.J., Jamous, A., Dawson, D., Sanders, R., Teddy, P.J. Moore, R.A. and Lloyd, J.W. (1987) The role of epidural clonidine in the treatment of patients with intractable pain. *Pain*, Suppl. 4, S84.

Gold, R.H. (1978) Treatment of low back syndrome with orphenadrine citrate. *Curr. Ther. Res.*, 23, 271–276.

Gomersall, J.D. and Stuart, A. (1973) Amitryptiline in migraine prophylaxis. Changes in pattern of attacks during a controlled clinical trial. *J. Neurol. Neurosurg. Psychiatry*, 36, 684–690.

Gomez-Perez, F.J., Rull, J.A., Dies, H., Rodriguez-Rivera, J.G., Gonzalez-Barranco, J. and Lozano-Castaneda, O. (1985) Nortryptiline and fluphenazine in the symptomatic treatment of diabetic neuropathy. A double-blind cross-over study. *Pain*, 23, 395–400.

Gorski, D.W., Chinthagada, M., Rao, T.L.K. and Shah, K. (1982) Epidural meperidine for phantom limb pain. *Reg. Anesth.*, 7, 39–41.

Gourlay, G.K., Wilson, P.R. and Glynn, C.J. (1982a) Pharmacodynamics and pharmacokinetics of methadone during the perioperative period. *Anesthesiology*, 57, 458–467.

Gourlay, G.K., Wilson, P.R. and Glynn, C.J. (1982b) Methadone produces prolonged post-operative analgesia. *Br. Med. J.*, 284, 630–631.

Gourlay, G.K., Willis, R.J. and Wilson, P.R. (1984) Post-operative pain control with methadone: influence of supplementary methadone doses and blood concentration-response relationships. *Anesthesiology*, 61, 19–26.

Gourlay, G.K. and Cousins, M.J. (1984) Strong analgesics in severe pain. *Drugs*, 28, 79–91.

Gourlay, G.K., Cherry, D.A. and Cousins, M.J. (1986) A comparative study of the efficacy and pharmacokinetics of oral methadone and morphine in the treatment of severe pain in patients with cancer. *Pain*, 25, 297–312.

Gustafsson, L.L., Ackerman, S., Adamson, H., Garle, M., Rane, A. and Schildt, B. (1982a) Disposition of morphine in cerebrospinal fluid after epidural administration. *Lancet*, i. 796.

Gustafsson, L.L., Schildt, B. and Jacobsen, K. (1982b) Adverse effects of extradural and intrathecal opiates: report of a nationwide survey in Sweden. *Br. J. Anaesth.*, 54, 479–486.

Gustafsson, L.L., Grell, A.-M., Garle, A., Rane, A. and Schildt, B. (1984) Kinetics of morphine in cerebrospinal fluid after epidural administration. *Acta Anaesth. Scand.*, 28, 535–539.

Hameroff, S.R., Crago, B.R., Cork, R.C., Scherer, K. and Leeman, E. (1982) Doxepin effects upon chronic pain, depression and serum opioids. *Anesth. Analg.*, 61, 187.

Hanks, G.W. and Trueman, T. (1984) Controlled-release tablets are effective in twice-daily dosage in chronic cancer pain. *R. Soc. Med. Internat. Congr. Ser.*, 64, 103–105.

Hannington-Kiff, J.G. (1974) Intravenous regional sympathetic block with guanethidine. *Lancet*, i, 1019–1020.

Hannington-Kiff, J.G. (1984) Antisympathetic drugs in limbs. In: *Textbook of Pain*. Chapter 3.B.3. pp. 566–573. Editors: P.D. Wall and R. Melzack. Churchill Livingstone, Edinburgh.

Harmer, M., Slattery, P.J. Rosen, M. and Vickers, M.D. (1983) Intramuscular on-demand analgesia: double blind controlled trial of pethidine, buprenorphine, morphine and meptazinol. *Br. Med. J.*, 286, 680–682.

Heel, R.C., Brogden, R.N., Speight, T.M. and Avery, G.S. (1979) Buprenorphine: a review of its pharmacologic properties and therapeutic efficacy. *Drugs*, 17, 81–110.

Heel, R.C., Brogden, R.N., Pakes, G.E., Speight, T.M. and Avery, G.S. (1980) Nefopam: a review of its pharmacological properties and therapeutic efficacy. *Drugs*, 19, 249–267.

Henry, D.A., Johnston, A., Dobson, A. and Duggan, J. (1987) Fatal peptic ulcer complications and the use of non-steroidal anti-inflammatory drugs, aspirin and corticosteroids. *Br. Med. J.*, 295, 1227–1229.

Holmes, A.H. (1978) Morphine IV infusion for chronic pain. *Drug Intell. Clin. Pharm.*, 12, 556–557.

Hoskin, P.J., Hanks, G.W., Omar, O.A., Filshie, J., Johnston, A. and Turner, P. (1987) The bioavailability and pharmacokinetics of buccal, oral and oral controlled release morphine in healthy volunteers. *Pain* (Suppl.), 4, 189.

Hosobuchi, Y., Lamb, S. and Bascom, D. (1980) Tryptophan loading may reverse tolerance to opiate analgesics in humans: a preliminary report. *Pain*, 9, 161–169.

Houde, R.W. (1974) The use and misuse of narcotics in the treatment of chronic pain. In: *Advances in Neurology, Vol. 4*. pp. 527–536. Editor: J.J. Bonica. Raven Press. New York.

Howard, R.P., Milne, L.A. and Williams, N.E. (1981) Epidural morphine in terminal care. *Anaesthesia*, 36, 51–53.

Hughes, J. and Kosterlitz, H.W. (1983) Introduction. *Br. Med. Bull.*, 39, 1–3.

Hupert, C., Yacoub, M. and Turgeon, L.R. (1980) Effect of hydroxyzine on morphine analgesia for the treatment of postoperative pain. *Anesth. Analg.*, 59, 690–696.

Huskisson, E.C. (1984) Non-narcotic analgesics. In: *Textbook of Pain*. Chapter 3.A.1. pp. 505–513. Editors: P.D. Wall and R. Melzack. Churchill Livingstone, Edinburgh.

Hwang, A.S. and Wilcox, G.L. (1987) Analgesic properties of intrathecally administered heterocyclic antidepressants. *Pain*, 28, 343–355.

Inturrisi, C.E. (1982) Narcotic drugs. *Med. Clin. North Am.*, 66, 1061–1071.

Inturrisi, C.E. (1984) Role of opioid analgesics. *Am. J. Med.*, 77 (Suppl. 3A) 27–36.

Inturrisi, C.E., Schultz, M., Shin, S-U., Umans, J.G., Angel, L. and Simon, E.J. (1983) Evidence from opiate binding studies that heroin acts through its metabolites. *Life Sci.*, 33 (Suppl. II) 773–776.

Inturrisi, C.E., Max, M.B., Foley, K.M., Schultz, M., Shin, S-U. and Houde, R.W. (1984) The pharmacokinetics of heroin in patients with chronic pain. *N. Engl. J. Med.*, 310, 1213–1217.

Ivey, K.J. (1975) Are anticholinergics of use in the irritable bowel syndrome? *Gastroenterology* 68, 1300–1307.

Jacobson, L. (1984) Intrathecal and extradural narcotics. In: *Advances in Pain Research and Therapy. Vol. 7*. pp. 199–236. Editors: C. Benedetti, C.R. Chapman and G. Moricca. Raven Press, New York.

Jaffe, J.H. and Martin, W.R. (1985) Opioid analgesics and antagonists. In: *The Pharmacologic Basis of Therapeutics. 7th Edition*. Chapter 22. pp. 491–531. Editors: A.G. Gilman, L.S. Goodman, T. W. Rall and F. Murad. Macmillan, New York.

Janssen, P.A.J. (1982) Potent, new analgesics, tailor-made for different purposes. *Acta Anaesth. Scand.*, 26, 262–268.

Jaspan, J., Herold, K., Maselli, R. and Bartkus, C. (1983) Treatment of severely painful diabetic neuropathy with an aldose reductase inhibitor: relief of pain and improved somatic and autonomic nerve function. *Lancet*, ii, 758–762.

Jenkins, D.G., Ebbut, A.F. and Evans, C.D. (1976) Imipramine in treatment of low back pain. *J. Internat. Med. Res.*, 4, (Suppl. 2) 28–40.

Jick, H. and Porter, J. (1978) Drug-induced gastrointestinal bleeding. *Lancet*, ii, 87–89.

Kafer, E.R., Brown, J.T., Scott, D., Findlay, J.W.A., Butz, R.F., Teeple, E. and Ghia, J.N. (1983) Biphasic depression of ventilatory response to CO_2 following epidural morphine. *Anesthesiology*, 58, 418–422.

Kaiko, R.F., Stanley, L., Wallenstein, M.S., Rogers, A.G., Grabinski, P.Y. and Houde, R.W. (1981) Analgesic and mood effects of heroin and morphine in cancer patients with postoperative pain. *N. Engl. J. Med.*, 304, 1501–1505.

Kaiko, R.F., Kanner, R., Foley, K.M., Wallenstein, S.L., Canel, A.M., Rogers, A.G. and Houde, R.W. (1987) Cocaine and morphine interaction in acute and chronic cancer pain. *Pain*, 31, 35–45.

Kantor, T.G. (1986) Ketoprofen: a review of its pharmacologic and clinical properties. *Pharmacotherapy*, 6, 93–103.

Kantor, T.G. (1988) New strategies for the use of anti-inflammatory agents. In: *Proceedings of the Vth World Congress on Pain. Pain Research and Clinical Management, Vol. 3.* pp. 80–86. Editors: R. Dubner, G.F. Gebhart and M.R. Bond. Elsevier, Amsterdam.

Kantor, T.G. and Steinberg, F.P. (1976) Studies of tranquilizing agents and meperidine in clinical pain. In: *Advances in Pain Research and Therapy, Vol. 1.* pp. 567–572. Editors: J.J. Bonica and D. Albe-Fessard. Raven Press, New York.

Kastrup, J., Petersen, P., Dejgard, A., Angelo, H.R. and Hilsted, J. (1987) Intravenous lidocaine infusion – a new treatment of chronic painful diabetic neuropathy? *Pain*, 28, 69–75.

Kessel, C. and Worz, R. (1987) Immediate response of phantom limb pain to calcitonin. *Pain*, 30, 79–87.

King, R.B. (1958) The medical control of tic douloureux. *J. Neurosurg.*, 15, 290–298.

King, R.B. (1980) Pain and tryptophan. *J. Neurosurg.*, 53, 44–52.

Kjaer, M., Henricksen, H. and Kundesen, J. (1982) A comparative study of intramuscular buprenorphine and morphine in the treatment of chronic pain of malignant origin. *Br. J. Clin. Pharmacol.*, 13, 487–492.

Kleibel, F. and Schmidt, G. (1978) Salm-calcitonin bei metastatischen Knockenschmerzen. *Dtsch. Med. Wockenschr.*, 109, 104.

Knill, R.L., Clement, J.L. and Thompson, W.R. (1981) Epidural morphine causes delayed and prolonged ventilatory depression. *Can. Anaesth. Soc. J.*, 29, 537–543.

Knivesdal, B., Molin, J., Froland, A. and Gram, L.F. (1984) Imipramine treatment of painful diabetic neuropathy. *J. Am. Med. Assoc.*, 251, 1727–1730.

Kocher, R. (1979) The use of psychotropic drugs in the treatment of cancer pain. In: *Advances in Pain Research and Therapy. Vol. 2.* pp. 285–289. Editors: J.J. Bonica and V. Ventafridda. Raven Press, New York.

Korbon, G.A., James, D.J., Verlander, J.M., DiFazio, C.A., Rosenblum, S.M., Levy, S.J. and Perry, P.C. (1985) Intramuscular naloxone reverses the side effects of epidural morphine while preserving analgesia. *Reg. Anesth.*, 10, 16–20.

Kozin, F., McCarthy, D.J., Sims, J. and Genant, H. (1976) The reflex sympathetic dystrophy syndrome. I. Clinical and histologic studies: evidence for bilaterality, response to corticosteroids and articular involvement. *Am. J. Med.*, 60, 321–331.

Krabbe, A.A. and Olesen, J. (1980) Headache provocation by continuous intravenous infusion of histamine. Clinical results and receptor mechanism. *Pain*, 8, 253–259.

Krames, E.S., Wilkie, D.J. and Gershow, J. (1986) Intrathecal D-Ala2-D-Leu5 enkephalin (DADL) restores analgesia in a patient analgetically tolerant to intrathecal morphine sulfate. *Pain*, 24, 205–209.

Krames, E.S., Gershow, J., Glassberg, A., Kenefick, T., Lyons, A., Taylor, P. and Wilkie, D. (1985) Continuous infusion of spinally administered narcotics for the relief of pain due to malignant disorders. *Cancer*, 56, 696–702.

Kudrow, L. (1980) Lithium prophylaxis for chronic cluster headache. *Headache*, 17, 15–18.

Kuipers, R.K.W. (1962) Imipramine in the treatment of rheumatic patients. *Acta Rheumatol. Scand.*, 8, 45–51.

Lagas, H.M. and Meijer, J. (1987) Ketanserin: IV vs. RIV in SRD. *Pain*, Suppl. 4, 548.

Laidlaw, J., Read, A.E. and Sherlock, S. (1981) Morphine tolerance in hepatic cirrhosis. *Gastroenterology*, 40, 389–396.

Lake, C.L., Duckworth, E.N., DiFazio, C.A., Durbin, C.G. and Magruder, M.R. (1982) Cardiovascular effects of nalbuphine in patients with coronary or valvular heart disease. *Anesthesiology*, 57, 498–503.

Lance, J.W. and Curran, D.A. (1964) Treatment of chronic tension headache. *Lancet*, i, 1236–1239.

Landow, L. (1985) An apparent seizure following inadvertent intrathecal morphine. *Anesthesiology*, 62, 545–546.

Langman, M.J.S. (1986) Peptic ulcer complications and the use of non-aspirin non-steroidal anti-inflammatory drugs. *Advers. Drug React. Bull.*, 120, 448–451.

Lascelles, R.G. (1966) Atypical facial pain and depression. *Br. J. Psychiatry*, 122, 651–659.

Laska, E.M., Sunshine, A., Mueller, F., Elevers, W.B., Siegel, C. and Rubin, A. (1984) Caffeine as an analgesic adjuvant. *J. Am. Med. Assoc.*, 251, 1711–1718.

Lee, I., Chalon, J., Ramanathan, S., Gross, S. and Turndorff, H. (1983) Analgesic properties of meperidine, amitriptyline and phenelzine in mice. *Can. Anaesth. Soc. J.*, 30, 501–505.

Levine, J.D., Gordon, N.C., Smith, R. and McBryde, R. (1986) Desipramine enhances postoperative analgesia. *Pain*, 27, 45–49.

Lief, P.A., Reisman, R., Rocco, A., McKay, W., Kaul, A. and Benfell, K. (1987) IV regional guanethidine vs. reserpine for pain relief in reflex sympathetic dystrophy (RSD): a controlled, randomized, double-blind, crossover study. *Pain*, Suppl. 4, 398.

Lindstrom, P. and Linblom, U. (1987) The analgesic effect of tocainide in trigeminal neuralgia. *Pain*, 28, 45–50.

Lockman, L.A., Hunninghake, D.B., Krivit, W. and Desnick, R.J. (1973) Relief of pain of Fabry's disease by diphenylhydantoin. *Neurology* (*NY*), 23, 871–875.

Loeser, J.D. (1989) Tic douloureux and atypical facial pain. In: *Textbook of Pain*. Chapter 38 pp. 535–543. Editors: P.D. Wall and R. Melzack. Churchill Livingstone, Edinburgh.

Loh, L., Nathan, P.W., Schott, G.D. and Wilson, P.G. (1980) Effects of regional guanethidine infusion in certain painful states. *J. Neurol. Neurosurg. Psychiatry*, 43, 446–451.

Lossius, R., Dietrichson, P. and Lunde, P.K.M. (1980) Effect of diazepam and desmethyl-diazepam in spasticity and rigidity: a quantitative study of reflexes and plasma concentrations. *Acta Neurol. Scand.*, 61, 378–383.

Maciewicz, R., Bouckoms, A. and Martin, J.B. (1985) Drug therapy of neuropathic pain. *Clin. J. Pain*, 1, 39–49.

Magni, G., Arsie, D. and De Leo, D. (1987) Antidepressants in the treatment of cancer pain. A survey in Italy. *Pain*, 29, 347–353.

Magora, F., Olshwang, D., Eimerl, D., Shorr, J., Katzenelson, R., Cotev, S. and Davidson, J.T. (1980) Observations on extradural morphine in various pain conditions. *Br. J. Anaesth.*, 52, 247–252.

Maltbie, A.A. and Cavenar, J.O. (1977) Haloperidol and analgesia: case reports. *Mil. Med.*, 142, 946–948.

Maltbie, A.A., Cavenar, J.O., Sullivan, J.L., Hammett, X.X. and Zung, W.W.K. (1979) Analgesia and haloperidol: a hypothesis. *J. Clin. Psychiatry*, 40, 323–326.

Marsland, A.R., Weekes, J.N.W., Atkinson, R.L. and Leong, M.G. (1982) Phantom limb pain: a case for beta blockers? *Pain*, 12, 295–297.

Martin, R., Salbaing, J., Blaise, G., Tetrault, J.-P. and Tetreault, L. (1982) Epidural morphine for postoperative pain relief: a dose-response curve. *Anesthesiology*, 56, 423–426.

Maruta, T. and Swanson, D.W. (1981) Problems with the use of oxycodone compound in patients with chronic pain. *Pain*, 11, 389–396.

Mather, L.E. (1983) Clinical pharmacokinetics of fentanyl and its newer derivatives. Clin. Pharmacokinetics, 8, 422–446.

Mather, L.E. (1985) A pharmacokineticist in pain. *Reg. Anesth.*, 10, 110–118.

Mather, L.E. and Denson, D.D. (1986) Clinical pharmacokinetics of analgesic drugs. In: *Practical Management of Pain*. Chapter 28. pp. 503–520. Editor: P.P. Raj. Year Book Medical Publishers, Chicago.

Mather, L.E. and Glynn, C.J. (1982) The minimum effective analgetic blood concentration of pethidine in patients with intractable pain: studies with pethidine. *Br. J. Clin. Pharmacol.*, 14, 385–390.

Mather, L.E. and Raj, P.P. (1986) Spinal opiates. In: *Practical Management of Pain*. Chapter 38. pp. 709–727. Editor: P.P. Raj. Year Book Medical Publishers. Chicago.

Mathew, N.T. (1978) Clinical subtypes of cluster headache and response to lithium therapy. *Headache*, 18, 26–30.

McCoy, D.D. and Miller, M.G. (1982) Epidural morphine in a terminally ill patient. *Anesthesiology*, 57, 427.

McDonald Scott, W.A. (1969) The relief of pain with an antidepressant in arthritis. *Practitioner*, 202, 802–807.

McGee, J.L. and Alexander, M.R. (1979) Phenothiazine analgesia – fact or fantasy? *Am. J. Hosp. Pharm.*, 36, 633–640.

McQuay, H.J., Moore, R.A., Poppleton, P., Bullingham, R.E.S. and Lloyd, J.W. (1986) Nefopam in chronic back pain: analgesic efficacy and plasma concentration after single and multiple dose use. *The Pain Clinic* 1, 117–124.

Medina, J.L. and Diamond, S. (1977) Drug dependence in patients with chronic headache. *Headache*, 17, 12–14.

Melzack, R., Ofiesh, J.G. and Mount, B.M. (1976) The Brompton mixture: effects on pain in cancer patients. *Can. Med. Assoc. J.*, 115, 125–129.

Melzack, R., Mount, B.M. and Gordon, J.M. (1979) The Brompton mixture versus morphine solution given orally: effects on pain. *Can. Med. Assoc., J.*, 120, 435–438.

Millan, M.J. (1986) Multiple opioid systems and pain. *Pain*, 27, 303–347.

Miller, R.R., Feingold, A. and Paxinos, J. (1970) Propoxyphene hydrochloride. A critical review. *J. Am. Med. Assoc.*, 213, 996–1006.

Miser, A.W., Miser, J.S. and Clark, B.S. (1980) Continuous intravenous infusion of morphine sulfate for control of severe pain in children with terminal malignancy. *J. Pediatr.*, 96, 930–932.

Miser, A.W., Davis, D.M., Hughes, C.S., Mulne, A.F. and Miser, J.S. (1983) Continuous subcutaneous infusion of morphine in children with cancer. *Am. J. Dis. Child.*, 137, 383–385.

Mitchell, J.R., Thorgeirsson, S.S. and Potter, W.Z. (1974) Acetaminophen induced hepatic injury: protective role of glutathione in man and rationale for therapy. *Clin. Pharmacol. Ther.*, 16, 676–684.

Mok, M.S., Lippmann, M. and Steen, S.N. (1979) Drug combinations with orphenadrine. *Clin. Ther.*, 2, 188–193.

Monks, R. and Merskey, H. (1989) Psychotropic drugs In: *Textbook of Pain*. Chapter 39, pp. 702–721. Editors: P.D. Wall and R. Melzack. Churchill Livingstone, Edinburgh.

Moore, J. and Dundee, J.W. (1961) Alterations in response to somatic pain associated with anaesthesia, Part VII: the effects of nine phenothiazine derivatives. *Br. J. Anaesth.*, 33, 422–431.

Moore, R.A., Bullingham, R.E.S., McQuay, H.J., Hand, C.W., Aspel, J.B., Allen, M.C. and Thomas, D. (1982) Dural permeability to narcotics: in vitro determination and application to extradural administration. *Br. J. Anaesth.*, 54, 210–214.

Mount, B.M., Ajemian, I. and Scott, J.F. (1976) Use of the Brompton mixture in treating the chronic pain of malignant disease. *Can. Med. Assoc. J.*, 115, 122–124.

Nahata, M.C., Miser, A.W., Miser, J.S. and Reuning, R.H. (1984) Analgesic plasma concentrations of morphine in children with terminal malignancy receiving a continuous subcutaneous infusion of morphine sulfate to control severe pain. *Pain*, 18, 109–114.

Neal, E.A., Meffin, P.J., Gregory, P.B. and Blaschke, T.F. (1979) Enhanced bioavailability and decreased clearance of analgesics in patients with cirrhosis. *Gastroenterology*, 77, 96–102.

Ness, T.J. and Gebhart, G.F. (1988) Inhibition of visceral and cutaneous spinal nociceptive transmission by morphine and clonidine: differential effects on intensity coding. In: *Proceedings of the Vth World Congress* on *Pain. Pain Research and Therapy, Vol. 3.* Chapter 49. pp. 442–448. Editors: R. Dubner, G.F. Gebhart and M.R. Bond. Elsevier, Amsterdam.

Neumann, P.B., Henricksen, H., Grosman, N. and Christensen, C.B. (1982) Plasma morphine concentrations during chronic oral administration in patients with cancer pain. *Pain*, 13, 247–252.

Nilsson, M.I., Meresaar, U. and Anggard, E. (1982) Clinical pharmacokinetics of methadone. *Acta Anaesth. Scand.*, 74 (Suppl. 2) 66–69.

Nordberg, G. (1984) Pharmacokinetic aspects of spinal morphine analgesia. *Acta Anaesth. Scand.*, 28 (Suppl. 79), 1–38.

Nordberg, G., Hedner, T., Mellstrand, T. and Dahlstrom, B. (1984) Pharmacokinetic aspects of epidural morphine analgesia. *Anesthesiology*, 60, 448–454.

Okasha, A., Ghaleb, H.A. and Sadek, A. (1973) A double-blind trial for the clinical management of psychogenic headache. *Br. J. Psychiatry* 122, 181–183.

Olsen, G.D. (1975) Morphine binding to human plasma proteins. *Clin. Pharmacol. Ther.*, 16, 1125–1130.

Orme, M. L'E. (1986) Non-steroidal anti-inflammatory drugs and the kidney. *Br. Med. J.*, 292, 1621–1622.

Osborne, R.J., Joel, S.P. and Sleven, M.L. (1986) Morphine intoxification in renal failure: the role of morphine-6-glucuronide. *Br. Med. J.*, 292, 1548–1549.

Osborne, R.J., Joel, S.P., Trew, D. and Sleven, M.L. (1988) Analgesic activity of morphine-6-glucuronide. *Lancet, i*, 828.

Oxman, T. and Denson, D.D. (1986) Antidepressants and adjunctive psychotropic drugs. In: *Practical Management of Pain.* Chapter 30. pp. 528–538. Editor: P.P. Raj. Year Book Medical Publishers, Chicago.

Paalzow, L.K. (1982) Pharmacokinetic aspects of optimal pain treatment. *Acta Anaesth. Scand.*, 74, (Suppl. 2) 37–43.

Paalzow, L.K., Nielsson, L. and Stenberg, P. (1982) Pharmacokinetic basis for optimal methadone treatment of pain in cancer patients. *Acta Anaesth. Scand.* 74, (Suppl. 2) 55–58.

Paoli, F., Darcourt, G. and Cossa, P. (1960) Note preliminaire sur l'action de l'Imipramine dans les etats douloureux. *Rev. Neurolog.*, 102, 503–504.

Parris, W.C.V., Harris, R. and Lindsey, K. (1987) Use of intravenous regional labetalol in treating resistant reflex sympathetic dystrophy. *Pain*, Suppl. 4, 399.

Pasqualucci, V., Tantucci, C., Paoletti, F., Dottorini, M.L., Bifarini, G., Belfiori, R., Berioloi, M.B., Grassi, V. and Sorbini, C.A. (1987) Buprenorphine vs. morphine via the epidural route: a controlled comparative study of respiratory effects and analgesic activity. *Pain*, 29, 273–286.

Paterson, S.J., Rodson, L.E. and Kosterlitz, H.W. (1983) Classification of opioid receptors. *Br. Med. Bull.*, 39, 31–36.

Patwardhan, R.V., Johnson, R.F., Hoyumpa, A. Jr., Sheehan, J.J., Desmond, P.V., Wilkinson, G.R., Branch, R.A. and Schenker, S. (1981) Normal metabolism of morphine in cirrhosis. *Gastroenterology*, 81, 1006–1011.

164

Pearce, J.M.S. (1980) Chronic migrainous neuralgia, a variant of cluster headache. *Brain*, 103, 149–159.

Peatfield, R.C. (1981) Lithium in migraine and cluster headache: a review. *J. R. Soc. Med.*, 74, 432–436.

Peatfield, R. (1983) Migraine: current concepts of pathogenesis and treatment. *Drugs*, 26, 364–371.

Peiris, J.B., Perera, G.L.S., Devendra, S.V. and Lionel, N.D.W. (1980) Sodium valproate in trigeminal neuralgia. *Med. J. Austral.* 2, 278.

Pedersen, J. and Madsen, M.R. (1985) Metastatic carcinoma in the epidural space. *Br. J. Anaesth.*, 57, 935.

Peroutka, S.J. (1983) The pharmacology of calcium channel antagonists: a novel class of anti-migraine agents? *Headache*, 23, 278–283.

Peroutka, S.J., Banghart, S.B. and Allen, G.S. (1984) Relative potency and selectivity of calcium antagonists used in the treatment of migraine. *Headache*, 24, 55–58.

Petersen, P. and Kastrup, J. (1987) Dercum's disease (adiposa dolorosa). Treatment of the severe pain with intravenous lidocaine. *Pain*, 28, 77–80.

Petts, H.V. and Pleuvry, B.J. (1983) Interactions of morphine and methotrimeprazine in mouse and man with respect to analgesia, respiration and sedation. *Br. J. Anaesth.*, 55, 437–441.

Phero, J.C., De Jong, R.H., Denson, D.D., McDonald, J.S. and Raj, P.P. (1983) Intravenous chlorprocaine for intractable pain. *Reg. Anesth.*, 8, 41.

Pickles, H. (1986) Prescriptions, adverse reactions and the elderly. *Lancet*, ii. 40–41.

Pilowsky, I., Hallett, E.C., Bassett, D.L., Thomas, P.G. and Penhall, R.K. (1982) A controlled study of amitriptyline in the treatment of chronic pain. *Pain*, 14, 169–179.

Plummer, J.L., Gourlay, G.K., Cherry, D.A., and Cousins, M.J. (1988) Estimation of methadone clearance: application in the management of cancer pain. *Pain*, 33, 313–322.

Portenoy, R.K. and Foley, K.M. (1986) Chronic use of opioid analgesics in non-malignant pain: report of 38 cases. *Pain*, 25, 171–186.

Porter, J. and Jick, H. (1980) Addiction rare in patients treated with narcotics. *N. Engl. J. Med.*, 302, 123.

Raftery, H. (1979) The management of post herpetic pain using sodium valproate and amitriptyline. *J. Irish Med. Assoc.*, 72, 399–401.

Raskin, N.H. (1981) Pharmacology of migraine. *Annu. Rev. Pharmacol. Toxicol.*, 21, 463–478.

Rasmussen, P. and Riishede, J. (1970) Facial pain treated with carbamazepine (Tegretol). *Acta Neurol. Scand.*, 46, 385–408.

Ray, D.A.A. and Tai, Y.M.A. (1988) Increasing doses of naloxone hydrochloride by infusion to treat pain due to thalamic syndrome. *Br. Med. J.*, 296, 969–970.

Regalado, R.G. (1977) Clomipramine (anafranil) and musculoskeletal pain in general practice: a pilot, open, non-comparative study of long-standing rheumatoid pain. *J. Internat. Med. Res.*, 5 (Suppl. 1) 72–77.

Regnard, C.F.B., Edwards, S. and Badger, C. (1984) Chloroform in morphine sulphate solutions. *Pharmaceutic. J.*, 233, 745–746.

Regnard, C.F.B. and Davies, A. (1986) *A guide to symptom relief in advanced cancer* (2nd Edition). Haigh and Hochland, Manchester.

Rice-Oxley, C.P. (1986) The limited list: clobazam for phantom limb pain. *Br. Med. J.*, 293, 1309.

Richens, A. and Dunlop, A. (1975) Serum phenytoin levels in the management of epilepsy. *Lancet*, ii, 247–248.

Rigal, F., Eschalier, A., Devoize, J.-L. and Pechadre, J-C. (1983) Activities of five antidepressants in a behavioural pain test in rats. *Life Sci.*, 32, 2965–2971.

Rompel, H. and Baurermeister, P.W. (1970) Aetiology of migraine and prevention with carbamazepine (Tegretol). *J. Neurol. Neurosurg. Psychiatry*, 33, 528–531.

Rosenblatt, R.M., Reich, J. and Dehring, D. (1984) Tricyclic antidepressants in treatment of depression and chronic pain: analysis of the supporting evidence. *Anesth. Analg.*, 63, 1025–1032.

Ross, E.M. and Gilman, A.G. (1985) Pharmacodynamics: mechanisms of drug action and the relationship between drug concentration and effect. In: *The Pharmacological Basis of Therapeutics. 7th Edition*. Chapter 2, pp. 35–48. Editors: A.G. Gilman, L.S. Goodman, T.W. Rall and F. Murad. Macmillan, New York.

Ross, S.B. and Reny, A.L. (1975) Tricyclic antidepressant agents. *Acta Pharmacol. Toxicol., (Copenhagen)* 36, 382–408.

Rossi, A.C., Hsu, J.P. and Faich, G.A. (1987) Ulcerogenicity of piroxicam: an analysis of spontaneously reported data. *Br. Med. J.*, 294, 147–150.

Roth, G.J. and Boost, G. (1975) An open trial of naproxen in rheumatoid arthritis patients with significant esophageal gastric and duodenal lesions. *J. Clin. Pharmacol.*, 15, 378–381.

Rumore, M.M. and Schlichting, D.A. (1985) Analgesic effects of antihistaminics. *Life Sci.*, 36, 403–416.

Rumore, M.M. and Schlichting, D.A. (1986) Clinical efficacy of antihistamines as analgesics. *Pain*, 25, 7–22.

Ryan, R.E., Sr., Ryan, R.E., Jr. and Sudilovsky, A. (1983) Nadolol: its use in the prophylactic treatment of migraine. *Headache*, 23, 26–31.

Samuelsson, H., Nordberg, G., Hedner, T. and Lindqvist, J. (1987) CSF and plasma morphine concentrations in cancer patients during chronic epidural morphine therapy and its relation to pain relief. *Pain*, 30, 303–310.

Saper, J.R. (1978) Migraine. II. Treatment. *J. Am. Med. Assoc.*, 239, 2480–2484.

Saunders, C. (1963) The treatment of intractable pain in terminal cancer. *Proc. R. Soc. Med.*, 56, 195–198.

Sawe, J., Dahlstrom, B., Paalzow, L.K. and Rane, A. (1981a) Morphine kinetics in cancer patients. *Clin. Pharmacol. Ther.*, 36, 629–635.

Sawe, J., Hansen, J., Ginman, C., Hartvig, P., Jakobsson, P.A., Nilsson. M-J., Rane, A. and Anggord, E. (1981b) Patient-controlled dose regimen of methadone for chronic cancer pain. *Br. Med. J.*, 282, 771–773.

Sawe, J., Svensson, J.O. and Rane, A. (1983) Morphine metabolism in cancer patients on increasing oral doses – no evidence for autoinduction or dose-dependence. *Br. J. Clin. Pharmacol.*, 16, 85–93.

Scadding, J.W., Wall, P.D., Wynn Parry, C.B. and Brooks, D.M. (1982) Clinical trial of propanolol in post-traumatic neuralgia. *Pain*, 14, 283–292.

Schnapp, M., Mays, K.S. and North, W.C. (1981) Intravenous 2-chloroprocaine in treatment of chronic pain. *Anesth. Analg.*, 60, 844–845.

Schott, G.D. and Loh, L. (1984) Anticholinesterase drugs in the treatment of chronic pain. *Pain*, 20, 201–206.

Schwartzman, R.J. and McLelland, T.L. (1987) Reflex sympathetic dystrophy. A review. *Arch. Neurol.*, 44, 555–561.

Seymour, R.A., Rawlins, M.D. and Rowell, F.J. (1982) Dihydrocodeine-induced hyperalgesia in postoperative dental pain. *Lancet*, i, 1425–1426.

Sharav, Y., Singer, E., Schmidt, E., Dionne, R.A. and Dubner, R. (1987) The analgesic effect of amitriptyline on chronic facial pain. *Pain*, 31, 199–209.

Shelly, M.P., Cory, E.P. and Park, G.R. (1986) Pharmacokinetics of morphine in two children before and after liver transplantation. *Br. J. Anaesth.*, 58, 1218–1223.

Sherlock, C.H. and Corey, L. (1985) Adenosine monophosphate for the treatment of varicella zoster infections: a large dose of caution. *J. Am. Med. Assoc.*, 253, 1444–1445.

Shetter, A.G., Hadley, M.N. and Wilkinson, E. (1986) Administration of intraspinal morphine sulfate for the treatment of intractable cancer pain. *Neurosurgery*, 18, 740–747.

166

Sicuteri, F., Geppetti, P., Marabini, S. and Lembeck, F. (1984) Pain relief by somatosta'ir ' attacks of cluster headache. *Pain*, 18, 359–365.

Sillanpaa, M. (1981) Carbamazepine. Pharmacology and clinical uses. *Acta Neurol. Scand.*, (Suppl. 88) 64, 1–202.

Simson, G. (1974) Propranolol for causalgia and Sudek's atrophy. *J. Am. Med. Assoc.*, 227, 327.

Sjostrom, S., Hartvig, P., Persson, P. and Tamsen, A. (1987a) Pharmacokinetics of epidural morphine and meperidine in humans. *Anesthesiology*, 67, 877–888.

Sjostrom, S., Tamsen, A., Persson, P. and Hartvig, P. (1987b) Pharmacokinetics of intrathecal morphine and meperidine in humans. *Anesthesiology*, 67, 889–895.

Sklar, S.H., Blue, W.T., Alexander, E.J. and Bodian, C.A. (1985) Herpes Zoster. The treatment and prevention of neuralgia with adenosine monophosphate. *J. Am. Med. Assoc.*, 253, 1427–1430.

Smith, R.J. (1971) Federal government faces painful decision on Darvon. *Science*, 203, 857–858.

Stambaugh, J.E. and Lane, C. (1983) Analgesic efficacy and pharmacokinetic evaluation of meperidine and hydroxyzine, alone and in combination. *Cancer Invest.*, 1, 111–117.

Steardo, L., Leo, A. and Marano, E. (1984) Efficacy of baclofen in trigeminal neuralgia and some other painful conditions. *Eur. Neurol.*, 23, 51–55.

Sunshine, A., Eighelboim, I., Olson, N. and Laska, E. (1987) Flurbiprofen, flurbiprofen dextrorotatory component (BTS 24332) and placebo in post-episiotomy pain. *Clin. Pharmacol. Ther.*, 41, 162.

Swerdlow, M. (1984) Anticonvulsant drugs and chronic pain. *Clin. Neuropharmacol.*, 7, 51–82.

Swerdlow, M. (1986) Anticonvulsants in the therapy of neuralgic pain. *The Pain Clinic*, 1, 9–19.

Swerdlow, M. and Cundill, J.G. (1981) Anticonvulsant drugs in the treatment of lancinating pain. *Anaesthesia.*, 36, 1129–1132.

Swerdlow, M. and Stjernsward, J. (1982) Cancer pain relief – an urgent problem. *World Health Forum*, 3, 325–330.

Taiwo, Y.O., Fabian, A., Pazoles, C.J. and Fields, H.L. (1985) Potentiation of morphine antinociception by monoamine reuptake inhibitors in the rat spinal cord. *Pain*, 21, 329–337.

Takeda, F. (1986) Results of field-testing in Japan of the WHO Draft Interim Guidelines on Relief of Cancer Pain. *The Pain Clinic*, 1, 83–89.

Tfelt-Hansen, P., Standnes, B., Kangasneimi, P., Hakkarainen, H. and Olesen, J. (1984) Timolol vs. propranolol vs. placebo in common migraine prophylaxis: a double-blind multicenter trial. *Acta Neurol. Scand.*, 69, 1–8.

Thoren, P., Asberg, M., Cronholm, B., Jornestedt, L. and Traskman L. (1980) Clomipramine treatment of obsessive-compulsive disorder. 1. A controlled clinical trial. *Arch. Gen. Psychiatry*, 37, 1281–1285.

Turkington, R.W. (1980) Depression masquerading as diabetic neuropathy. *J. Am. Med. Assoc.*, 243, 1147–1150.

Twycross, R.G. (1977) Choice of strong analgesics in terminal cancer: diamorphine or morphine? *Pain*, 3, 93–104.

Twycross, R.G. (1978) Relief of pain in advanced cancer. *Prescribers J.*, 18, 117–124.

Twycross, R.G. (1984) Narcotics. In: *Textbook of Pain*. Chapter 3.A.2. pp. 514–525. Editors: P.D. Wall and R. Melzack. Churchill Livingstone, Edinburgh.

Twycross, R.G. and Dewhurst, J.K. (1981) Controlled release morphine tablets. *Lancet*, i, 892.

Tyber, M.A. (1974) Treatment of the painful shoulder syndrome with amitriptyline and lithium carbonate. *Can. Med. Assoc. J.*, 111, 137–140.

Tyrer, P.J. (1984) Benzodiazepines on trial. *Br. Med. J.*, 288, 1101–1102.

Tyrer, S.P. and Matthews, J.N.S. (1988) Trazodone in dysaesthesia. *Pain*, 33, 132.

Urban, B.J., France, R.D., Steinberger, E.K., Scott, D.I. and Maltbie, A.A. (1986) Long-term use of narcotic/antidepressant medication in the management of phantom limb pain. *Pain*, 24, 191–203.

Vane, J.R. (1972) Prostaglandins and the aspirin-like drugs. *Hosp. Pract.*, 7, 61–71.

Van Winkle, W.B. (1976) Calcium release from skeletal muscle sarcoplasmic reticulum: site of action of dantrolene sodium? *Science*, 193, 1130–1131.

Ventafridda, V., Spoldi, E., Caraceni, A., Tamburini, M. and De Conno, F. (1986) The importance of continuous subcutaneous morphine administration for cancer pain control. *The Pain Clinic*, 1, 47–55.

Vilming, S.T., Lyberg, T. and Lataste, X. (1986) Tizanidine in the management of trigeminal neuralgia. *Cephalgia*, 6, 181–182.

Visitunthorn, U. and Prete, P. (1981) Reflex sympathetic dystrophy of the lower extremity: a complication of herpes zoster with dramatic response to propranolol. *West. J. Med.*, 135, 62–66.

Walsh, N.E., Ramamurthy, S., Schoenfeld, L. and Hoffman, H. (1986) Analgesic effectiveness of D-phenylalanine in chronic pain patients. *Arch. Physic. Med. Rehabil.*, 67, 436–439.

Walsh, T.D. (1984a) Oral morphine in chronic cancer pain. *Pain*, 18, 1–11.

Walsh, T.D. (1984b) A controlled study of MST Continus tablets for chronic pain in advanced cancer. *R. Soc. Med. Internat. Congr. Ser.*, 64, 99–102.

Walt, R., Katschinski, B., Logan, R., Ashley, J. and Langman, M.J.S. (1986) Rising frequency of ulcer perforation in elderly people in the United Kingdom. *Lancet*, i. 489–492.

Wang, J.K., Nauss, L.A. and Thomas, J.E. (1979) Pain relief by intrathecally applied morphine in man. *Anesthesiology*, 50, 149–151.

Wang, J.K. (1985) Intrathecal morphine for intractable pain secondary to cancer of pelvic organs. *Pain*, 21, 99–102.

Ward, N.G., Bloom, V.L. and Friedel, R.O. (1979) The effectiveness of tricyclic antidepressants in the treatment of coexisting pain and depression. *Pain*, 7, 331–341.

Watson, C.P.N., Evans, R.J., Reed, K., Merskey, H., Goldsmith, L. and Warsh, J. (1982) Amitriptyline versus placebo in postherpetic neuralgia. *Neurology*, 32, 671–673.

Watson, C.P.N. and Evans, R.J. (1985) A comparative trial of amitriptyline and zimelidine in postherpetic neuralgia. *Pain*, 23, 387–394.

Watson, C.P.N., Evans, R.J. and Watt, V.R. (1988) Post-herpetic neuralgia and topical capsaicin. *Pain*, 33, 333–340.

Watson, J., Moore, A., McQuay, H., Teddy, P., Baldwin, D., Allen, M. and Bullingham, R. (1984) Plasma morphine concentrations and analgesic effects of lumbar extradural morphine and heroin. *Anesth. Analg.*, 63, 629–634.

Weber, J.C.P. and Griffin, J.P. (1986) Prescription, adverse reactions in the elderly. *Lancet*, i, 1220.

Weddel, S.J. and Ritter, R.R. (1981) Serum levels following epidural administration of morphine and correlation with relief of postsurgical pain. *Anesthesiology*, 54, 210–214.

Weerasuriya, K., Patel, K. and Turner, P. (1982) Beta-adrenoreceptor blockade and migraine. *Cephalgia*, 2, 33–45.

Williams, N.E. (1986) Current views on the pharmacological management of pain. In: *The Therapy of Pain. 2nd Edition*. Chapter 5. pp. 91–114. Editor: M. Swerdlow. MTP Press, Lancaster.

Wilton, T.D. (1974) Tegretol in the treatment of diabetic neuropathy. *South African Med. J.*, 48, 869–872.

World Health Organization. (1986) Cancer Pain Relief. World Health Organization. Geneva.

Yaksh, T.L. (1981) Spinal opiate analgesia: characteristics and principles of action. *Pain*, 11, 293–346.

Yaksh, T.L. and Rudy, T.A. (1976) Analgesia mediated by a direct spinal action of narcotics. *Science*, 192, 1357–1358.

Yaksh, T.L. and Onofrio, B.M. (1987) Retrospective consideration of the doses of morphine given intrathecally by chronic infusion in 163 patients by 19 physicians. *Pain*, 31, 211–223.

Young, R.R. and Delwaide, P.J. (1981) Drug therapy: spasticity. *N. Engl. J. Med.*, 304, 28–33, 96–99.

Zaualeta, C. (1976) Study of a new analgesic compound in the treatment of tension headache. *J. Internat. Med. Res.*, 4, 67–72.

Zenz, M., Schappler-Scheele, B., Neuhans, R., Piepenbrock, S. and Hilfrich, J. (1981) Long-term peridural morphine analgesia in cancer pain. *Lancet*, i, 91.

M. Swerdlow and J.E. Charlton (eds.) Relief of Intractable Pain
© 1989, Elsevier Science Publishers B.V. (Biomedical Division)

6

Non-invasive and other simple physical methods

Gordon M. Wyant

This chapter comprises a number of clinical modalities in common use in many pain treatment facilities. They have all been studied to a greater or lesser extent and have been the subject of detailed descriptions. In the context of this chapter it will be possible only to describe the basic properties of each modality, its physiological potential, mode of action and treatment implications. While some of the subjects discussed are invasive in a minor sense, other non-invasive procedures, such as transcutaneous electrical nerve stimulation (TENS) and psychological management, are not included, as they are the subjects of separate chapters.

ACUPUNCTURE

The history of acupuncture is intimately bound to the history of China and the Orient. The first recorded text, the Canon of Medicine, goes back to the year 475 BC and contains a basic description of acupuncture points and meridians, indications for and contra-indications to treatment. Its practice in China was discouraged during the Ching Dynasty between 1644 and 1911 and during the days of the republic, only to be re-introduced and given the stamp of official approval and even encouragement with the coming to power of the Mao regime. Traditional Chinese medicine, which comprises both acupuncture, moxibustion and herbal medicine, was then accorded equal place with western medicine, and indeed at one time its use was publicized and encouraged even for pain control during surgical operations.

Classical Chinese acupuncture is based on the general concept of Yin and Yang, two opposite life forces which normally are in complete balance. They are likened to the contrast between night and day, motion and immobility, earth and sky. The

life energy Ch'i is believed to flow through the body in a network of 14 main channels or meridians. Imbalance between Yin and Yang results in excess or deficit
of Ch'i and this produces pain and disease. By applying acupuncture along traditional concepts of Chinese physiology, the equilibrium is restored and with it
health and well-being. A vast number of acupuncture points have been identified
through the centuries, most but by no means all of which are located on meridians, many of which bear the names of internal organs to which are ascribed Yin
or Yang properties. Other points of more recent origin and which do not fit into
the scheme of meridians are identified as extra points (Academy of Traditional
Chinese Medicine, 1975). The entire system of treatment is based on the traditional Chinese concept of the function of internal organs which in many instances is
quite alien to western physiological thought. No scientific or experimental basis
exists to substantiate the theories on which these practices are based.

The modern Chinese, although still adhering to the basic principles of classical
acupuncture, have attempted to explain it and in a rather tentative way have
started to conduct animal experiments in order to reproduce and understand the
phenomenon. They had shown in the early '70s that acupuncture can interfere with
conduction of painful stimuli at several levels of the spinal cord, and have theo-
rized that there might be interference with the functioning of transmitter substances within the central nervous system.

Their studies had suggested that an anti-pain factor might be produced in the
brain by acupuncture, as it had been shown in rabbits that cross-circulation per-
mitted analgesia to be transferred from one animal to the other. This at a time
when encephalins had not yet been discovered.

Acupuncture, as practised in China for the treatment of symptoms, has had
considerable success, although perhaps not to the same extent as claimed when
measured by Western standards (Wyant and Camerlain, 1977). Less known in the
West than body acupuncture is the very widespread practice of ear acupuncture
which is based on the belief that the outer ear represents the foetus in utero and
treatment of various organs is effected by needling the appropriate area. The re-
markable fact here is that changes in skin resistance similar to those noted in body
acupuncture can be clearly demonstrated as the exploring probe approaches the
representative area of a particular diseased portion of the body.

With the increasing interest in acupuncture for pain relief in Western countries,
there has developed a desire to submit its mechanism of action to scientific
scrutiny. There is little doubt that in some individuals, given the right circumstances, analgesia can be produced by acupuncture and that its incidence exceeds
that which one would expect from a mere placebo effect. However, emotional control and cultural factors, as well as expectations, enter heavily into the picture.
It has proved entirely impossible to duplicate in the Western population the success rate which this kind of treatment has enjoyed in Oriental societies. Whether

the stimulus by the needle evokes a response which can be explained by the 'gate control theory' and is due to presynaptic inhibition in the substantia gelatinosa, or whether it is due to the mobilization of endorphins, or both, remains a matter of speculation. However, it has been shown that naloxone decreases or eliminates the analgesia produced by classical needle acupuncture in healthy subjects (Mayer et al., 1977) and inhibits pain relief elicited by low frequency electrical stimulation in patients with chronic pain (Sjölund et al., 1977). This would seem to implicate at least in part morphine-like substances in the analgesic process (Sjölund and Eriksson, 1976); indeed, these same workers have shown that the CNS concentration of endorphins increases in response to pain-relieving low frequency electrical stimulation. The counteraction by naloxone of pain relief after acupuncture would thus be due to its effect on the endorphins or their receptors. Indeed, Lovacky and co-workers (1987) have shown an increase of beta-endorphins 30–60 min after onset of treatment in the 75% of patients with low back pain who had relief from the treatment. The increase in endorphins was seen only when true acupuncture points were used and could not be demonstrated in individuals who were not suffering from low back pain. The D-amino acids, namely D-phenylalanine and D-leucine, produce naloxone-reversible analgesia, similar to electro-acupuncture. Combining the two modalities is claimed to produce an additive effect (Cheng and Pomeranz, 1980).

Liu (1980) has pointed out that acupuncture deals with both the perceptional and the emotional aspects of pain. The acupuncture process induces a sensation which is carried by large-size fibres into the thalamus. Endorphins are liberated which block the transmission of nociceptive impulses at the synapses, so that pain is no longer perceived. Meanwhile, the endorphins also act on the limbic system, thus submerging the emotional aspects of pain. The musculoskeletal system is the first buffer of stress and by relieving stress, acupuncture is said to exert some of its beneficial effects on the somatic component of pain (Jacobs, 1985).

Another hypothetical explanation of the mechanism of acupuncture is based on its antiprostaglandin effect (Frost et al., 1976). Earlier, Melzack (1973) had suggested that acupuncture, like TENS, might act through a process of hypersensitivity. There is good evidence, however, that the acupuncture effect is mediated through afferent nervous impulses, since analgesia fails to develop on the hypaesthetic side in hemiplegic patients or when the nerves innervating the acupuncture site are blocked by local anaesthetic. Activation of high threshold afferents is a common feature of needle manipulation or electrical low frequency stimulation. Needle stimulation, however, affects only receptors and afferents in a limited region, whereas electrical stimulation must activate receptors in a much larger area in order to influence the pain. The site of production of electroacupuncture analgesia is believed to reside in the lower brainstem structures involving the raphe nuclei, the locus ceruleus and other reticular cells (Takeda et al., 1979). Ding et al. (1983) brought yet another perspective to the same question by showing that there was a clear increase in lymphocyte transformation 3 h post-acupuncture as compared to the pre-acupuncture state in eight of nine volunteers, while Sin (1983) demonstrated enhanced phagocytic activity of the reticuloendothelial system in mice following electric acupuncture. The same author then showed in 1984 that acupuncture suppresses the early phase of increased vascular permeability in rats exposed to thermal and histamine-induced injury. This is in agreement with the Eastern concept of the promotion of self-defence and homeostasis in the restoration of health, rather than the Western emphasis on the elimination of pathogens (Dingzong, 1986). Takase (1983) has injected trace amounts of sodium hydroxide into meridian points without needling and found this effective in 'neuralgia' without an organic cause. He showed that pain always originated in a region of sodium deficiency.

There is evidence that low frequency stimulation such as is used in acupuncture activates descending control systems (Anderson, 1979). High frequency electrical stimulation, on the other hand, is believed to interfere with transmission in the primary pain afferents, producing fatigue and conduction block (Callaghan et al., 1978). Frost et al. (1976) report that the duration of pain relief from analgesia averages 1 month, while Spoerel et al. (1976) believe that daily treatments are no more effective than weekly or bi-weekly ones, and that acupuncture is most effective in painful conditions of neck, shoulder, knee and low back. In Yamauchi's experience (1976) with 72 chronic pain patients who had undergone 660 acupuncture treatments in 1 year, only 11 showed marked improvement 4 months after treatment. Few studies are available on the effect of acupuncture on body function, but Wong and Brayton (1982) have determined by means of electrocapacitance plethysmography that blood flow in the forearm during acupuncture is reduced by an average of 33%.

From clinical experience, it is clear that in most instances, the intensity of the analgesia is insufficient to block severe painful stimuli and that in this respect it shares with other treatment modalities the property of an inverse ratio of stimulus to analgesic effects.

There are many different ways in which acupuncture stimulation can be applied. In the classical treatment, the needle is twirled manually in a clockwise and anti-clockwise fashion rotating it between the thumb and index finger and at the same time thrusting it up and down in a slow or rapid movement. This is usually carried on for a few minutes and the needle is then left in situ and the twirling repeated after a pause. A less intense stimulation would consist of inserting the needle and leaving it in place without any manipulation whatsoever. Electrical stimulation by an alternating current is the most commonly used stimulation in the West. Santiestebau (1984), comparing electroacupuncture to selected physical therapy for acute spine pain, has come to the conclusion that the acupuncture initially reduced the pain and increased the range of movement, thus laying the groundwork for better response to exercise and mobilization.

Acupuncture has been used in a wide variety of pain conditions, both acute and chronic. Introduced at the correct location, the acupuncture needle produces a characteristic sensation of heaviness and a sickening dull ache at the site of insertion and its immediate surrounding: indeed, Chinese acupuncturists believe that if no such feeling is experienced, the treatment will not be successful and that the proper acupuncture point has been missed. Studies have indicated that the analgesic effects of acupuncture are related to deep afferents rather than to cutaneous ones. In contrast to Chinese practices, many physicians in the West rely on the identification of areas of lowered electrical resistance in the skin surface by passing an exploring electrode over the skin until a point of lowered skin resistance is identified by alteration in the pitch of sound in the exploring instrument. Treatments usually extend over a period of about half an hour and might be repeated every other day. One of the major disadvantages is that even when pain relief is achieved, its duration is usually limited and rarely is the pain abolished permanently. It is a common experience that the longer the pain has existed the more treatments are required to subdue it and the greater are the chances of failure.

Acupuncture has been recommended at one time or another for the treatment of all sorts and manner of disease and conditions, and indeed enjoys universal application in China to this day. By and large, acupuncture in the West is restricted to the treatment of chronic pain with particular emphasis on the musculoskeletal system. It has also been used to assist in weight reduction and in withdrawal from smoking, drugs, alcohol and in the control of withdrawal symptoms. For many of the longer term treatments, insertion of staples into the ear is the preferred stimulation (Sacks, 1975; Sadowsky, 1982). Reports of the success rate in these endeavours vary widely (Cox, 1975; Gilbey, 1977; Giller, 1976; Lau, 1975; Leung, 1977; Parker, 1977; Requena, 1980). The application of acupuncture in the treatment of a large variety of disease, sometimes in conjunction with other modalities, is more restricted, although sporadic recommendations to that effect surface regularly in the acupuncture literature. Such recommendations encompass almost every disease state imaginable, ranging across the entire spectrum from relatively minor ailments to severe and potentially lethal diseases. These recommendations emanate from the writings of a limited number of authors and are hardly ever confirmed by the experiences of others.

The entire system of traditional Chinese acupuncture is a complicated one which requires intensive study. It is natural therefore that many different adaptations have been promoted to enhance the scope of acupuncture in clinical practice. *Acupressure* is a system which uses conventional meridians and acupuncture points, but instead of needles employs digital pressure only (Beggs, 1980). On the other hand, the refinement of electrical and electronic instrumentation has left its imprint also on acupuncture. The use of *ultrasound* (Khoe, 1975, 1977) and *electromagnetism* (Tany and Sawatsuga, 1975) are cases in point. *Ryodoraku*, a Japanese modification of acupuncture is a more lasting example. The method involves the use of a 'Neurometer', an instrument which by emission of a 12 V, 150–200 μA current was used initially merely to locate acupuncture points. Later, the output of the instrument was found capable of reinforcing the acupuncture effects when applied to the needle (Lowenschuss, 1975). Ryodoraku has also been recommended for the diagnosis of cancer and for evaluating the effectiveness or otherwise of treatment as the disease is said to produce specific patterns on Ryodoraku charts (Kobayashi, 1984).

Another modification of classical acupuncture is the method advocated by Voll. By means of an instrument called the 'Dermatron', a system has been developed in which the change of resistance at acupuncture points is related to various pathological states in particular organs and in which each point is directly related to a specific structure or function. It is claimed that in this way early diagnosis of disease is made possible, long before clinical or laboratory signs can be elicited. It is further claimed that when medicine is introduced into the circuit during point measurements, the correct medicine will bring readings to more normal levels, permitting one not only to establish the kind of drug which is indicated, but also its potency and dosage (Voll, 1975, 1980). *Laser* acupuncture using a low energy beam aimed at acupuncture points has enjoyed considerable vogue during the last few years. Its effectiveness in physical therapy has been attributed to depolarization and repolarization of contracted muscle fibres and to the relief of arteriolar muscle spasm with consequent reactive vasodilation. It has been postulated that the electron excitation of the myochondral membrane leads to changes in metabolic processes resulting in ATP formation and stimulation of enzyme activity, thus restoring normal properties at cell and organ levels (Kleinkort and Foley, 1984). The increase of muscle strength engendered by these processes has been confirmed by Sopler (1984), who found a 12.8% increase in the ability of a healthy individual for weight lifting. Even more recent than *laser* acupuncture is the use of low strength *magnets* in the treatment of dental pain, headache and back pain, and one author has even recommended it for the treatment of the common cold (Prince, 1983a,b; Ludwig, 1984; Shapiro, 1987). Finally, mention must be made of *colour* acupuncture. This modality which uses six main colours is said to have virtually unlimited power of penetration in contrast to *lasers*, the potential for penetration of which is limited to 0.1 inch (Ludwig, 1986). However, the work on the use of magnets and colour is quite new and so far remains uncorroborated.

In Chinese and other oriental practice, acupuncture is frequently associated with *Moxibustion*, the burning of the dried and shredded leaves of *Artemis vulgaris*, which emits an aromatic odour and has warming properties even if waved several centimetres above the skin surface or is burned at the free end of the acupuncture needle.

The Chinese also like to combine acupuncture with *cupping*, a procedure in which a bamboo or glass container is applied to the skin while a partial vacuum has been created within it by a flame which has consumed the oxygen in the air. The container thus adheres firmly to the skin surface and the vacuum causes local hyperaemia. The treatment is effective in conditions affecting superficial muscles and other tissues, but has the disadvantage of causing ecchymoses with discoloration which is slow to subside.

Akin in concept to ear acupuncture, *reflexology* is based on the assumption that the human body and each organ has its representation in a specific location on the sole of the foot. Paired organs are projected in mirror image positions, while single organs are represented only on the ipsilateral sole. By firmly rubbing the representation of the affected part with the thumb in a back and forth motion, relief from pain in the appropriate organ or part of the body is claimed to be achieved. No scientific evidence has been advanced for reflexology, nor for many of the assumptions of traditional Chinese medicine.

CLINICAL IMPLICATIONS

Richardson and Vincent (1986) have reviewed reports of controlled studies that are available in the literature and have found evidence for the short-term effectiveness of acupuncture in relieving pain arising from a large array of clinical conditions. They found that about 50–80% of patients are usually helped, with wide variations from study to study, but that about half the patients suffer relapses. In the majority of instances there has been no statistical difference between acupuncture and other treatment modalities, such as TENS, physiotherapy, etc. On the other hand, Lehmann and co-workers (1986), limiting themselves to the study of chronic low back pain treated with electroacupuncture, found that their patients experienced less pain when assessed on a return visit than those who had been treated with TENS. This observation would tend to support the clinical impression of the usefulness of acupuncture in the treatment of musculoskeletal disorders, especially in combination with other treatment modalities.

Perusal of the available acupuncture literature reveals that this treatment has been used in a wide variety of conditions, but reports for the most part are anecdotal and lack convincing scientific evidence. Nevertheless, there might be no harm in many instances in trying acupuncture as an alternative if other more traditional methods have failed, provided, of course, that correctable organic lesions have been ruled out.

TRIGGER POINTS

References in the literature to trigger points go back as far as 1843. Their distribution, origin and pathology were first described by Lange (1931) and the present term 'trigger point' was applied to them later by Steindler (1959). Since then a large body of literature has developed to which Travell has been one of the most prolific contributors. The entire subject has been extensively reviewed by Simons (1975, 1976).

Trigger points can be found in muscles, ligaments, joint capsules or bursae, but they are by far most common in muscle, and indeed can affect any striated muscle in the body. The importance of trigger points lies not so much in the existence of localized painful areas in muscle as in the referred pain with which they are associated. Trigger points can be produced experimentally by exposure to cold and exertion, and Kellgren (1938) was able to produce localized pain and radiation patterns simulating trigger points by injection of hypertonic saline. Clinically, they are most commonly due to trauma, chronic muscle strain, ischaemia or emotional tension; in fact, anything that produces muscle spasm can also cause trigger points. The radiation patterns of trigger points are quite typical and have been well mapped out (Travell and Rinzler, 1952; Kraus, 1973). The clinical importance of the reproducibility of referral or target zones lies in the fact that unless these patterns are known, the origin of the pain in the relatively distant trigger point might not be suspected, and specific treatment may therefore not be instituted (Figs. 6.1–6.4).

Trigger points can be either active or latent. Active trigger points are identified by the fact that pressure upon them is not only locally painful, but will also reproduce in many instances the referred pain. They can frequently be identified by palpation as firm bands and might under certain circumstances exhibit the 'jump sign', which is elicited by applying moderate tension to the relaxed muscle and snapping the band briskly with a palpating finger. Latent trigger points, on the other hand, can be identified only by deep pressure and a positive 'jump sign', and produce only soreness, but not pain, in the reference zone; they can be activated by stress. If trigger points are allowed to exist for any length of time, satellite triggers will develop, which give rise to overlapping pain patterns.

Sustained pressure on a trigger point might cause pain in the referral zone provided the threshold is not too high. The reference areas also exhibit vasomotor, secretory and other autonomic changes, but after the trigger point has been obliterated, vasodilation replaces vasoconstriction. Characteristically, there is no neurological deficit in the painful affected areas. Symptoms tend to outlast the precipitating event which had caused the trigger point in the first instance, probably because persisting mechanical stresses continue to affect the underlying somatic structures causing muscle guarding, limitation of movement and impairment of circulation (Travell, 1976). Melzack et al. (1977) have found a high correlation between trigger points and acupuncture points and believe that both represent the same phenomenon; they explain this in terms of an underlying neural mechanism.

No precise explanation is given for the specificity of the reference zone which they believe represents complicated interactions in the central nervous system. Quite recently, Fine et al. (1988), in a double-blind cross-over study, have shown that the effects of trigger point injections with bupivacaine can be reversed by injecting 10 mg naloxone intravenously, but not by placebo. They conclude that this suggests an endogenous opioid mediator for the decreased pain, increased range of motion and reduction of palpable bands. These findings would tend to support the similarity between trigger points and acupuncture, as it is known that naloxone can reverse also the effects of acupuncture.

Histologically, trigger points present as loci of myofibrositis characterized by a metachromatic substance with platelet aggregation and localized oedema in the interfibrillar connective tissue. It has been postulated that trauma is the reason for the extravasation of platelets which release serotonin and that this causes vasoconstriction, hence the oedema. This, in turn, results in degranulation of mast cells with consequent liberation of histamine and heparin. The histamine counteracts the vasoconstriction and the heparin prevents clotting of extravasated blood and lymph (Brendstrup et al., 1975).

While trigger points can occur in any muscle, they tend to be more common in some areas than in others and some are more interesting than others. Dorigo et al. (1979) have found that trigger points develop in intermittent claudication, and that exercise tolerance improves after they are injected. They postulate that activities from the trigger points are added to the contraction from tissue hypoxia and that the injection interrupts a vicious cycle of abnormal input for muscles, thus increasing the exercise tolerance without increasing blood flow. Another interesting trigger point is occasionally seen in the piriformis muscle, which, being situated deep in the pelvis, is somewhat difficult to locate. Pain from this muscle is referred down in the sciatic distribution, which is explained by the close anatomical relation between the muscle, the sacro-iliac joints and the roots of the sciatic nerve (Wyant, 1979). Another important trigger is at the posterior arch of the atlas, which should be sought in headaches originating in the cervical region.

Treatment consists essentially of attempts to eradicate the trigger itself. This is most frequently achieved by needle puncture, but may also be carried out by vapocoolant sprays to the overlying skin or other counter-irritants. There is no unanimity as to whether injection should be with a small amount of local anaesthetic with or without the addition of steroids, whether injection of normal saline alone might be preferable, or whether dry needling alone suffices. Lewit (1979) considers that the needle puncture is the essential part of the procedure and he has achieved immediate analgesia without hypaesthesia in 86.6% of cases. He emphasizes that the effectiveness of the procedure depends on the intensity of the pain produced by the trigger zone and the precision with which the exact point of tenderness is located by the needle. He calls this the 'needle effect'. Brief intensive stimulation

178

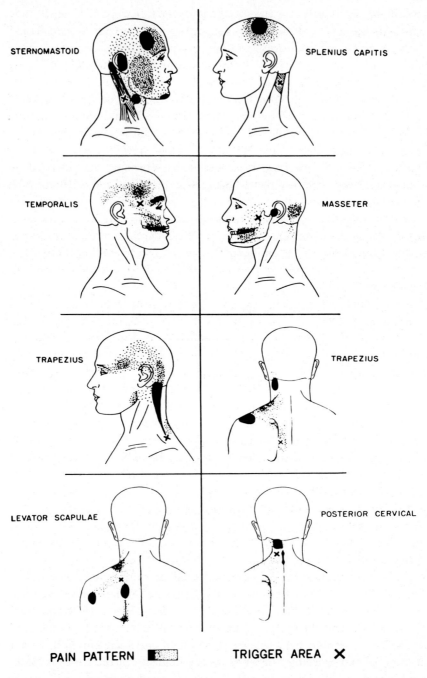

STERNOMASTOID

SPLENIUS CAPITIS

TEMPORALIS

MASSETER

TRAPEZIUS

TRAPEZIUS

LEVATOR SCAPULAE

POSTERIOR CERVICAL

PAIN PATTERN ▮▤▢   TRIGGER AREA ✕

Figs. 6.1–6.4. Trigger points and associated pain patterns (reproduced from *Postgraduate Medicine*, by kind permission of the Editor).

179

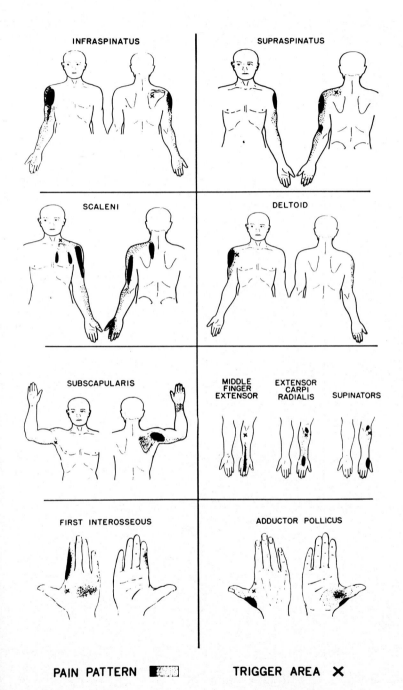

PAIN PATTERN ▮▬░   TRIGGER AREA ✖

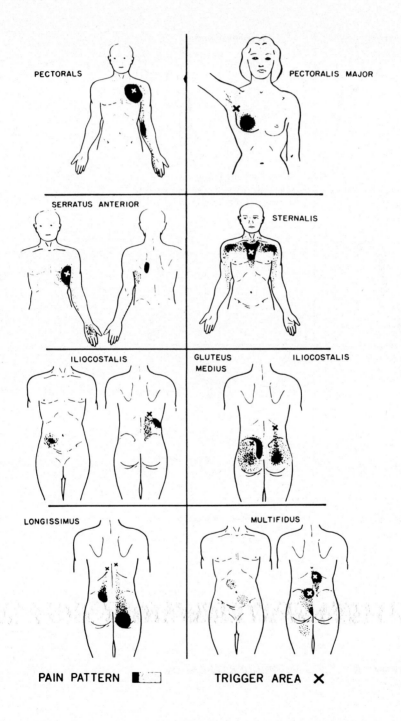

PECTORALS

PECTORALIS MAJOR

SERRATUS ANTERIOR

STERNALIS

ILIOCOSTALIS

GLUTEUS
MEDIUS

ILIOCOSTALIS

LONGISSIMUS

MULTIFIDUS

PAIN PATTERN ▮▯   TRIGGER AREA ✕

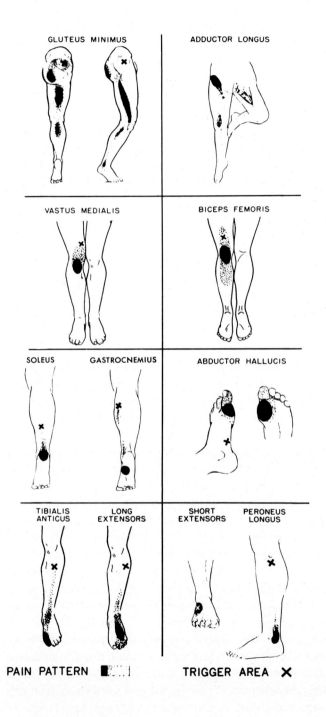

GLUTEUS MINIMUS

ADDUCTOR LONGUS

VASTUS MEDIALIS

BICEPS FEMORIS

SOLEUS   GASTROCNEMIUS

ABDUCTOR HALLUCIS

TIBIALIS ANTICUS   LONG EXTENSORS

SHORT EXTENSORS   PERONEUS LONGUS

PAIN PATTERN ▓▒░   TRIGGER AREA ✕

frequently carried out in this way often produces long pain relief (Melzack et al., 1977). Since the injection of saline is painful, Travell recommends that local anaesthetics be used for the purpose, unless non-invasive modalities are applied. Ready and associates (1983) have found that local anaesthetics applied by jet injection are less painful and give results as satisfactory as those obtained by injections by hypodermic syringe. The choice of local anaesthetic lies with any of the commercially available substances, as long as they do not contain vasoconstrictors and the most dilute concentration is employed. As for steroid additions, the choice is between triamcinolone suspension, 20–40 mg, or methylprednisolone solution. Jaeger and Reeves (1986) have been able to decrease myofascial trigger point sensitivity in 20 subjects with myofascial head and neck pain by using passive stretch, and they have recorded the response objectively by means of the pressure algometer. They have also been able to demonstrate a relationship between trigger point sensitivity and the intensity of the referred pain. Thus, experimental proof has been offered for the clinical benefit of the 'stretch and ice' or 'stretch and spray' technique in which a surface coolant, such as ethyl chloride, is employed.

VIBRATORS AND PERCUSSION

Vibrators have been widely used in the control of certain kinds of pain. It is believed that mechanical vibratory stimulation activates the large diameter afferent fibres and it is known that Pacinian corpuscles and other cutaneous receptors such as primary endings of muscle spindles are activated by vibration. Peripheral impulses of this nature reach the spinal cord and initiate a complex sequence of events which results in inhibition of pain transmission, of which Melzack and Wall's gate control concept (1965) is only one. Bini and associates (1984), on the other hand, have postulated that the pain suppression occurs at central levels, since vibration within an area of projected pain, and to a lesser extent even outside that area, reduced the pain caused by 2 Hz stimulation within cutaneous fascicles of the median nerve at the wrist of 16 volunteers. They had to come to that conclusion since stimulation was applied at the nerve trunks, not from nociceptors. Ottoson et al. (1981) have reported the use of vibration at 100 Hz to various points in the face and skull for control of postoperative pain after extraction of impacted wisdom teeth. They remark, however, that in a small number of patients, vibration actually increases the pain, and it is well known that initially this kind of treatment tends to be quite painful. However, it can be made more tolerable by the application of a tourniquet proximal to the area to be treated until numbness supervenes. Lundeberg and associates (1984) and Lundeberg (1984), in two large clinical series of patients with chronic pain of neurogenic and musculoskeletal origin, have shown pain relief in over half of the individuals, with significant increase in social activities and decrease in drug intake. Other indications for vibration therapy have been myofascial conditions, postherpetic neuralgia (Matthews and Miller, 1975) and amputation stump neuromata (Swerdlow, 1979).

Russell and Spalding (1950) have reported the treatment of painful amputation stumps by *percussion* and have achieved good results from this modality of treatment. A rubber hammer is commonly used for that purpose, but the Chinese, to whom this treatment has been known for a long time, use a small hammer with short blunt spikes.

SHORTWAVE DIATHERMY

Shortwave diathermy is produced by utilising the effect of a high frequency (27 million per second) alternating current. A high frequency current is one that exceeds 500 000 cycles and thus provides 1 000 000 impulses per second, each of which therefore lasts 0.001 milliseconds. This is too short to cause nerve stimulation and consequently there is no discomfort or muscle contraction as the current passes through the body. Heat is produced in the tissue by the conversion of electrical to thermal energy due to the movement of charged particles. This is achieved by placing the tissues into a rapidly varying electrostatic or electromagnetic field, depending on the technique used. A circuit in the machine which produces a high frequency current is coupled to the patient circuit by induction. The intensity used depends entirely on the individual patient response of 'feeling a comfortable warmth'. The main physical effect of shortwave diathermy is the production of heat. The response to the heat produced is responsible for the physiological effect of increased blood flow. There are generally two methods of application:

(a) Condensor field technique – Makes use of a rapidly varying electrostatic field.

(b) Inductothermy technique – With the use of an inductothermy cable, there are two fields: a rapidly varying electromagnetic field and an electrostatic field between different parts of the cable.

It is beyond the scope of this description to discuss in detail the various indications for diathermy in medicine; suffice to say that for purposes of pain management, the heat produced reduces the excitability of nerves; this in turn induces muscle relaxation resulting in relief of spasm and pain. Other effects include reduction of chronic inflammation, promotion of healing, control of chronic infection and increased extensibility of connective tissue. Therapeutic uses of shortwave diathermy may include non-infective inflammatory conditions, such as arthritis and fibrositis, and infective processes, such as sinusitis and gynaecological conditions. In the early stages of inflammation, it is best not to treat directly the inflamed area as this might increase tension from exudate or bacterial activity. It is better to give a mild dose to neighbouring anatomical areas. The increased blood supply which accompanies the rise in tissue temperature also results in acceleration of all metabolic processes, vasodilation and removal of waste products. Stronger heating, in addition, might also act through the mechanism of counterirritation.

Side effects include an increase in body temperature, reduction in blood pressure and increase in the secretion of sweat. In the acute stages of an inflammatory condition, caution must be exercised or indeed treatment entirely avoided to prevent an increase in the inflammatory response. In a subacute stage, with the condition subsiding, a mild dose may be given, gradually increasing to a full thermal dose in the chronic stages.

There are many conditions in which application of shortwave diathermy is contraindicated or potentially dangerous; these are:
- vascular disease with decreased arterial supply, thrombosis or phlebitis where a danger of embolus formation exists;
- recent radiotherapy or haemorrhage (including pelvic treatment during menstruation);
- lack of sensation of the part;
- malignancy;
- pregnancy;
- lack of understanding on the part of the patient or inability to report the sensations experienced;
- metallic implants;
- pacemakers;
- ischaemic tissues;
- marked oedema;
- over-wet dressings or towels;
- tuberculosis of joints;
- acute infection or inflammation;
- severe cardiac abnormalities;
- abnormal blood pressure, high or low.

Extreme caution is necessary because the only guideline to intensity of treatment is the patients' perception of heating effects. There are no objective measurements. The many contraindications coupled with the possible hazardous side effects and dangers, such as burns, scalds, hypotension and electrical shock, have resulted in more frequent usage of other safer, but just as effective methods or modalities of treatment.

ULTRASOUND

Medical therapeutics can employ ultrasonic waves which are mechanical acoustic waves. The therapeutic use of ultrasound waves was first introduced by Wood and Loomis in 1927. The human ear can detect sound waves within a frequency range of 30–20 000 cycles per second, while those of higher frequency are referred to as ultrasonic waves. In contrast to diathermy, sound waves are longitudinal waves in matter and consist of to-and-fro movements of particles in the direction in which the rays are travelling. Thus, they differ from the electromagnetic waves of diathermy, which consist of an up-and-down movement and can be transmitted through space, whereas sound waves require particles of substance through which to travel. The most widely used treatment frequencies in medical practice are in the vicinity of 1 000 000 cycles per second (1 MHz), but may be 750 000 to 3 000 000 cycles per second (0.75–3 MHz).

In order to produce waves of the high frequency needed for ultrasound therapy, vibration is induced in a crystal quartz or similar material. Rapidly varying voltage is applied across the crystal which changes shape, expands and contracts, and produces an oscillating surface.

Ultrasonic waves, being vibrations in matter, follow well-known, recognized laws of physics. They travel more easily in media of higher density than in other media, and when a wave encounters a different medium from that in which it is presently travelling, it might be reflected, refracted, transmitted or absorbed. In the course of these distortions, energy in the form of heat is released. This heat reaches deeper tissues than that produced by diathermy, because of their greater density. In addition to the thermal effect, a second mechanical effect is achieved which can disrupt adhesions or increase the elasticity of scar tissue. This is often called the 'micromassage' effect. The setting of the instrument is determined by the desired effect. The depth of the structure at fault and the relative density of the tissue to be treated help to determine the effective dose. The operator can alter the intensity, which represents the amount of energy which crosses a unit area in a unit of time, and can choose continuous or pulsed waves; the duration of application can be changed, and the application can be either fixed or mobile. The pulsing frequency will determine the depth of penetration. In addition, a specific ultrasound coupling agent is utilized to allow efficient transmission of the waves from the sound head to the tissue across the air interface. These are various commercial gels, oils or water.

The basic usefulness of ultrasound in pain control is as a deep heating modality. The thermal effect causes vasodilation and enhances lymphatic flow. It selectively heats superficial cortical bone, periosteum, joint structures, muscle tendon sheaths and major nerve trunks. This results in an increase in collagen tissue elasticity, decrease in joint stiffness and pain, reduction in muscle spasm and increase in local blood flow. Due to the mechanical and electromechanical effects, ultrasound reduces nerve conduction velocities. Hence, ultrasound is useful in the treatment of the pain from osteoarthritis, rheumatoid arthritis and deep sprains and strains, in particular those affecting the hip joint capsule. Success has also been reported in causalgia, ankle sprains, varicose ulcers, intercostal neuralgia, tendinitis, tenosynovitis, fasciitis, especially those of a superficial nature, bursitis and painful amputation stumps, in the treatment of phantom limb and neuromata (Schwartz, 1954; Rubin and Kuifert, 1955). It is reportedly successful in the breakdown or 'softening' of scar tissue adhesions during immature or mature stages. Ultrasound is frequently most effective when used with deep friction massage, flexibility exercises and mobilizing exercises where indicated.

Like all modalities of treatment, harmful effects can result also from the use of ultrasound. There is evidence that it can initiate blood coagulation and thrombus formation, and damaging effects, such as burns and cavitation of bone, can be increased when a technique of stationary application is used. Contraindications are vascular afflictions, such as emboli or haemorrhage, advanced heart or vascular disease, anaesthetic areas, application to bone prominences and very acute inflammatory conditions. It may be used with care in acute soft tissue injury or during stages of acute inflammation, if pulsed; low intensities with a mobile treatment head are used for periods of brief duration (2–3 min). It is preferable to treat the surrounding area and not the lesion directly in these instances.

HEAT AND COLD

Heat and cold can be used interchangeably and are especially useful in the treatment of muscle spasm as they decrease the sensitivity of muscle to stretch.

Heat raises the threshold to pain whether applied directly to the skin or to nervous tissue. It can be useful in alleviating both acute and chronic pain, but like other modalities of heat applications, it too must be of mild degree or used with caution in acute painful conditions. Superficial heat is applied by means of hotpacks, whirlpool and hot sawdust, paraffin, heating pads, infrared radiation, hot air baths and immersion into hot water. When it is intended to reach deeper layers, other modalities, such as diathermy and ultrasound, are more useful.

Cold exerts an anaesthetic effect, reduces muscle spasm, initially reduces blood flow, and so decreases the local inflammatory response, oedema and haemorrhage. One of the characteristics of prolonged application of cold in excess of 20 min is its long latency response ('hunting'), in which vasoconstriction is followed by vasodilation, which then in turn is followed again by vasoconstriction. This can continue in series as long as the cold is applied. Cold therapy has been shown to be beneficial in increasing mobility and decreasing pain and oedema, but usually only when combined with an active therapeutic exercise program. Means of applying cold therapy consist of cold water immersion, ice massage and contrast baths and application of icepacks and spray, such as, for instance, with ethyl chloride and other substances with a low boiling point. Cold may appropriately be applied by two different methods:

- short-term cooling during the stage of acute inflammation or about 48–72 h following trauma, as in acute sprains. It is applied for a maximum of 10–15 min, with at least 30 min off, and reapplied frequently in this manner, once each hour if possible. The physiological effect is primarily one of vasoconstriction and the inhibition of exudate production.
- In subacute and chronic stages, prolonged cooling of 20–30 min each is more appropriately used once or twice a day to obtain the same effects.

COMPARISON OF HEAT AND COLD (Tepperman and Devlin, 1983)

	Heat	Cold
Cell metabolism	increase	decrease
Vascular response	dilatation	constriction
Inflammatory response	increase	decrease
Skin vessels	dilatation	constriction
Connective tissue distensibility	increase	decrease
Synovial fluid viscosity	decrease	increase
Nerve conduction	increase	decrease
Muscle spindle activity	increase	decrease
Muscle contractility	increase	decrease

Cryotherapy is the method of choice when there is an acute injury or an acute inflammatory response. For chronic conditions, heat or cold may be used interchangeably or together as contrast baths.

COUNTER-IRRITANTS

Stroking and rubbing of a painful area is an instinctive response to pain of any kind and, like chemical counter-irritation, activates afferent fibres, the result being a 'closing of the gate'. Many chemical counter-irritants are available, of which Bengues Balsam (20% menthol and 20% methyl salicylate) or Betnovate 0.1% cream have been recommended in postherpetic neuralgia. The application of cold sprays, with ethyl chloride, for instance, probably serves a similar purpose and this is an alternative physical modality recommended for postherpetic neuralgia by Matthews and Miller (1975). More recently, DMSO (dimethylsulphoxide) has been advocated for muscle aches and arthritic pain, and a number of propietary preparations are available over the counter for similar purposes with such high-sounding names as 'Heet', a combination containing methyl salicylate and camphor, and 'Absorbine Jr.', the active component of which is chloroxylenol. The popularity of these remedies lends credence to the mustard plaster so loved by our grandmothers.

MASSAGE

The benefits of massage reside primarily in the indication of muscle relaxation and increased perfusion with the secondary effects of increasing muscle temperature and of removal of waste products of metabolism, both being soothing effects. There are essentially two techniques of applying massage: one is a deep relaxing massage using a broad surface area and applying slow stroking motions. Deep friction massage consists of localized cross-friction over small areas located at the exact point of the lesion. From a physiological point of view, massage provides analgesia mediated either through the nervous system or through local input, prevents or reduces adhesions, increases local circulation and relaxes muscle spasm by increasing the tone in individual muscle spindles. Deep friction massage is primarily used in ligamentous and tendinous lesions and can be useful in local muscle belly lesions. Massage should always be combined with therapeutic exercise to enhance its effect and to utilize periods of decreased muscle spasm, relaxation and enhanced mobility. Massage is primarily a means to an end by first inducing relaxation and pain relief, allowing otherwise difficult or painful exercise and functional activity. With the independent use of exercise and activity, the strength and movement achieved will usually result in long-term pain relief.

MOBILIZATIONS

Mobilization can be defined as passive movement of a joint within its physiological range. It is used when specific movement dysfunction on passive and active movement testing is demonstrated. The movement dysfunction can be defined as 'an altered state of mechanics demonstrating either an aberrant motion or an increase or decrease from the expected range' (Paris, 1979). Characteristics of mobilization are small amplitude movements applied in an oscillating fashion. They are applied very specifically to certain joints or specific parts of the movement. Mobilizations are primarily used to produce the passive accessory movement which is necessary for full pain-free voluntary gross movement and which is frequently lost following trauma, swelling, or periods of relative joint immobilization (exogenous or endogenous). These may be reproduced in various segments of the gross active range of motion or range of accessory joint motion. The effects can be considered as neurophysiological (sensory input) and mechanical. They enhance joint lubrication and decrease elastic recoil of soft tissue structures. Once these purposes have been achieved, a specific active exercise program, considering the particular movement requirements, should be supplemented.

THERAPEUTIC EXERCISES

Therapeutic exercises can best be defined as a specifically prescribed modality, used on an individual basis designed to effect a change in physical and at times also in the psychological status of the patient. Embodied in this definition is the two-fold concept of prevention and rehabilitation. A suitable program is developed from the clinical assessment and from data collected by examination of the involved anatomy, the existing pathology and biochemical changes, and from movement dysfunction. The essential element of therapeutic exercises is that they must be made to fit the individual for whom they are designed and the prescription must be sufficiently exact to be effective and efficient. Therapeutic exercises in the pain patient might involve instruction in activity modification, relaxation, changes in postural and in specific movement patterns, factors often referred to as 'body mechanics'. An exercise program must be regularly reassessed and progressed or modified to meet the changing physical and occupational needs of the patient. The major variables used in a therapeutic exercise regime include intensity, duration, frequency, number of sets, repetitions, type and duration of rest period, type of exercises (isometric, isotonic, isokinetic), specific range of motion used, positioning (gravity-assisted or -resisted, for example), positioning of resistance, use of diagonal or straight patterns of movement.

THERMOGRAPHY

Thermography differs from all other modalities described in this chapter in that it is a diagnostic, not a therapeutic tool. Tissue temperature is related to vascularity, since increased blood supply results in increased local metabolism. It is the purpose of thermography to map out such areas of increased heat production. Early work in this area involved the use of liquid crystals, unique substances which exhibit the mechanical properties of liquid with the optical properties of solids. The colour changes resulting from varying temperatures can be recorded on colour film (Lee et al., 1976). Newman, Seres and Miller (1984) found the method reliable when compared with physical examination and electromyelography. They concluded that it appeared to be promising in the assessment of chronic back pain in patients with radicular symptoms, especially when CT scanning and myelography might give false positives as the result of previous back operations.

190

Another method of assessing temperature changes in superficial tissues is one of recording the infrared emission created by heat patterns radiating from the skin (Davy, 1977). The method is sensitive enough to determine the presence of soft tissue injury, but whether thermographic changes are synonymous with pain remains to be established. As opposed to heat patterns, diminished or absent blood flow presents itself as a 'cold patch'. Such cold patches have been equated, for instance, with vascular headache (Swerdlow and Dieter, 1986) and are reported to be useful in differentiating between vascular or cluster headache on the one hand and muscle contraction headache on the other (Edmeads, 1986). However, it is by no means clear that the absence of heat patterns or cold patches necessarily rules out an organic cause for pain.

REFERENCES

Acupuncture

Academy of Traditional Chinese Medicine (1975) *An Outline of Chinese Acupuncture*. Foreign Languages Press, Peking.

Anderson, S.A. (1979) Pain control by sensory stimulation. In: *Advances in Pain Research and Therapy, Vol. 3*. Editors: J.J. Bonica, J.C. Lieberskind and D. Albe-Fessard, Raven Press, New York, pp. 569–585.

Beggs, D.M. (1980) Acupressure as preventive measure, diagnostic aid and treatment modality. *Am. J. Acupunct.*, 8, 341–347.

Callaghan, M., Sternback, R.A., Nyquist, J.K. and Timmermans, G. (1978) Changes in the somatic sensitivity to transcutaneous electrical analgesia. *Pain*, 5, 115–127.

Cheng, R.S.S. and Pomeranz, B. (1980) A combined treatment with D-amino acids and electroacupuncture produces greater analgesia than either treatment alone; naloxone reverses these effects. *Pain*, 8, 231–236.

Cox, B.G. (1975) Patient motivation: a factor in weight reduction with auricular acupuncture. *Am. J. Acupunct.*, 3, 339–341.

Ding, V., Roath, S. and Lewith, G.T. (1983) The effect of acupuncture in lymphocyte behavior. *Am. J. Acupunct.*, 11, 51–57.

Dingzong, W. (1986) Acupuncture in the body's promotion of self-defense and homeostasis. *Am. J. Acupunct.*, 14, 123–126.

Frost, E.A.M., Hsu, C.Y. and Sadowsky, D. (1976) Acupuncture therapy. *N.Y. State J. Med.*, 76, 695–697.

Gilbey, V. and Neuman, B. (1977) Auricular acupuncture for smoking withdrawal. *Am. J. Acupunct.*, 5, 239–247.

Giller, R.M. (1976) Auricular acupuncture and weight reduction. *Am. J. Acupunct.*, 4, 33–36.

Jacobs, H.B. (1985) Acupuncture modalities function by relieving stress and its symptoms. *Am. J. Acupunct.*, 13, 163–164.

Khoe, W.H. (1975) Ultrasound acupuncture in low back pain and sciatic neuralgia caused by piriformis: muscle spasm. *Am. J. Acupunct.*, 3, 53–57.

Khoe, W.H. (1977) Ultrasound acupuncture: effective treatment modality for various diseases. *Am. J. Acupunct.*, 5, 31–34.

Kleinkort, J.A. and Foley, R.A. (1984) Laser acupuncture. Its use in physical therapy. *Am. J. Acupunct.*, 12, 51–56.

Kobayashi, T. (1984) Cancer diagnosis by means of Ryodoraku neurometric patterns. *Am. J. Acupunct.*, 12, 305–312.

Lau, B.H.S., Wang, W. and Wong, D.S. (1975) Effect of acupuncture on weight reduction. *Am. J. Acupunct.*, 3, 335–338.

Lehmann, T.R., Russell, D.W., Spratt, G.F., Colby, H., Liu, Y.K., Fairchild, M.L. and Christensen, S. (1986) Efficacy of electroacupuncture and TENS in the rehabilitation of chronic low back pain patients. *Pain*, 26, 277–290.

Leung, A.S. (1977) Acupuncture treatment of withdrawal symptoms. *Am. J. Acupunct.*, 5, 43–50.

Liu, Z.Y. (1980) Acupuncture for chronic pain: practice and mechanism of action. *Am. J. Acupunct.*, 8, 313–317.

Lovacky, S., Lodin, Z., Tauber, O., Thomae, K., Zizkowsky, J., Dvorak, P. and Srajer, J. (1987) Acupuncture treatment and its effect on low back pain: correlation with β-endorphin immunoreactivity. *Am. J. Acupunct.*, 15, 245–249.

Lowenschuss, O. (1975) Electroacupuncture progress and effectiveness. *Am. J. Acupunct.*, 3, 347–351.

Ludwig, W. (1984) What is Indupoint acupuncture therapy? *Am. J. Acupunct.*, 12, 153–156.

Ludwig, W. (1986) A new method of color acupuncture therapy. *Am. J. Acupunct.*, 14, 35–38.

Mayer, D.J., Price, D.O. and Rafii, A. (1977) Antagonism of acupuncture analgesia in man by the narcotic antagonist naloxone. *Brain Res.*, 121, 368–372.

Melzack, R. (1973) *The Puzzle of Pain*. Penguin Books, London.

Parker, L.N. and Mok, M.S. (1977) The use of acupuncture for smoking withdrawal. *Am. J. Acupunct.*, 5, 363–366.

Prince, J.P. (1983) The use of low strength magnets of EAV points. *Am. J. Acupunct.*, 11, 125–130.

Prince, J.P. (1983) Further experience with low strength magnets applied to EAV acupuncture points. *Am. J. Acupunct.*, 11, 249–254.

Requena, Y., Michel, D., Fabre, J., Pernice, C. and Nguyen (1980) Smoking withdrawal therapy by acupuncture. *Am. J. Acupunct.*, 8, 57–63.

Richardson, P.H. and Vincent, C.A. (1986) Acupuncture for the treatment of pain: A review of evaluative research. *Pain*, 24, 16–40.

Sacks, L.L. (1975) Drug addiction, alcoholism, obesity treated by auricular staplepuncture. *Am. J. Acupunct.*, 3, 147–150.

Sadowsky, H. (1982) Weight control in obesity: a simple, effective and practical approach. *Am. J. Acupunct.*, 10, 53–58.

Santiestebau, A.J. (1984) Comparison of electroacupuncture and selected physical therapy for acute spine pain. *Am. J. Acupunct.*, 12, 257–261.

Shapiro, R.S. (1987) Rapid, effective, non-invasive treatment of pain and disease with acupuncture magnets. *Am. J. Acupunct.*, 15, 43–47.

Sin, Y.M. (1983) Effect of electric acupuncture and moxibustion on phagocytic activity of the reticuloendothelial system of mice. *Am. J. Acupunct.*, 11, 237–241.

Sin, Y.M. (1984) Acupuncture and thermal injury. *Am. J. Acupunct.*, 12, 133–138.

Sjölund, B.H. and Eriksson, M.B.E. (1976) Electro-acupuncture and endogenous morphines. *Lancet*, 2, 1085.

Sjölund, B.H., Terenius, L. and Eriksson, M.B.E. (1977) Increased cerebrospinal fluid levels of endorphines after electro-acupuncture. *Acta Physiol. Scand.*, 100, 382–384.

Sopler, D. (1984) Effect of cranial laser acupuncture on muscle strength in healthy individuals. *Am. J. Acupunct.*, 12, 117–124.

Spoerel, W.E., Varkey, M. and Leung, C.Y. (1976) Acupuncture and chronic pain. *Am. J. Chin. Med.*, 4, 267–279.

Takase, K. (1983) Revolutionary new pain theory and acupuncture treatment procedure based on new theory of acupuncture mechanism. *Am. J. Acupunct.*, 11, 305–323.

192

Takeda, K., Taniguchi, N., Kuriyama, H. and Matsushita, A. (1979) Experimental study on the mechanism of acupuncture anaesthesia. In: *Advances in Pain Research and Therapy, Vol. 3*. Editors: J.J. Bonica, J.C. Lieberskind and D. Albe-Fessard. Raven Press, New York, pp. 623–628.

Tany, M. and Sawatsuga, S. (1975) New development: electromagnetic acupuncture. *Am. J. Acupunct.*, 3, 58–66.

Voll, R. (1975) Twenty years of electroacupuncture diagnosis in Germany. A progress report. *Am. J. Acupunct.*, 3, 7–17.

Voll, R. (1980) The phenomenon of medicine testing in electroacupuncture according to Voll. *Am. J. Acupunct.*, 8, 97–104.

Wong, W.H. and Brayton, D. (1982) The physiology of acupuncture: effects of acupuncture on peripheral circulation. *Am. J. Acupunct.*, 10, 59–63.

Wyant, G.M. and Camerlain, M. (1977) Chinese acupuncture. *Can. Anaesth. Soc. J.*, 24, 75–89.

Yamauchi, N. (1976) The results of therapeutic acupuncture in a pain clinic. *Can. Anaesth. Soc. J.*, 23, 196–206.

Trigger points

Brendstrup, P., Jespersen, K. and Asboe-Hansen, G. (1975) Morphological and chemical connective tissue changes in fibrositic muscles. *Ann. Rheum. Dis.*, 16, 438–440.

Dorigo, B., Bartoli, V., Grisillo, D. and Belopi, D. (1979) Fibrositic myofascial pain in intermittent claudication; effect of anesthetic block of trigger points on exercise tolerance. *Pain*, 6, 183–190.

Fine, P.G., Milano, R. and Hare, B.D. (1988) The effects of myofascial trigger point injections are naloxone reversible. *Pain*, 32, 15–20.

Jaeger, B. (1986) Quantification of changes in myofascial trigger point sensitivity with the pressure algometer following passive stretch. *Pain*, 27, 203–210.

Kellgren, H.H. (1938) Observations on referred pain arising from muscle. *Clin. Science*, 3, 175–190.

Kraus, H. (1973) Trigger points. *N.Y. St. J. Med.*, 1310–1314.

Lange, M. (1931) *Die Muskelharten (Myogelosen)*. J.F. Lehman Verlag, Munchen.

Lewit, K. (1979) The needle effect in the relief of myofascial pain. *Pain*, 6, 83–90.

Melzack, R., Stillwell, D.M. and Fox, E.D. (1977) Trigger points and acupuncture points for pain: correlation and implications. *Pain*, 3, 3–23.

Ready, L.B., Kozody, R., Barsa, J.E. and Murphy, T.M. (1983) Trigger point injections vs. jet injection in the treatment of myofascial pain. *Pain*, 15, 201–206.

Simons, D.G. (1975, 1976) Muscle pain syndromes. Parts I and II. *Am. J. Phys. Med.*, 54, 289–310, and 55, 15–42.

Steindler, A. (1959) *Lectures on the Interpretation of Pain in Orthopaedic Practice*. C.C. Thomas, Springfield.

Travell, J. (1976) Myofascial trigger points – clinical view. *Adv. Pain Res. Ther.* Editors: J.J. Bonica and D. Albe-Fessard, Raven Press, New York 1, 919–926.

Travell, J. and Rinzler, S.H. (1952) The myofascial genesis of pain. *Postgrad. Med.*, 11, 425–434.

Wyant, G.M. (1979) Chronic pain syndromes and their treatment: II Trigger points. *Can. Anaesth. Soc. J.*, 26, 216–219.

Suggested further reading:

Travell, J.G. and Simons, D.G. (1983) *Myofascial Pain and Dysfunction. The Trigger Point Manual*. Williams & Wilkins, Baltimore/London.

Vibration and percussion

Bini, G., Cruccu, G., Hagbarth, K.-E., Schady, W. and Torebjörk, E. (1984) Analgesic effect of vibration and cooling on pain induced by intraneural electrical stimulation. *Pain*, 18, 239–248.

Lundeberg, T. (1984) Long-term results of vibratory stimulation as a pain relieving measure for chronic pain. *Pain*, 20, 13–23.

Lundeberg, T., Nordemar, R. and Ottoson, D. (1984) Pain alleviation by vibratory stimulation. *Pain*, 20, 25–44.

Matthews, W.B. and Miller, H. (1975) *Diseases of the Nervous System, 2nd Edn.* Blackwell, Oxford, p. 191.

Melzack, R. and Wall, P.D. (1965) Pain mechanisms: a new theory. *Science*, 150, 971–979.

Ottoson, D., Ekblom, A. and Hansson, P. (1981) Vibratory stimulation for the relief of pain of dental origin. *Pain*, 10, 37–45.

Russell, W.R. and Spalding, D.M.K. (1950) Treatment of painful amputation stumps. *Br. Med. J.*, 2, 68–73.

Swerdlow, M. (1979) Personal Communication.

Ultrasound

Rubin, D. and Kuifert, J.H. (1955) Use of ultrasonic vibration in the treatment of pain arising from phantom limbs, scars and neuromas; a preliminary report. *Arch. Phys. Med. Rehab.*, 36, 445.

Schwartz, F.F. (1954) Indications and contraindications therapy. *South. Med. J.*, 47, 854–858.

Wood, R.W. and Loomis, A.L. (1927) Physical and biological effects of high frequency sound waves of great intensity. *Philos. Mag.*, 7, 417–436.

Heat and Cold

Tepperman, P.S. and Devlin, M. (1983) Therapeutic heat and cold. A practitioner's guide. *Postgrad. Med.*, 73(1), 69–76.

Mobilizations

Paris, S.V. (1979) Mobilization of the spine. *Phys. Ther.*, 59, 988–995.

Suggested further reading:

Wadsworth, H. and Chanmugan, A. (1983) *Electrophysical Agents in Physiotherapy*. Science Press, Marrickville, NSW, Australia.

Thermography

Davy, J.R. (1977) *Phys. Techn.*, 8, 54–61.

Edmeads, J. (1986) Is thermography a marker for vascular headache? Editorial. *Headache*, 26, 47.

Lee, M.H., Sadove, M.S. and Kim, S.I. (1976) Liquid crystal thermography in acupuncture therapy. *Am. J. Acupunct.*, 4, 145–148.

Newman, R.I., Seres, J.L. and Miller, E.B. (1984) Liquid crystal thermography in the evaluation of chronic back pain: A comparative study. *Pain*, 20, 293–305.

Swerdlow, B. and Dieter, J.H. (1986) The validity of the vascular 'cold patch' in the diagnosis of chronic headache. *Headache*, 26, 22–26.

M. Swerdlow and J.E. Charlton (eds.) Relief of Intractable Pain
© 1989, Elsevier Science Publishers B.V. (Biomedical Division)

7

Peripheral nerve blocks in relief of intractable pain

Mark Churcher

Peripheral nerve blocks with local anaesthetics are of both diagnostic and therapeutic value in the management of patients with chronic pain. The relief of pain following a nerve block often outlasts the length of action of the local anaesthetic. The 'gate theory' of Melzack and Wall can be used to explain this observation. Anaesthetic blocks diminish the sensory input acting on T cells so reducing T cell output to below the critical level evoking pain. They may also inhibit the activity of neuron feedback loops producing a segmental damping effect.

The response of patients to needle puncture gives the operator a useful insight into the patient's psychological make-up. A lack of reaction is seen in both the stoic and hysteric, whilst an exaggerated response may be found in those demoralized by long-term pain and in the neurotic. Many patients with pain will have a placebo response to injection which complicates the interpretation of diagnostic blocks (Papper, 1967). The true nature of the patient's response can be elucidated by alternating injections of local anaesthetic with those of saline.

The place of neurolytic solutions in the treatment of chronic pain is contentious. Advances in pharmacology, intrathecal injections, stimulation techniques and thermocoagulation are all responsible for a decline in enthusiasm for peripheral neurolytic injections. Perhaps both an increase in reported complications and an unfavourable medico-legal climate are significant contributory factors.

Neurolytic blocks should only be performed by an experienced operator after a definite diagnosis has been made. A preliminary local anaesthetic block prior to chemical block is important. It: (a) shows that blocking that particular nerve at that site will, in fact, produce pain relief; (b) demonstrates to the patient what it will feel like after neurolysis has been carried out and may show up complications involved; and (c) occasionally produces long-lasting freedom from pain. A full explanation should be given to the patient and a consent form obtained before proceeding. A sterile technique should be used and sedation given if necessary.

This chapter attempts to put the place of peripheral somatic nerve blocks into clinical perspective and includes a description of various painful conditions which are helped by this form of treatment.

NERVE BLOCKING AIDS

X-Ray facilities are necessary for checking the position of needles during sensory root injection of the trigeminal nerve. Biplane screening is useful for hip blocks, and small amounts of contrast medium are helpful when injections are technically difficult.

Nerve stimulation with block aid monitors (Greenblatt and Denson, 1962) or modified transcutaneous stimulators is a useful aid to performing nerve blocks and invaluable when neurolytic solutions are injected in sites where there are no bony landmarks; however, nerve blocking aids will not compensate for anatomical ignorance. Success in nerve blocking depends on getting the conscious patient's confidence, accurate identification of bony landmarks and the production of paraesthesiae.

Agents and compounds

The most reliable agent for peripheral nerve neurolysis is ethyl alcohol. This is normally used in concentrations of 80–100%. Pitres and Vaillard (1888) were the first workers to use alcohol injections in the treatment of trigeminal neuralgia. Finkelnburg (1907) showed that when 60–80% alcohol solution was injected beneath the sheath of the sciatic nerve of dogs, they invariably developed paralysis of the leg and foot which lasted weeks or months. Microscopically, the nerves were almost completely degenerate. When alcohol was injected in the immediate vicinity of the sciatic nerve, paralysis occurred with demonstrable degeneration of the most superficial fibres. These results were later confirmed by Labat (1933). Many experimental investigations have shown the neurolytic action of concentrated ethyl alcohol. May (1912) found that besides neurolysis, the injections caused severe adhesions – these may partly explain the diminishing effects of successive alcohol injections in patients with trigeminal neuralgia. Penman and Smith (1950) gave a histological description of total neurolysis of the trigeminal nerve 3 months after alcohol injection.

According to Pizzolato and Mannheimer (1961), 95–100% ethyl alcohol, when injected intraneurally or perineurally, gave fourth degree injury of nerves; coagulation necrosis characterized by a diffuse eosinophilic staining, with complete loss of detail in axons, myelin sheath, nodes of Ranvier and Schwann cells. They found that under the same conditions, phenol produced fourth degree nerve damage, with regeneration of the axon 68 days later. Sunderland (1968) states that the neural damage sustained by injection of sclerosing substances varies in severity from rapidly reversible changes, causing only transient loss of function, to permanent constrictive scarring in and about the nerve sufficient to prevent recovery in the affected fibres. The extent and severity of damage are influenced by such factors as the internal structure of the nerve at the site of injection, the volume of solution injected, and its concentration and sclerosing properties. Histological studies show that aqueous phenol causes chemical destruction of and changes in the nerve which are indistinguishable from those caused by alcohol (Adriani, 1967). Alcohol injections are usually painful and may cause nausea and vomiting. The incidence of post-injection neuritis following neurolytic injections varies with both agent and site of injection and is greatest with alcohol (Adriani, 1967).

Phenol has a local anaesthetic action and Khalili and Ditzler (1968) report few complications from neuritis. Solutions of phenol in water are unstable in concentrations above 7.5% and higher concentrations are used in combination with glycerine. Concentrations as low as 1% are neurolytic (Mehta, 1973), but the clinical effect of such weak solutions is transitory. Stronger solutions of phenol produce a more prolonged block and 8–12% phenol in glycerine/water mixture is used for peripheral blocks. (Phenol in pure glycerine is viscid and difficult to inject through fine gauge needles.) Aqueous phenol is widely used and the nerve destruction produced is followed by fibre regeneration within 2 weeks (Khalili and Ditzler, 1968). Pain relief often outlasts this period by several months. Intravascular injection of small volumes of phenol may cause transient tinnitus and flushing (Reid et al., 1970) whilst larger volumes act as a CNS stimulant causing muscle tremors leading to convulsions (Felsenthal, 1974). Absorption of large amounts of phenol will depress consciousness, reduce blood pressure and cause renal damage (Goodman and Gilman, 1980). Patients injected with phenol in doses near the upper limit (600 mg, Bryce-Smith, 1966) often feel unwell for 24 h. Phenol has been shown to have a greater affinity for blood vessels than for nerve tissue (Nour-Eldin, 1970), and this could explain why many of the serious complications caused by 'overspill' or inaccurate placement are due to blood vessel damage.

Some authors report useful results using ammonium sulphate solution as a neurolytic agent (Dam, 1965; Davies et al., 1967; Miller et al., 1975; Brechner et al., 1977). Others note its irritant nature and find any pain relief produced to be short-lived (Katz, 1974). Proctocaine (Adriani, 1967), benzyl alcohol (5% and 7.5%) and chlorocresol (1 in 15) (Swerdlow, 1972) are other less frequently used neurolytics.

All neurolytic agents produce an inflammatory response and injection under the skin can cause ulceration. Fig. 7.1 shows skin ulceration following an infraorbital alcohol injection. This patient rapidly developed a haematoma after a second in-

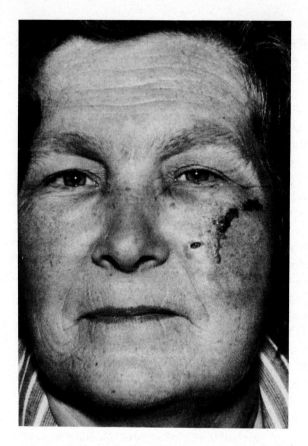

Fig. 7.1. Skin ulceration following infraorbital alcohol injection.

jection for trigeminal neuralgia. Following injection, the needle track should be cleared with saline or air as the needle is being withdrawn to prevent sinus formation.

The indications, methods and agents for peripheral somatic nerve block are discussed under the headings 'Cancer' and 'Non-cancer' pain. Although this is a practical classification with obvious advantages, the reader should appreciate that the allocation of blocks to these two groups is somewhat arbitrary.

NERVE BLOCKS IN CANCER PAIN

The patient with cancer pain is often seen when hope of a cure has passed. Specific cancer treatment with radiotherapy, oncolytics or hormones does not always relieve the pain and exacerbation of pain does not always indicate extension of the disease; indeed, there are occasions when pain is a complication of therapy rather than a sign of tumour spread. The pathophysiology of tumour spread and the mechanism whereby pain is produced should be understood before relief is attempted, so it is important to take a careful history before physical examination to elucidate the exact distribution, quality and other features of the pain. Thus, pain of a burning or aching nature, relieved by limb elevation, is more likely to be reduced by sympathetic than by somatic nerve block. Clinical examination should include a search for evidence of motor paralysis, sensory impairment or abnormal autonomic function.

The methods and agents selected for pain relief should take into account the needs and wishes of the patient. They should not depend solely on technical skills or available facilities. Cancer pain usually involves several segments and it is often possible to provide good pain relief without motor paralysis by intrathecal rather than peripheral nerve block.

Fig. 7.2 shows the dermatome skin innervation and is helpful in determining the roots responsible for pain transmission.

Peripheral somatic nerve block is ideal for some patients with cancer pain of the head and neck; it is also useful in chest wall pain.

Cancer pain in the head and neck

Malignant disease in the area of distribution of the *trigeminal nerve* can give localized or widespread pain which may be accompanied by trismus, dysphagia and halitosis. Local or metastatic spread to cervical glands or the cervical plexus can produce pain behind the angle of the jaw, down into the neck and shoulder, or upwards behind the ear. Pain control may be obtained initially by blocking the main nerve or one of its branches. Local spread and distant metastases, however, may give rise to pain which can only be relieved by injecting neighbouring nerves, as carcinoma of the head and neck frequently spreads to involve tissues supplied by the glossopharyngeal, vagus and cervical nerves. *Trigeminal sensory root* injection (see p. 206) should be performed when pain involves the upper two divisions of this nerve. The deep injection of the *ophthalmic nerve*, from the lateral edge of the orbit into the nerve where it enters the orbit is rarely performed as it is considered too dangerous; it may be complicated by retrobulbar haematoma or lesions of the optic nerve. Pain involving the *maxillary nerve* is relieved by blocking the fibres as they cross the upper part of the pterygomaxillary fissure and may be performed as follows: A 7.5 cm, 22 S.W.G. short bevelled needle is advanced through the mandibular notch at a 45° angle to the skin and aimed at the junction of the optic nerve and sclera, to come in contact with the anterior edge of the lateral pterygoid plate at a depth of 4.5–5 cm. The needle is then withdrawn and rein-

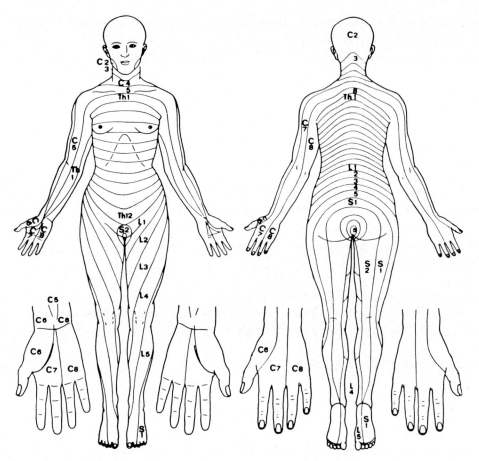

Fig. 7.2. Dermatome innervation chart.

serted anterior to the pterygoid plate into the pterygopalatine fossa for a further 0.5–1 cm, or until paraesthesiae result (see Fig. 7.3). When carrying out maxillary injection, it is important to have a marker on the needle, for if the needle is deeper than necessary it may penetrate the inferior orbital fissure producing a haematoma or abducens nerve palsy. Absolute alcohol (1–1.5 ml) is injected when definite paraesthesiae are reported; the operator must not be misled by reports of pain from periosteal probing.

In cases of maxillary carcinoma, it is as well, before performing maxillary neurolysis, to make sure by tomography that the disease has not already spread inside the skull.

Mandibular nerve block is performed at the base of the skull using the lateral approach (see Fig. 7.4). A mark is made on the skin over the middle of the mandi-

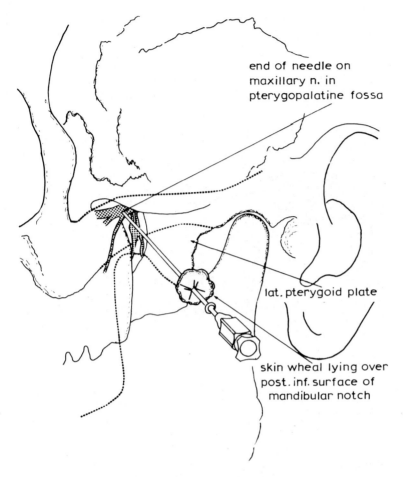

end of needle on
maxillary n. in
pterygopalatine fossa

lat. pterygoid plate

skin wheal lying over
post. inf. surface of
mandibular notch

Fig. 7.3. Anatomy of maxillary nerve in the pterygopalatine fossa with the needle in place for injection. (Modified from D.C. Moore, 1975. Courtesy of Charles C. Thomas, Springfield.)

bular notch below the zygomatic arch and a 5 cm 22 S.W.G. short bevelled needle is advanced to strike the lateral pterygoid plate at a depth of 3.8–4.5 cm. The needle is then partially withdrawn and redirected posteriorly 0.5 cm deeper. A test injection of local anaesthetic is given first. On a later occasion paraesthesiae are elicited before 1–1.5 ml of absolute alcohol is injected. Bilateral alcohol mandibular blocks may produce retraction of the mandible with airway obstruction (Moore, 1965).

When the effects of maxillary or mandibular block are wearing off (a few weeks to a year after injection), it is sometimes possible to repeat the injection; usually, however, spread of the disease makes satisfactory reblocking unlikely. These

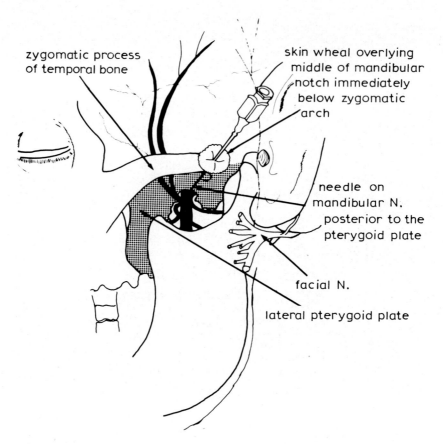

zygomatic process
of temporal bone

skin wheal overlying
middle of mandibular
notch immediately
below zygomatic
arch

needle on
mandibular N.
posterior to the
pterygoid plate

facial N.

lateral pterygoid plate

Fig. 7.4. Mandibular nerve block at the base of the skull. (Modified from D.C. Moore, 1975. Courtesy of Charles C. Thomas, Springfield.)

blocks are very painful and it is as well to have the patient heavily sedated before-hand.

Pain behind the angle of the jaw radiating to the middle ear and exacerbated by swallowing may be relieved by blocking the *glossopharyngeal nerve*. This nerve is injected below the jugular foramen as it lies in close relationship to the vagus, accessory and hypoglossal nerves (see Fig. 7.5). The glossopharyngeal nerve may be found midway between the mastoid process and the angle of the mandible, and just below the external auditory meatus.

Montgomery and Cousins (1972) describe injection using radiological control. They advance a 25 S.W.G. 5 cm needle until the tip lies posterior to the styloid process and close to the jugular foramen (see Fig. 7.6). The needle position is checked by both lateral and submental films. A preliminary test injection of 1 ml

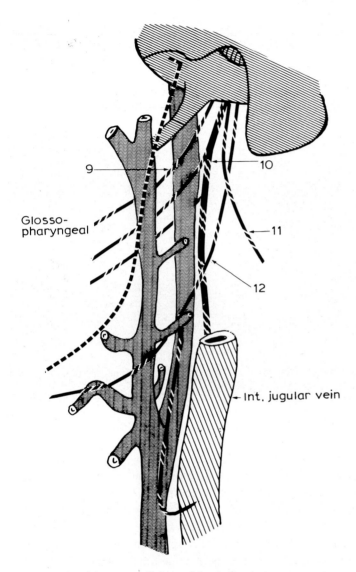

Fig. 7.5. Cranial nerves at the base of the skull.

of local anaesthetic is given to assess the degree of pain relief and the nature of any complications. Should this small volume of local prove satisfactory, an equivalent volume of absolute alcohol can be injected at a later occasion. Dwyer (1972) recommends joint glossopharyngeal and vagal block using larger volumes of alcohol (4–8 ml). In practice, it is difficult to differentiate glossopharyngeal from vagal pain, and even small amounts of solution may spread from the site of injection

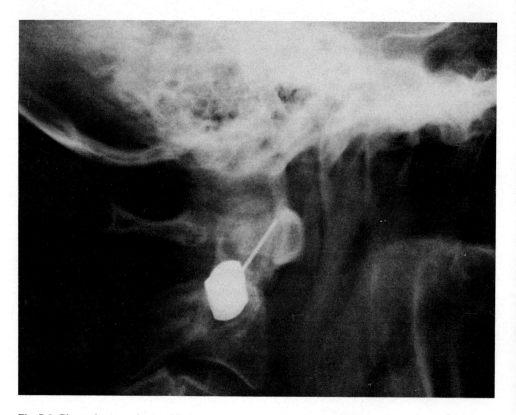

Fig. 7.6. Glossopharyngeal nerve block.

of the glossopharyngeal nerve to the vagus, hypoglossal and accessory nerves. Bonica (1954) injects at a slightly lower level and reports both hoarseness and dysphagia as complications, which may be a small price to pay for pain relief. Adriani (1967) advises against bilateral glossopharyngeal blocks.

Pain in the cervical region is often diffuse in nature; it radiates across dermatomes and may have both somatic and sympathetic components. In such difficult patients, the author prefers subdural injection of 7.5% phenol in contrast medium. Injections are contraindicated for cervical root pain associated with vertebral instability.

The *superior laryngeal* nerve may be injected for the pain of laryngeal carcinoma; the anterior approach is carried out as follows: with the patient supine and the head slightly extended, the hyoid cornua on the side to be injected are made prominent by gentle pressure with the free hand. A 5 cm needle is inserted at a point 1 cm below and 2 cm in front of the extremity of the greater cornu of the hyoid. The needle is advanced towards the cornu, passing between the cornua of the hyoid bone and thyroid cartilage. The point of the needle must not be allowed to go beyond the line joining these cornua, otherwise major vessels will be punctured. Paraesthesiae, if produced, characteristically radiate up towards the ear. Local anaesthetic (2 ml) should be injected and the results should be assessed before an equivalent volume of absolute alcohol is injected (Labat, 1930).

Patients with pain due to carcinomatous infiltration of the *brachial plexus* may get relief by plexus injection of 20 ml of 1–2% aqueous phenol (Brown, 1976). Severe lancinating pain may follow this injection, requiring a morphine cover for 48 h. Neill (1979) describes a technique using two injections of absolute alcohol diluted in an equivalent volume of 0.5% bupivacaine. His patient was relieved for the few remaining weeks of life from severe pain associated with a pathological fracture of the humerus.

Cancer pain in chest and abdomen

Tumour involvement of the chest wall or upper abdomen may result in pain which can be relieved by *intercostal blocks*. An injection of 2–3 ml of 6% aqueous phenol or 1–1.5 ml of 10% phenol in glycerine/water per intercostal nerve, using the technique described by Moore and Bridenbaugh (1962), is recommended. A repeat injection may be needed the following week. This pain is often better treated by intrathecal or subdural injection.

NON-CANCER PAIN

Treatment of patients with intractable pain of non-malignant origin should be planned in relation to a normal life expectancy, and the philosophy of 'relief at any price' may court disaster. A joint examination and discussion of the patient with a surgeon or physician in another discipline is a medically useful and legally valuable safeguard.

Trigeminal neuralgia

Tic douloureux is a disease of the elderly and must be differentiated from other causes of facial pain before initiating treatment. The diagnosis is made on a characteristic history coupled with negative neurological findings. The pain is unilateral, lancinating in nature and comes with lightning suddenness in a series of rapidly recurring spasms. The distribution and precipitation are characteristic, for pain commonly starts in the upper lip and radiates to the orbit or ear, and is precipitated by light touch, eating or temperature changes. Periodic attacks with spasms of pain are characteristic of the condition. Unfortunately, the intensity and frequency of attacks increases with time (Stookey and Ransohoff, 1959; Rasmussen, 1965). Carbamazepine controls the pain in 75–85% of cases (Arieff and Wetzel, 1967). It is wise to start with a dose of 100 mg b.d., increasing this to 200 mg t.d.s., if necessary. Patients sometimes report both giddiness and gastrointestinal disturbances with high initial doses, and skin rashes progressing to exfoliation and blood dyscrasias are known complications of drug therapy. Phenytoin (Epanutin) 100 mg t.d.s. should be given in addition if high doses of carbamazepine fail to control symptoms. Patients not responding or sensitive to these drugs are faced with the alternative of some form of surgery, electrocoagulation or fifth nerve injection. Different methods of treatment vary in recurrence rate and degrees of anaesthesia and the correct treatment for any specific patient will depend not only on the available skills and facilities, but also on the wishes of the patient and his general medical condition.

Peripheral trigeminal nerve alcohol block is often useful when drug treatment fails. Patients may have pain relief for 6 months to a year (occasionally longer), and this gives them a protracted trial of the sensations which accompany numbness. They are then better able to give informed consent to further more permanent procedures, when sensation returns or pain spreads to other parts of the face. Alcohol blocks of the peripheral branches of the trigeminal nerve supplying trigger spots are of particular value in patients where there is some doubt about the diagnosis. The supraorbital, infraorbital and mental nerves are injected in their respective foramina as they lie on a line drawn parallel to and 2.5 cm from the sagittal plane. Small volumes of absolute alcohol (0.2–0.3 ml), accurately placed, will suffice. The supraorbital notch or foramen is approached at right angles to the face, whilst the infraorbital foramen is reached through a low medial insertion of the needle. When performing infraorbital nerve block, the needle tip should not be advanced further than 0.5 cm past the foramen, for the roof of the infraorbital canal is sometimes deficient, allowing solution to diffuse into the orbit. The mental foramen points up in the direction of the ear, approaches the alveolar margin in the elderly, and is not always as easy to enter with the needle as a study of the skull might suggest. The techniques of mandibular and maxillary nerve block are briefly described on pp. 199–201. The complications of peripheral alcohol block are: pain at the injection site, haematoma and sloughing of the mucous membrane and skin. Maxillary alcohol block is not recommended for trigeminal neuralgia, because blindness can follow, even in the best hands (Moore, 1965).

Gasserian ganglion and sensory root injection are indicated (a) in those whose pain can no longer be controlled for a reasonable length of time by blocking the II or III divisions or one of the more peripheral branches of the trigeminal nerve and (b) in distressed elderly patients where the provision of immediate permanent pain relief has overriding consideration.

The anterior approach, described by Härtel (1914), is recommended by Adriani

(1967) and White and Sweet (1969). The lateral method which was first described by Levy and Baudoin (1906), and was used extensively by Harris (1926), is less satisfactory as injections tend to be too peripheral. The surface markings using Härtel's technique are as follows: a line is drawn from the external angular process of the orbit, parallel with the sagittal plane. A cross is made on this line above the lateral margin of the mouth at the level of the second upper molar tooth, indicating the needle puncture point. The horizontal plane, along which the needle must travel to enter the foramen ovale, is shown by a line joining the cross to the top of the root of the ear. A size 21 S.W.G. 10 cm short bevelled needle is advanced, aimed at the pupil in the vertical plane and just in front of the root of the ear in the horizontal plane. The infratemporal surface of the greater wing of the sphenoid is struck at a depth of 5–7 cm. The needle tip should now lie near the anterior lip of the foramen ovale. The needle is then half withdrawn and reinserted along the line leading to the root of the ear. Should the needle fail to pass through the foramen using these surface markings, the procedure is repeated using a lower lateral skin puncture and identical aiming points. When the needle slips past the foramen, the stylet is withdrawn and the hub observed and aspirated for cerebrospinal fluid (CSF) or blood. Aspiration of CSF indicates that the needle has reached Meckel's cave. Fig. 7.7 shows the relationship of the needle to both bony structures and the trigeminal nerve.

Useful information is gleaned from three standard radiological views: lateral, submentovertical and transorbital. A needle near the trigeminal notch, 5 mm from the clivus of the skull on the lateral view and at least 3 mm below the crest of the petrous temporal bone is in a good position for a test injection (see Fig. 7.8). Following the aspiration of CSF from Meckel's cave, Penman (1958) has perfected a technique using small increments of absolute alcohol with the head extended. The author, however, prefers to use a heavy solution of phenol in glycerine with the patient sitting and the head flexed in these circumstances (see below) and uses alcohol when CSF fails to flow.

Preliminary injections of local anaesthetic were used by earlier workers in this field, but such injections sometimes confuse rather than clarify; they also reduce the effect of alcohol by dilution. The response of the conscious sedated patient to 0.1 ml of absolute alcohol injected drop by drop through a 1 ml syringe is more helpful. Alcohol injected into the sensory root or ganglion gives burning pain and flushing of the face. Total sensory anaesthesia can be produced with 0.25 ml of alcohol. Henderson (1967) noted that the position of the gasserian ganglion relative to the foramen ovale varies over a 10 mm range and that it may be necessary to inject 25 mm posterior to the foramen to produce a good result. He also correlated the results of alcohol injections with anatomical variants by dye studies and dissections (Henderson, 1965).

A method has been introduced by Jefferson (1963) which is easier to master,

208

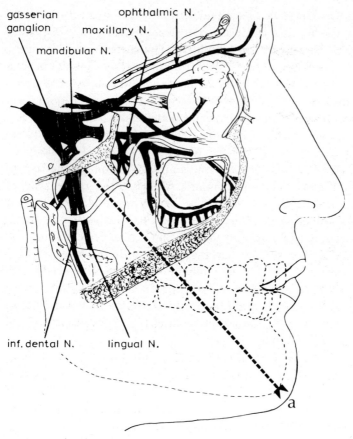

gasserian
ganglion

ophthalmic N.

maxillary N.

mandibular N.

inf. dental N.   lingual N.

a

Fig. 7.7. Gasserian ganglion block by Härtel's route; (a) indicates the needle position. (Modified from Labat, 1930. W.B. Saunders Co., Philadelphia.)

less painful on administration and followed by fewer complications. Furthermore, this method seems to enable a more controlled spread of neurotoxic agent. A 10 cm needle is inserted, using Härtel's approach, deep enough to reach the subarachnoid space in Meckel's cave. X-Rays are then taken to find the relationship of the needle tip to the petrous temporal bone. The needle should be below the superior border of the petrous temporal on the lateral and transorbital views. The patient is then sat up and the head flexed before injection, to prevent the solution spreading into the posterior cranial fossa. An injection of 0.25–0.5 ml of 5% phenol in glycerine gives complete sensory loss with corneal anaesthesia. The patient is kept in the injecting position for 15 min and the sensory loss produced is usually permanent. Jefferson (1966) aspirated CSF in less than half his patients and found that 72% of them remained pain-free for up to 4 years.

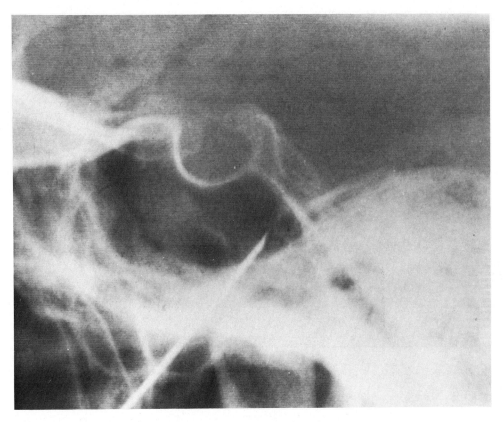

Fig. 7.8. The relation of the needle tip to the clivus of the skull.

Häkanson (1981) reports good pain relief with no serious complications or undesirable side effects following the injection of small volumes of glycerol into the trigeminal cistern. A needle is introduced into the trigeminal cistern by the anterior percutaneous route with the premedicated patient in the sitting position. Following spontaneous CSF drainage, metrizamide is injected to assure an intracisternal position of the tip of the needle. A small volume of glycerol (0.3 ml) is injected after removal of the contrast medium and the patient is kept in the sitting position for 1 h. Pain relief may take 5 days to develop and although no sensory disturbance can be demonstrated by clinical examination, most patients notice a slight numbness. Häkanson, in a series of 130 patients, reports that over 90% of his patients were pain-free following one, or in a few cases, two, injections during a mean follow-up period of about 2 years. This technique has been used extensively with variable results. Waltz and Copland (1986) showed that different preparations of glycerol could account for the poor results in some of his patients.

210

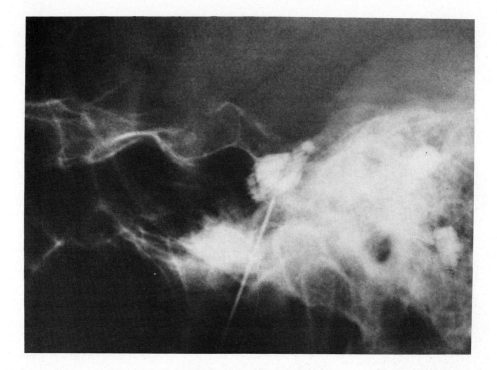

Fig. 7.9. Contrast medium in the trigeminal cistern.

When he used glycerol with a high viscosity, he reported an 85% success rate (Waltz et al., 1985). Sweet (1986) virtually discontinued using the technique because of too many initial failures, late recurrences, and major sensory losses or dysesthesiae. He reviews the subject in *'Operative Neurosurgical Techniques'* (Sweet, 1988).

Ecker (1976) described an injection technique, using small amounts of alcohol (0.1 ml). Corneal sensation was preserved in approximately 85% of the cases. He found that 81% of his patients followed-up had either died pain-free or were still comfortable 7 years after injection. These results of individual treatments should be compared with those of Ruge et al. (1958), who reviewed 821 alcohol injections by different specialists into the trigeminal nerve or its branches and noted an average duration of relief of only 7.23 months.

Many complications of injections have been described. The most common are in consequence of facial anaesthesia and can be minimized by good management. The incidence of neuropathic keratitis may be reduced by giving patients strict instructions over care of the eye and fixing a shield at the side of their glasses. A lack of tear formation (due to the paralysis of the greater superficial petrosal nerve) may contribute to post-injection conjunctivitis (Davies, 1970). Paraffin eye drops will help with lubrication and a tarsorrhaphy should rarely be necessary. Anaesthesia dolorosa is the most distressing complication from injection; unfortunately, it is not possible to predict which patients will develop symptoms. Paraesthesiae following injection are more common and patients are often helped by reassurance that the severe pain will not return. Stender (1961) reports a 16% incidence of paraesthesiae and a 3.3% incidence of anaesthesia dolorosa following surgery. Trophic ulcers on the face are self-inflicted and patients are warned about the hazards of habits such as scratching the side of the nose (it may be necessary for them to wear gloves at night). Facial haematoma is commoner when patients are injected during a painful spell, and a palsy of the oculomotor, trochlear or abducens nerves lasting beyond the third post-injection day may persist for 6 months. Henderson (1967) reviewed 88 patients and found six slight palsies of the oculomotor and two of the abducens nerve; the weakness was usually transient and all recovered completely.

Nerve entrapment

Peripheral nerves may be trapped at a number of sites in the body, giving rise to an intractable syndrome of intermittent and even continuous pain, accompanied sometimes by numbness, paraesthesiae and other sensory abnormalities. Pain due to entrapment of the lateral cutaneous nerve of the thigh has been known for many years and has been given the title of 'meralgia paraesthetica'. Similar symptoms following inguinal herniorrhaphy, caused by nerves fixed in scar tissue, are a well recognized surgical complication. The clinical manifestations of entrapments of the segmental nerves of the thorax and abdomen have been described more recently (Kopel and Thompson, 1963). Applegate (1972a) mentions sites where nerves are stretched or compressed, and explains some of the mechanisms. The intercostal nerves turn sharply at the lateral border of the rectus sheath, pass through a fibromuscular ring and terminate as anterior cutaneous nerves (see Fig. 7.10). They are fixed posteriorly at the site of the right angled turn and in the skin, and are probably subjected to a stretching and compression in the ring associated with the herniation of extraperitoneal fat. Patients have both sharp intermittent pain and constant burning discomfort, often related to changes in posture. Finger-point tenderness is found at the point of entrapment in the lateral margin of the rectus sheath when the patient tenses his abdominal muscles. Mehta and Ranger (1971) injected 2–3 ml of 5% aqueous phenol into the tender places deep to the anterior wall of the rectus sheath. Approximately 60% of their patients were pain-free 2–3 weeks after injection. The majority of these had no recurrence of symptoms when reviewed 3.5 years later. They advise using a nerve stimulator when injecting obese patients. The lateral cutaneous branches of the intercostal nerves

212

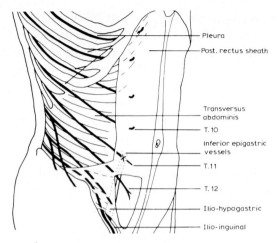

Fig. 7.10. The relation of intercostal nerves to rectus sheath. (From *Intractable Pain*, M. Mehta (Ed.) 1973, courtesy W.B. Saunders Co., Philadelphia.)

and cutaneous branches of the posterior primary rami are liable to entrapment where they pierce muscles. Patients may have symptoms similar to those with abdominal wall entrapment and respond equally well to treatment. Applegate (1972b) notes that many of these sites correspond to acupuncture points. Injections of local anaesthetic alone coupled with an explanation of pain mechanisms may be all that is needed for relief.

Coccydynia

This painful condition is commoner in women, who may give a history of trauma from injury or childbirth. Although it is sometimes associated with subluxation of the sacrococcygeal joint, excision of the coccyx is not always curative. In most patients, pain tends to lessen with time, and three or four caudal blocks at weekly intervals with 5 ml of 0.5% bupivacaine may be helpful.

A few patients have persistent pain on sitting and lying supine, and can be helped by neurolytic blocks. Bilateral injection into the fifth sacral and coccygeal nerves is performed with the patient in the prone position. Skin wheals are raised laterally and caudally to the sacrococcygeal joints, and a 5 cm needle is inserted at the side of the proximal part of the body of the coccyx. 0.5–0.75 ml of 10% phenol in glycerine/water is injected at each site. Swerdlow (1977) finds that sometimes patients get good relief on one side only, and require reinjection of the other side. Three or four blocks may be necessary before pain relief lasting 6–12 months is achieved. Care must be taken to avoid the subcutaneous injection of the neurolytic solution in this site; otherwise a tissue slough may result.

Postherpetic neuralgia

Herpes zoster is an infectious disease caused by the varicella-zoster (V.Z.) virus. The infection is usually localized in the sensory root ganglia. Most zosters are caused by spontaneous reactivation of a latent virus when body defences are low, as for example in old age and in patients receiving immunosuppressive therapy. The incidence of development of postherpetic neuralgia is related to age, and De Moragas and Kierland (1957) have shown that with age an increasing number of patients will develop the postherpetic syndrome. In the sixth decade, more than 50% of all patients with herpes zoster will develop postherpetic neuralgia, whereas this is very rare in the age group of 20–30 years.

The symptoms of postherpetic neuralgia can be explained by damage to afferent fibres. With advancing age, there is normally a progressive loss of large fibres, and this change is more marked in those with postherpetic neuralgia. The damage in herpes zoster is caused by acute inflammation which does most injury to the large fast-conducting fibres. Moreover, the small fibres regenerate faster than the larger ones, and many of the latter become slow-conducting when they regenerate. The majority of the nerve fibres left have a diameter of about 5 μm instead of 13 μm. When the inhibitory influence of the faster large fibres is lacking, burning pains of long duration result, mediated via the small fibres (Noordenbos, 1959).

The pains of herpes zoster are of three types: burning pain with cutaneous hyper-aesthesiae, sharp shooting intermittent pain and a continual background ache. During the acute phase, pain can be of such severity that control is difficult to achieve, even with regular doses of narcotics. Systemic steroid therapy may reduce the inflammatory response and ease the pain (Elliot, 1964). Unfortunately, one of the complications of zoster is a generalised fatal encephalitis which may be encouraged by steroids.

In established postherpetic neuralgia, nerve blocks play a secondary place to general supportive therapy, antidepressants and transcutaneous stimulation (Nathan and Wall, 1974). Intercostal injections with local anaesthetics give a characteristic reponse; the pain is often worse for 48 h after the local has worn off, the patient then experiencing several relatively pain-free days. However, a course of intercostal blocks produces no dramatic improvement, and neurolytic blocks for chest wall postherpetic neuralgia are singularly unrewarding.

Patients with extensive facial herpes zoster who show no improvement within a week merit a gasserian ganglion injection with steroids, as the results are dramatic; the pain rapidly settles and the rash clears. The gasserian ganglion is injected in the heavily sedated patient using Härtel's anterior approach (see p. 208). Pain relief follows the injection of 0.5 ml (20 mg) methylprednisolone acetate.

The patient with intense scalp sensitivity should have an trial supraorbital nerve block with a local anaesthetic. This can be followed by alcohol at a later date.

Neurolytic gasserian ganglion injections with 5% phenol in glycerine or absolute alcohol are contraindicated, for they fail to relieve the aching or shooting pains. If, however, the main complaint is of hyperaesthesiae, a gasserian ganglion injection using 0.2 ml of 3% aqueous phenol may prove worthwhile.

Intercostal neuralgia

Intercostal neuralgia may follow rib fractures or chest surgery and is a frequent manifestation of spinal deformity and degeneration. A diagnosis must be made before starting treatment, as many different medical and surgical conditions will present as chest wall pain. Intercostal blocks a hand's breadth from the spine, using 5 ml of 0.25% bupivacaine per space, will give short-term pain relief. Success depends on blocking not only the affected segment but also the nerves above and below. Neurolytics have good long-term results in certain authors' hands. Dam (1965) reports pain relief in 109 out of 162 patients injected with solutions containing Mepivacaine and 10% ammonium sulphate. Miller et al. (1975) treated 41 patients with over 6 months pain with intercostal blocks of 5–10 ml of 10% ammonium sulphate. Sixty percent of the treatments produced complete or nearly complete relief of pain. The author uses 2–3 ml of 6% aqueous phenol or 1 ml of 10% phenol in glycerine/water when neurolytics are required for intercostal neuralgia. The use of both TENS for rib fractures and local injections of steroids (for pain from secondary tumour in the ribs) has reduced the need for intercostal blocks.

Hip pain

Pain relief in the arthritic hip by surgical section of the obturator nerve and the nerve to quadratus femoris has been demonstrated by Tavernier (1948). Ergenbright and Lowry (1949), after injecting these two nerves with local anaesthetic, found that some patients had a pain-free period lasting some months. James and Little (1976) perform the two nerve blocks with 0.5% bupivacaine. The obturator nerve is first injected with 10 ml at the obturator foramen and this is followed by a 15 ml injection deep on the posterior surface of the body of the ischium. Over half their patients had benefit. An image intensifier is helpful when injecting the obese and it is not unusual to find the increase in mobility more marked than the analgesia. (Sometimes the pain relief is achieved on the anterior but not the posterior aspect, and vice versa.) Active physiotherapy is an important part of the management and the injection allows some patients to be tided over until a 'hip replacement' operation is available. However, a recent study casts some doubt on the effectiveness of this therapy (Edmonds-Seal et al., 1982).

A parallel procedure has been suggested for shoulder pain due to chronic osteoarthritis. This involves blocking the suprascapular nerve (Moore, 1965; Adriani, 1967).

Occipital neuralgia and neck pain

Occipital neuralgia is a troublesome manifestation of degenerative disease of the cervical spine. It also occurs following injury in association with pain in the neck and reflex muscle spasm. Occipital nerve block is performed in the sub-occipital triangle by injection of 2–3 ml 0.5% bupivacaine a finger-breadth lateral to the external occipital protuberance and just below the superior nuchal line. Some patients are helped by weekly injections of local anaesthetic; others improve following an injection of 1–2 ml 6% aqueous phenol.

Pain in the neck is a common manifestation of cervical spondylosis and may follow hyperextension injuries from sport or road accidents. Cervical nerve block is indicated if the pain does not settle with conservative treatment and is performed as follows: the patient lies supine with his face turned away from the painful side and the neck slightly extended. The transverse processes of the cervical vertebrae are palpated in a line passing through the tip of the mastoid process down to the base of the posterior triangle. The tip of the transverse process of C_2 can be felt 1.5 cm below the mastoid process. The skin is infiltrated over the appropriate transverse process and a 5 cm needle is advanced at right angles to the neck until the transverse process is felt. Aspiration before injection of 5 ml 0.5% bupivacaine is mandatory; both intravascular and intrathecal injection are a possibility in this site. Neurolytic agents should probably be confined to patients with cancer and only given after a test dose of 1 ml local anaesthetic has proved effective. The needle is left in situ when testing, and 1 ml of 10% phenol in glycerine/water is injected later. Cervical sympathetic block, hoarseness due to vagal block, and phrenic paralysis are some of the reported complications (Moore, 1965). Local anaesthetics can also diffuse through the dura (Foldes et al., 1956), producing cranial nerve complications (Kepes and Foldes, 1973).

Detrusor dysfunction and the contracted bladder

Detrusor instability may be either idiopathic or secondary to chronic infection, interstitial cystitis, radiotherapy or neurological disorders. Patients present with urgency, frequency of micturition, incontinence and pain. The diagnosis rests on a characteristic urodynamic picture (reduced bladder capacity with large pressure waves).

Psychological factors may play a part in the development of idiopathic detrusor instability and in some patients relaxation and bladder training procedures have produced good results (Frewin, 1978). The effects of sacral nerve block or section in this condition on bladder capacity and function have been described by Mierowsky (1969) and Rockswold et al. (1973). Torrens and Griffith (1976) supported their findings concerning the dominance of the S_3 nerve root in bladder function.

Alloussi et al. (1984) showed in patients with idiopathic instability that neither unilateral nor bilateral S_4 and S_2 block influenced detrusor activity; in contrast, a change in bladder configuration and detrusor activity followed S_3 blockade. Bilateral block of S_3 led to a complete but reversible paralysis of the bladder detrusor with increased bladder distensibility. Despite preservation of sensory function in the bladder, micturition could not be elicited either voluntarily or involuntarily during the time that the anaesthetic was exerting an effect. They reported a permanent improvement in 22 patients treated by reversible bilateral S_3 blockade.

The author recommends a course of bilateral S_3 blocks using 0.5% bupivacaine and has found that symptoms tend to recur, though to a lesser degree, after a month. Simon et al. (1982) reported encouraging results treating a mixed group

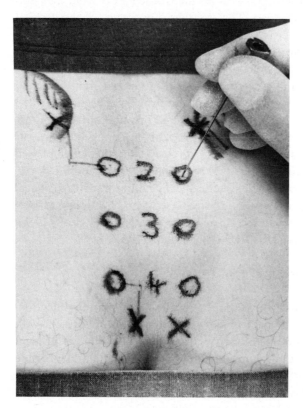

Fig. 7.11. Trans-sacral nerve block. Depth marker omitted.

of 15 patients, some of whom had secondary detrusor instability. They injected 2 ml of 6% aqueous phenol into the appropriate nerve root following test local anaesthetic blocks and reported a 53% incidence of pain relief lasting for an average 26.5 months. Essenhigh and Ryan (1982) have also had beneficial results from S_3 nerve root block in a group of patients having both idiopathic and secondary detrusor instability.

Post-amputation pain

Post-amputation pain is sometimes associated with painful stump neuromas which may press or rub against the prosthesis. Should infiltration with local anaesthetics make the patient more comfortable, surgery may be considered. Injection of the neuroma with a neurolytic solution is rarely successful.

Cryoanalgesia

Cryoanalgesia was introduced into pain clinic practice by Lloyd et al. (1976). Its use has been restricted by the size of the probe and by difficulties with accurate nerve localisation. Evans et al. (1981) mention its advantages when handling perineal pain whilst others have experience with various neuralgias (Mehta, 1982; Wang, 1985). There is a lack of consistency in the reported results. The ability to produce reliable reversible long-term transcutaneous nerve block still defeats the clinician.

Radiofrequency lesioning

The production of a controlled lesion following stimulation has obvious advantages over neurolytic injections. This is especially so with respect to trigeminal neuralgia (see p. 205, 309). Uematsu (1974) reports the advantages of radiofrequency rhizotomy for intractable pain by producing a selective denervation with a sparing of both touch and motor power. Using this technique, Sluiter and Mehta (1981) and Nash (1986) report good results in over half their patients.

Radiofrequency neurectomy for intercostal pain is described as effective by Tasker et al. (1980). Shealy (1975) reports his results from facet denervation in a series of 207 patients with back pain; he notes a 79% incidence of pain relief lasting for over 6 months for those patients with no previous surgery. The results of others in this field have been less satisfactory (Mehta, 1982). Factors responsible for inconsistent results are (1) patients with a combination of mechanical (facet joint) and nerve root pain, (2) incomplete nerve lesioning (Bogduk et al., 1987), and (3) untreated nerve filaments.

Miscellaneous

Paravertebral nerve root block is of diagnostic and therapeutic value in patients with chronic backache. Some patients with persistent pain have no evidence of organic disease, and management becomes easier if blocking a single nerve root gives relief. Paravertebral lumbar somatic block is performed with the patient in the lateral position. The transverse process, corresponding to the nerve to be blocked, is found at the level of the cephalad end of its spinous process. The skin is infiltrated with local anaesthetic over the appropriate transverse process and a 10 cm needle is advanced until the process is struck. The needle is then withdrawn and advanced a further 3 cm below the lower border of the process. The large lumbar nerves are often penetrated, producing painful paraesthesiae. An injection of 10 ml 0.5% bupivacaine should produce a satisfactory block. Puncture of large vessels or the dura are potential risks at this site, so aspiration before injection must be the rule.

Paravertebral neurolytic injections are rarely justified because of the risks involved. The solution may enter a prolonged dural cuff and spread to the spinal cord (Brittingham et al., 1954); it will produce a degree of motor block and may well cause a post-injection neuritis. Nerve root blocks must be avoided in patients on anticoagulants (Learned and Cahoon, 1951), and care must be taken not to produce a pneumothorax when the first lumbar nerve is injected.

Khalili and Ditzler (1968) report on the treatment of pain in spasticity by lumbar paravertebral injections of weak solutions of aqueous phenol. However, most experienced clinicians treating spasticity prefer to use small volumes of 10–20% phenol in glycerine intrathecally, and the future may well lie with partial thermal rhizotomy (Uematsu, 1974).

The treatment of perineal pain associated with carcinoma of the rectum by trans-sacral S_4 neurolytic blocks is described by Robertson (1983). He recommends injecting 2.5 ml 6% aqueous phenol after a satisfactory test block using local anaesthetic. Most patients required a second injection for pain relief. No disturbance of bladder or motor function followed treatment, and sensory effects were confined to the perineum.

CONCLUSIONS

Peripheral nerve blocks have valuable diagnostic, prognostic and therapeutic functions. However, caution is advocated with neurolytic solutions. The author still uses neurolytics in the elderly uncooperative or deaf patient with trigeminal neuralgia, for craniofacial cancer pain and for selected patients with bladder pain.

REFERENCES

Adriani, J. (1967) *Labat's Regional Anesthesia, 3rd Edn*. W.B. Saunders Co., Philadelphia.

Alloussi, S., Loew, F., Mast, G.J., Alzin, H. and Wolf. D. (1984) Treatment of detrusor instability of the urinary bladder by selective sacral blockade. *Br. J. Urol.*, 56, 464–467.

Applegate, W.V. (1972a) Abdominal cutaneous nerve entrapment syndrome. *Surgery*, 71, 118–124.

Applegate, W.V. (1972b) Correspondence. *Br. Med. J.*, 3, 351.

Arieff, A.S. and Wetzel, N. (1967) Tegretol in the treatment of neuralgias. *Dis. Nerv. Syst.*, 28, 820.

Bogduk, N., Macintosh, J. and Marsland, A. (1987) Technical limitations to the efficacy of radiofrequency neurotomy for spinal pain. *Neurosurgery*, 20:4, 529–534.

Bonica, J.J. (1954) In: *The Management of Pain*. Lea & Febiger, Philadelphia.

Brechner, V.L., Brechner, T.F. and Allen, G.D. (1977) Anaesthetic measures in management of pain associated with malignancy. *Semin. Oncol.*, 4, 99.

Brittingham, T.E., Berlin, L.N. and Wolff, H.G. (1954) Nervous system damage following paravertebral block with Efocaine. Report of three cases. *J. Am. Med. Assoc.*, 154, 329.

Brown, A. (1976) In: *Symposium on Malignant Disease*. Royal College of Physicians of Edinburgh, No. 47.

Bryce-Smith, R. (1966) Local and regional anaesthesia. *Postgrad. Med. J.*, 42, 367.

Dam, W.H. (1965) Therapeutic blockade. *Acta Chir. Scand.*, Suppl., 343, 89.

Davies, J.I., Stewart, P.B. and Fink, H.P. (1967) Prolonged sensory block using ammonium salts. *Anesthesiology*, 28, 244.

Davies, M.S. (1970) Corneal anaesthesia after alcohol injection of the trigeminal sensory root. *Br. J. Ophthal.*, 54, 577.

De Moragas, J.M. and Kierland, R.R. (1957) The outcome of patients with herpes zoster. *Arch. Dermatol.*, 75, 193.

Dwyer, B. (1972) Treatment of pain of carcinoma of the tongue and floor of the mouth. *Anaesth. Int. Care.*, 1, 59–64.

Ecker, A. (1976) Sensory loss and prolonged remission of tic douloureux after selective alcoholic gasserian injection. In: *Advances in Pain Research and Therapy, Vol. 1*. Editors: J.J. Bonica and D. Albe-Fessard. Raven Press, New York.

Edmonds-Seal, J., Turner, A., Khodadeh, S., Bader, D.L. and Fuller, D.S. (1982) Regional hip blockade in osteoarthritis. Effects on pain perception. Anaesthesia, 37, 147–151.

Elliot, F.A. (1964) In: *Clinical Neurology*. W.B. Saunders Co., Philadelphia.

Ergenbright, W.V. and Lowry, F.C. (1949) Procaine injection for relief of pain in the hip. *J. Bone Jt Surg.*, 31a, 820.

Essenhigh, D.M. and Ryan, D.W. (1982) An appraisal of S3 blocks in the management of incontinence. *Br. J. Urol.*, 54, 697–699.

Evans, P.J.D., Lloyd, J.W. and Jack, T.M. (1981) Cryoanalgesia for intractable perineal pain. *J. R. Soc. Med.*, 74, 804–809.

Felsenthal, G. (1974) Pharmacology of phenol in peripheral nerve blocks. A review. *Arch. Phys. Med. Rehabil.*, 55, 13–27.

Finkelnburg, S. (1907) Experimentelle Untersuchungen über den Einfluss von Alkohol Injektionen auf periferische Nerven. *Verh. Dtsch. Kongr. Inn. Med.*, 24, 75.

Foldes, F.F., Colavincenzo, J.W. and Birch, J.H. (1956) Epidural anaesthesia: a reappraisal. *Anesth. Analg. Curr. Res.*, 35, 33.

Frewin, W.K. (1978) An objective assessment of the unstable bladder of psychosomatic origin. *Br. J. Urol.*, 50, 249.

Goodman, L.S. and Gilman, A. (1980) *The Pharmacological Basis of Therapeutics, 6th Edn*. Macmillan, London.

Greenblatt, G.M. and Denson, J.S. (1962) Needle nerve stimulator locator: nerve blocks with a new instrument for locating nerves. *Anesth. Analg. Curr. Res.*, 41, 599.

Häkanson, S. (1981) Trigeminal Neuralgia Treated by the Injection of Glycerol into the Trigeminal Cistern. *Neurosurgery*, 9, 6, 638–645.

Harris, W. (1926) In: *Neuritis and Neuralgia*. Oxford University Press, London.

Härtel, F. (1914) Die Behandlung der Trigeminusneuralgie mit Intrakraniellen Alkoholeinspritzungen. *Dtsch. Z. Chir.*, 129, 429.

Henderson, W.R. (1965) Hunterian Lecture. *Ann. R. Coll. Surg. Engl.*, 37, 346.

Henderson, W.R. (1967) Trigeminal neuralgia; the pain and its treatment. *Br. Med. J.*, 1, 7.

James, C.D.T. and Little, T.F. (1976) Regional hip blockade. *Anaesthesia*, 31, 1060.

Jefferson, A. (1963) Trigeminal root and ganglion injections using phenol in glycerin for the relief of trigeminal neuralgia. *J. Neurol. Neurosurg. Psychiat.*, 26, 345.

Jefferson, A. (1966) Trigeminal neuralgia: trigeminal root and ganglion injections using phenol in glycerin. In: *Pain*. Editors: R.S. Knighton and P.R. Dumke. Little, Brown & Co., Boston.

Katz, J. (1974) In: *Advances in Neurology, Vol. 4*. Editor: J.J. Bonica. Raven Press, New York.

Kepes, E.R. and Foldes, F.F. (1973) Transient abducens paralysis following therapeutic nerve blocks of head and neck. *Anesthesiology*, 38, 393.

Khalili, A.A. and Ditzler, J.W. (1968) In: *Medical Clinics of North America*. Editor: J. Eckenhoff. W.B. Saunders Co., Philadelphia.

Kopel, H.P. and Thompson, W.A.L. (1963) *Peripheral Entrapment Neuropathies*. Williams & Wilkins, Baltimore.

Labat, G. (1930) In: *Regional Anaesthesia. Its technic and clinical applications. 2nd Edn*. Editor: J. Adriani. W.B. Saunders Co., Philadelphia.

Labat, G. (1933) The action of alcohol on the living nerve: experimental and clinical considerations. *Anesth. Analg. Curr. Res.*, 12, 190.

Learned, L.O. and Cahoon, F.R. (1951) Retroperitoneal haemorrhage as a complication of lumbar paravertebral injections. *Anesthesiology*, 12, 391.

Levy, F. and Baudoin, A. (1906) Les injections profondes dans le traitement de la neuralgie facile rebelle. *Presse Méd.*, 13, 108.

Lloyd, J.W., Barnard, J.D.W. and Glynn, C.J. (1976) Cryoanalgesia, a new approach to pain relief. *Lancet*, ii, 932–934.

May, O. (1912) The functional and histological effects of intraneural and intraganglionic injections of alcohol. *Br. Med. J.*, 2, 465.

Mehta, M. (1973) In: *Intractable Pain*. W.B. Saunders, Co., Philadelphia.

Mehta, M. (1982) Chronic pain. Editors: R.S. Atkinson and C.L. Hewer. *Recent Advances in Anaesthesia and Analgesia, Vol. 14*, 157–177. Churchill Livingstone, Edinburgh.

Mehta, M. and Ranger, I. (1971) Persistent abdominal pain. Treatment by nerve block. *Anaesthesia*, 26, 330.

Mierowsky, A.M. (1969) The management of chronic interstitial cystitis by differential sacral neurectomy. *J. Neurosurg.*, 30, 604.

Miller, R.D., Johnston, R.R. and Hosobuchi, Y. (1975) Treatment of intercostal neuralgia with 10 per cent ammonium sulfate. *J. Thorac. Surg.*, 69, 476.

Montgomery, W. and Cousins, M.J. (1972) Aspects of management of chronic pain illustrated by ninth nerve block. *Br. J. Anaesth.*, 44, 383–385.

Moore, D.C. (1965) In: *Regional Block (1975), 4th Edn*. C.C. Thomas, Springfield.

Moore, D.C. and Bridenbaugh, L.D. (1962) Intercostal nerve block in 4333 patients; indications, technique and complications. *Anesth. Analg. Curr. Res.*, 41, 1.

Nash, T.P. (1986) Percutaneous radiofrequency lesioning of dorsal root ganglia for intractable pain. *Pain*, 24, 67–73.

221

Nathan, P.W. and Wall, P.D. (1974) Treatment of post-herpetic neuralgia by prolonged electric stimulation. *Br. Med. J.*, 3, 645.

Neill, R.S. (1979) Ablation of the brachial plexus. *Anaesthesia*, 34, 1024–1027.

Noordenbos, W. (1959) *Pain*. Elsevier, Amsterdam.

Nour-Eldin, F. (1970) Preliminary Report: Uptake of phenol by vascular and brain tissue. *Microvasc. Res.*, 2, 224–225.

Papper, E.M. (1967) Rovenstine Memorial Lecture. *Anesthesiology*, 28, 1074.

Penman, J. (1958) In: *Operative Surgery, Vol. 8*. Editors: C. Rob and R. Smith. Butterworth, London.

Penman, J. and Smith, M.C. (1950) Degeneration of the primary and secondary neurons after trigeminal injection. *J. Neurol. Neurosurg. Psychiat.*, 13, 36.

Pitres, A. and Vaillard, L. (1888) Des Névrites Provoquées par le contact de l'alcool pur ou dilué avec les nerfs vivants. *C.R. Soc. Biol. (Paris)*, 5, 550.

Pizzolato, P. and Mannheimer, W.H. (1961) *Histopathologic Effects of Local Anaesthetic drugs*. C.C. Thomas, Springfield.

Rasmussen, P. (1965) Facial Pain. Thesis. Munksgaard, Copenhagen.

Reid, W., Watt, J.K. and Gray, T.G. (1970) Phenol injection of sympathetic chain. *Br. J. Surg.*, 47, 45–55.

Robertson, D.H. (1983) Transsacral neurolytic nerve block. *Br. J. Anaesth.*, 873–875.

Rockswold, G.L., Bradley, W.E. and Chou, S.N. (1973) Differential sacral rhizotomy in the treatment of neurogenic bladder dysfunction. *J. Neurosurg.*, 38, 748.

Ruge, D., Brochner, R. and Davis, L. (1958) A study of the treatment of 637 patients with trigeminal neuralgia. *J. Neurosurg.*, 17, 528.

Shealy, C.N. (1975) Percutaneous radiofrequency denervation of spinal facets. *J. Neurosurg.*, 43, 448.

Simon, D.L., Carron, H. and Rowlingson, J.C. (1982) Treatment of bladder pain with transsacral nerve block. *Anesth. Analg.*, 61, 46–48.

Sluiter, M. and Mehta, M. (1981) Treatment of chronic neck and back pain by percutaneous thermal lesions. In: *Persistent Pain: Modern Methods of Treatment, Vol. 3*. Editors: S. Lipton and J. Miles. Academic Press, London. pp. 141–179.

Stender, A. (1961) *Second Intern. Congr. Neurol. Surg.*, ICS No. 36, E25. Excerpta Medica, Amsterdam.

Stookey, B. and Ransohoff, J. (1959) *Trigeminal Neuralgia – Its History and Treatment*. C.C. Thomas, Springfield.

Sunderland, S. (1968) *Nerve and Nerve Injuries*. Livingstone Ltd., Edinburgh.

Sweet, W.H. (1986) The treatment of trigeminal neuralgia (tic douloureux). *N. Engl. J. Med.*, 315, 174–177.

Sweet, W.H. (1988) Retrogasserian glycerol injection for treatment of trigeminal neuralgia. In: *Operative Neurosurgical Techniques*. Grune and Stratton, New York.

Swerdlow, M. (1972) The Pain Clinic. *Br. J. Clin. Pract.*, 26, 403.

Swerdlow, M. (1977) In: *Persistent Pain. Modern Methods of Treatment, Vol. 1*. Editor: S. Lipton. Academic Press, London.

Tasker, R.R., Organ, L.W. and Hawrylyshyn, P. (1980) *Deafferentation and Causalgia Pain*. Editor: J.J. Bonica. Raven Press, New York.

Tavernier, L. (1948) Surgical treatment of degenerative arthritis of the hip. *Rheumatism*, 4, 176.

Torrens, M.J. and Griffith, H.B. (1976) Management of the uninhibited bladder by selective sacral neurectomy. *J. Neurosurg.*, 44, 176.

Uematsu, S. et al. (1974) Percutaneous radiofrequency rhizotomy. *Surg. Neurol.*, 2, 319–325.

Waltz, T.A., Dalessio, D.J., Ott, K.H., Copeland, B. and Abbott, G. (1985) Trigeminal cistern glycerol injections for facial pain. *Headache*, 25, 354–357.

Waltz, T.A. and Copeland, B. (1986) Correspondence. *N. Engl. J. Med.*, 316, 693.

Wang, J.K. (1985) Cryoanalgesia for painful peripheral nerve lesions. *Pain*, 22, 191–194.

White, J.C. and Sweet, W.H. (1969) In: *Pain and the Neurosurgeon*. C.C. Thomas, Springfield.

M. Swerdlow and J.E. Charlton (eds.) Relief of Intractable Pain

8

Intrathecal and extradural block in pain relief

Mark Swerdlow

The accessibility of the spinal cord offers a relatively easy means of producing spinal root block for diagnostic, prognostic or treatment purposes. Differential spinal block by subarachnoid injection of cerebrospinal fluid (CSF) or various concentrations of procaine has been much used to distinguish whether the pain is relieved by placebo, by sympathetic block or by somatic block (Ahlgren et al., 1966; Winnie and Collins, 1968). Therapeutically, the actual approach to the nerve roots may be by subarachnoid, subdural or extradural injection. Intrathecal and, to a lesser extent, extradural injections of neurolytic agents are among the most valuable methods available for the relief of some types of intractable pain.

The credit must go to Corning for being the first to attempt to relieve pain by subarachnoid medication. In 1894, he reported injecting cocaine intrathecally in two patients and obtaining pain relief for some hours. Tuffier (1899) administered subarachnoid cocaine to relieve pain in a young man with sarcoma of the leg and he too found that the results, although temporary, were most impressive. It was not until 1931, however, that a neurolytic agent (alcohol) was injected intrathecally for the relief of intractable pain (Dogliotti, 1931). The value of the method was soon appreciated and an increasing number of reports of its use followed, although for some time the incidence of complications acted as a deterrent (Hay, 1962). In 1955, Maher suggested that phenol in glycerine was more easily manageable than alcohol and produced better results, and this agent has since achieved widespread use. More recently, Maher (1963) introduced the intrathecal use of chlorocresol. The history of the use of neurolytic spinal block has been described in detail elsewhere (Swerdlow, 1988).

PRINCIPLES OF SUBARACHNOID NEUROLYTIC INJECTION

Pain impulses enter the spinal cord via the posterior roots, and the roots of any spinal nerve can be readily blocked by injecting a neurolytic solution within the theca. Lumbar puncture at the correct level and, to a lesser extent, appropriate positioning and tilting of the patient during injection, will help to ensure that the neurolytic agent will move towards the selected roots. Thus, with 'heavy' solutions (e.g., phenol in glycerine and chlorocresol in glycerine), the patient will be placed in the semisupine position for injection (Fig. 8.1), while with 'light' solutions (e.g., alcohol), a semiprone position will be used (Fig. 8.2).

The fact that cerebrospinal fluid drains away from the posterior roots may be a further factor in ensuring that the neurolytic agent produces an effective block. The use of glycerine prevents mixing with CSF and helps to localize the phenol or chlorocresol, which is gradually released from the glycerine. Nathan and Scott (1958) found that with phenol/Myodil mixtures, the phenol content of Myodil (io-phendylate) fell markedly within an hour, and Maher (1963) reported that 1 h after injection of chlorocresol/glycerine into the CSF, 43% of the chlorocresol had diffused out of the glycerine and that only 5% of the chlorocresol remained in the glycerine after 3 h. More recent studies (Matsuki et al., 1971; Ichiyanagi et al., 1975) suggest that both alcohol and phenol are released and dispersed in the CSF more quickly than was previously thought, although their conclusions have been questioned (Flanigan and Boop. 1974).

Following chemical neurolysis, there is a gradual regeneration of nerve fibres and as time goes by, little by little the pain might return.

There have been a number of studies on the effects of neurolytic agents on nerve tissue, both in experimental animals and on post-mortem specimens from patients who had previously received neurolytic injections.

It has been reported that a few days after subarachnoid injection of alcohol, there is demyelination and degeneration in the dorsal roots (Gallagher et al., 1961) and that the CSF shows an increase in pressure and a slight increase in the albumen and leucocyte levels, which returned to normal within 10 days. Derrick (1966) reports that following subarachnoid administration of alcohol (in three cases), there was degeneration of axis cylinders in the posterior roots. The posterior root ganglia near the injected level showed moderate swelling and chromatolysis, and the associated posterior roots showed severe demyelination.

Marion Smith (1964) studied the effects of phenol on spinal nerve roots and found degeneration changes consistently present in nerve roots and myelin sheaths; there was more extensive damage in the posterior than in the anterior roots. The degeneration was patchy, and cumulative damage sometimes gave rise to obvious secondary degeneration in the posterior columns. Variations in the concentration of phenol could result from pocketing due to surface tension in the

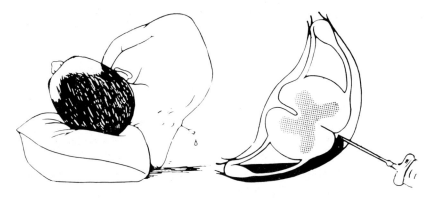

Fig. 8.1. Posterior nerve root block with hyperbaric neurolytic solution (from *Proceedings of the Fourth World Congress of Anaesthesiologists*, Excerpta Medica, Amsterdam).

dural cuffs (Wolman, 1966). Schaumburg and colleagues (1970) found that the amount of Wallerian degeneration produced by phenol was directly proportional to the strength of the solution and the duration of application to the nerve. Wilkinson et al. (1964) showed that in 10% concentration, phenol can cause serious interruption of motor fibres; and Berry and Olszewski (1963), Smith (1964), and Hansebout and Cosgrove (1966) all describe the indiscriminate toxic effect of phenol on all structures with which it comes into contact. The local effects of alcohol are not dissimilar (Hughes, 1966), but the damage is less localized.

Nathan et al. (1965) believe that alcohol and phenol derivatives exert both a

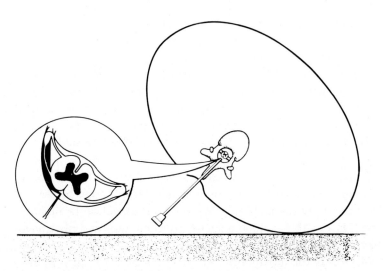

Fig. 8.2. Posterior nerve root block with hypobaric neurolytic solution.

local anaesthetic action (which differentiates between types of nerve fibres) and a destructive action (which is non-selective). Upon intrathecal injection of phenol, a block of a large number of fibres of many nerve roots rapidly develops. The majority of fibres soon recover the power to conduct impulses, but in some the recovery is only temporary. Nathan and co-workers consider that, with conventional concentrations of neurolytic agents, the number of nerve fibres which degenerate is insufficient to cause permanent weakness or loss of sensibility. In experiments with intrathecal phenol in cats, they found that even in 1% concentration, phenol caused destruction of nerve fibres of all sizes, both myelinated and non-myelinated. However, they did not find evidence of cord damage or of major meningeal changes, and rarely of massive degeneration of all the fibres of a nerve root. With higher concentrations, however, such serious destruction has been reported (Baxter and Schacherl, 1962). Nathan and his colleagues (1965) consider, therefore, that the clinical success of chemical rhizotomy is not due to the qualitative selective destruction of afferent fibres, but is quantitative, depending on the destruction of an adequate number of them.

CLINICAL

Subarachnoid neurolytic block should be used mainly for cancer pain, which is usually due to pressure on somatic nerve roots by secondaries in the vertebrae or tumours in the paravertebral region. In general, in patients with an anticipated long survival time, a surgical or percutaneous cordotomy will probably provide a longer period of pain relief. In patients with a shorter life expectancy, however, and in those who are unable, unfit or unwilling to undergo the surgical procedure, intrathecal neurolysis offers a good prospect of worthwhile pain relief so that the patient can remain ambulant and on minimal oral analgesic medication. Intrathecal neurolytic injection is also valuable in patients with extensive and bilateral cancer pain. Here, the risks of performing bilateral cordotomy can be avoided by performing cordotomy on the side with the most extensive pain and an intrathecal neurolysis on the other side. If the clinical findings suggest the possibility of a sympathetic aetiology for the pain, then diagnostic sympathetic block should be performed first.

Finally, it should be stated that when intrathecal neurolysis is the method of choice, it should be instituted at the earliest possible time when there is severe and persistent pain. Needless to say, spinal blockade is only one aspect of the management of a patient with intractable pain, and social, psychological and pharmacological support will also be needed.

Intrathecal neurolysis has the advantages that it is relatively simple, painless and free from serious complications; it can be carried out on patients in poor general condition and in the elderly. It involves only brief hospitalization and can be made available to and deal with relatively large numbers of patients, and it requires no special technical equipment or facilities. It can be repeated or extended if inadequate, and neurosurgical procedures can be performed at a later time if the patient's condition improves or if the pain state warrants it. In patients with terminal illness, the duration of pain relief is sufficient to afford a relatively comfortable end.

Opinions are divided on the use of intrathecal neurolytic agents in non-terminal disease. In general, this use of the technique is not recommended. In the author's opinion, justification of such use would depend on the cause, severity and duration of the pain, the age and mobility of the patient, the nature and results of treatments already received and the possibility of achieving adequate relief by other means.

The patient for intrathecal injection is admitted to hospital, preferably 24 h or more before injection, so that the ward staff can assess the amount of pain that he is suffering, his mobility and the state of his bodily functions. A note is also made of the medication which he is receiving and of any side effects or complications which are present. A detailed history will already have been taken and a full clinical examination carried out at the previous out-patient or domiciliary consultation (Swerdlow, 1968). Before commencement of treatment, it is important to tell the patient that nerve block may remove some but not all of the pain; that we are treating pain and not attempting to cure the causative disease; that he will be staying in hospital for a day or two so that the results of the injection can be assessed; and that it is possible that a second injection might be necessary. It is wiser not to inject unwilling patients or those who are in doubt. If there is pain in more than one place, the area of most severe pain is tackled first. If there is bilateral pain, the author treats the two sides separately, the more severe side first, although some (Derrick, 1966) perform bilateral block with alcohol, the patient lying in the prone position. The author prefers not to attempt to block both sides with one injection (involving as this does a larger dose of solution), but rather to concentrate the agent to the posterior nerve roots of one side and to block the other side at a subsequent session. The dosage recommended below should be strictly adhered to because, although an increase in dose may improve results (Lipton, 1981), it is likely to cause an increased incidence of complications.

Premedication should be avoided whenever possible because the full cooperation of the patient is necessary to decide on the immediate localization of the neurolytic solution. If the patient is unduly apprehensive and premedication is thought essential, it should be kept to a minimum and a small dose of tranquillizer mixture may be found useful (Swerdlow and Cockings, 1958). Further, it is better if the patient is not given any analgesic drugs in the 3 or 4 h before injection, as it is helpful if pain is present at the time the injection is performed. Good results

228

can be obtained by intrathecal injection of either alcohol or phenol, and the choice depends to some extent on personal experience and training and on whether one prefers to use a hyperbaric or a hypobaric solution. Occasionally, the condition of the patient will dictate whether a prone or supine position will be practical and hence which type of agent should be used (e.g., curvature of the spine, discomfort lying on the painful side, orthopnoea, etc.). In general, the earlier the patient is referred for treatment, the better the chance of achieving good relief (Swerdlow, 1967).

TECHNIQUE OF INTRATHECAL PHENOL INJECTION

Intrathecal injection should be carried out on an operating table or some such table which will permit easy and rapid tilting of the patient in any direction. Needless to say, a full aseptic technique must be observed. The patient is laid on his side on the half of the table furthest away from the operator and with the painful side underneath; he should be curled up around the assistant in the lumbar puncture position (Fig. 8.3). After producing a skin wheal with local anaesthetic, a 21

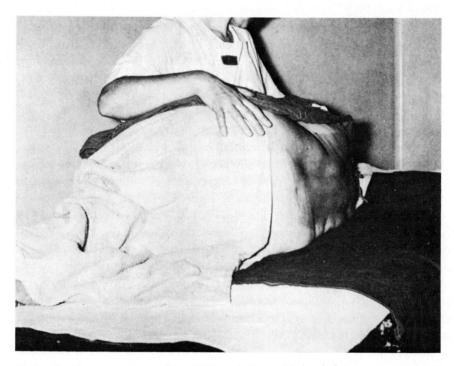

Fig. 8.3. Position for lumbar puncture with hyperbaric neurolytic solution.

gauge Howard Jones or other spinal needle is inserted into the interspace corresponding to the nerve root level (not the vertebral level) of the middle of the painful area. It should be remembered that, because of the slope of the vertebral spines, the trajectory of the needle will be approximately at right angles to the dorsal plane in the lumbar and cervical regions, but will be markedly oblique in the thoracic region (Fig. 8.4). When performing lumbar puncture at levels above the L_2 interspace, the greatest care should be taken to avoid puncturing the cord; furthermore, whenever neurolytic solutions are being injected, care should be taken that there is a free flow of fluid through the needle and that injection does not cause immediate pain. When lumbar puncture has been performed, the patient is tilted backwards so that his back is at approximately 45° to the table top (Fig. 8.5) and the legs are extended. Having confirmed that there is still a free flow of CSF, the syringe containing the neurolytic solution is attached to the lumbar puncture needle and a preliminary dose of 0.2 ml of solution is injected. Solutions in glycerine are very viscid and considerable force will be needed to inject through a 21 gauge spinal needle; the injection is made much easier if a 1 ml tuberculin-

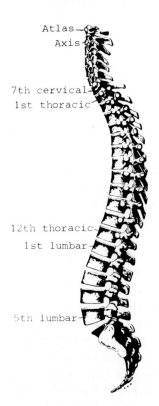

Fig. 8.4. Spinal column: lateral view (from Gray's Anatomy, 33rd Edn. Churchill Livingston, London).

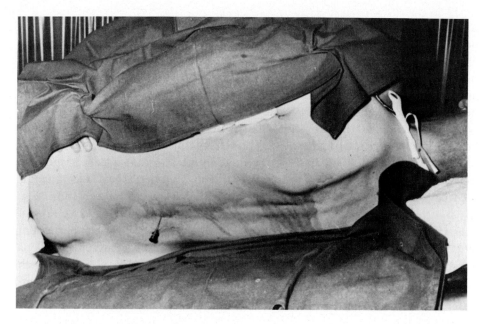

Fig. 8.5. Position for injection of hyperbaric solution for lower trunk pain.

type syringe is used. After 30–60 s, the patient is asked to indicate if he feels any sensations anywhere on the underside of his body. If the patient reports sensations on the upper side of the body, the bevel of the needle may have inadvertently been facing upwards and it should be turned facing down. The impact of phenol on the nerve roots frequently causes early onset of symptoms such as a feeling of warmth, tingling, prickling or pain. When such symptoms are reported, the operator decides whether the site of the sensation is caudad, cephalad or exactly in the site in which he aims to achieve nerve block, and if necessary the table is tilted to move the phenol to the desired nerve roots. (If the needle is found to be sited more than one segment away from the desired nerve level, it is probably better to remove the needle and re-introduce it at the correct level, if this can be easily done.) A further 0.1 ml of solution is now injected and once again the patient is asked to indicate where sensations are felt; further tilting may be necessary before a good apposition is achieved. Once the sensations are being felt in the place where analgesia is desired, the remainder of the dose is given. The total dose of phenol or chlorocresol in glycerine ranges from 0.5 to 1 ml depending chiefly on the number of nerve roots being treated, the length of the spine and the part of the spine being injected, sacral sites being given least and thoracic most. The spinal needle is then removed and a small dressing applied to the point of puncture. By this time, the patient should be reporting a feeling of numbness in the area of analgesia and this numbness may become very intense within minutes. After completion of the injection, pillows or some other form of support are put under the patient to make it more comfortable for him to lie in the 45° position and he remains so for about 20 min.

The method described above is for subarachnoid injection of phenol or of chlorocresol in glycerine. Phenol, 5–7% and chlorocresol, 1 in 50 or 1 in 40 behave as 'heavy' solutions relative to the CSF, and the glycerine allows for easy positioning of the small volume of solution injected. Following injection of phenol, the patient almost invariably can easily describe the nature and location of symptoms caused by the initial injection; this is not so after chlorocresol, when sometimes he states that there are no symptoms or sensations at all. When this occurs, it is more difficult to decide just where the chlorocresol is having impact, and one may have to rely on whether or not the patient reports that his pain is disappearing and that numbness develops. It is difficult under these conditions to get any useful information by pinprick or cotton wool testing; sometimes there are already deficiencies in skin sensation and moreover the patient finds it difficult to give clear-cut answers about such testing when he is undergoing the mental strain of the injection. Mehta (1973) uses a mixture of equal parts of phenol and chlorocresol in the hope of obtaining the ease of localization of phenol together with the longer duration of chlorocresol. Papo and Visca (1976) use a mixture of 2.5% phenol with 2% chlorocresol in glycerine.

TECHNIQUE OF SUBARACHNOID ALCOHOL INJECTION

Absolute ethyl alcohol is hypobaric (SG 0.806) and the patient must, therefore, be placed with the side to be blocked elevated in the 45° position and with the table split, so that the relevant dorsal roots are at the highest point (Fig. 8.6). A 22 gauge needle may be used. With the patient lying prone or semiprone, the CSF pressure may be too low for free flow of fluid to occur and it may be necessary to aspirate CSF with a syringe to confirm thecal puncture.

When alcohol is injected intrathecally and contacts the sensory nerve roots, it causes severe burning pain or paraesthesiae which last a few seconds and then gradually fade; the patient must be warned of this beforehand, so that he does not move unduly. A dose of 0.5 ml alcohol is injected through the spinal needle, paraesthesiae sought and appropriate tilting carried out if necessary. Further 0.5 ml increments are given at 5–10 min intervals, the injection in each case being made slowly to reduce the amount of turbulence and dilution with its spread in the CSF. Sensory level and motor function should be tested between injections and if motor involvement becomes apparent, the injection should be stopped. Most workers consider that 2 ml is about the uppermost limit of dosage of alcohol

232

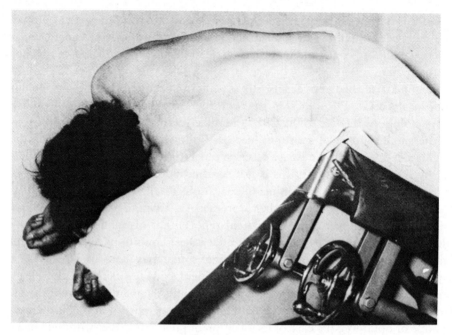

Fig. 8.6. Position for intrathecal injection of alcohol for thoracic pain.

at any one treatment. Alcohol is fixed fairly rapidly and the level of analgesia cannot then be changed much despite tilting of the table; the same is true of phenol and chlorocresol. The duration of relief varies from weeks to a year or more and averages 3 months.

Post-injection management

After injection, the patient is returned to the ward; it is advisable to keep him in bed for the remainder of the day to minimize the risk of headache. He should be encouraged to drink as much as possible. Following the injection, he should be watched for the occurrence of headache and note should also be made that he passes urine and has normal bowel activity. Furthermore, it is important to observe whether any sensory or motor defects develop following the block.

After a difficult block, it is helpful to tell the patient that he may have some soreness or aching in the back for a little while; this may spare him a period of apprehension, worrying whether something has gone wrong. Following the intrathecal injection, patients, particularly those who have been suffering severe pain for a long time, may complain of new, different sensations – intensification of pain, intense numbness, paraesthesiae, etc. – and require some reassurance that all is well.

If good pain relief is obtained, a careful watch must be kept on patients who have been on opioid analgesics for some time. It is advisable in such cases to reduce gradually the amount of opioid the patient is receiving and this will require cooperation with the patient's family doctor when he returns home (Swerdlow, 1967). Sometimes no worthwhile degree of relief is obtained after the block. Not infrequently good pain relief is achieved on the day of the block, but within a day or two it is clear that relief is either greatly or somewhat inadequate and a further injection is required before a satisfactory result is obtained. Furthermore, relief of pain may be satisfactory while the patient is in hospital but inadequate when he returns home.

After phenol or chlorocresol block, a fair assessment of results can be obtained within a day or two, but after alcohol, the maximum effect of the block may not be obvious for a few days. In assessing results, the patient's own opinion is, of course, the key one and if he considers that the relief is inadequate, further blocking must be considered. However, the opinion of the nursing staff who are constantly in contact with the patient is of considerable value. Frequently the initial injection gives inadequate relief. In such cases it is usually worth repeating the injection. Gerbershagen (1981) reports that 20% of patients required a second injection after intrathecal alcohol neurolysis. If the second injection is unsuccessful, the present author considers that a third injection would be unlikely to succeed and would involve an increased risk of complications.

In patients suffering from visceral abdominal as well as from somatic pain, a bilateral coeliac plexus block will be required in addition to intrathecal injection (see Chapter 9).

Pain involving the nerve distribution from the two extremes of the spinal cord can be dealt with by intrathecal methods, but each of these areas involves special problems and difficulties.

(1) Block of the *upper thoracic and cervical segments* may result in paralysis of cranial nerves or of the arm, as well as in severe headache. Furthermore, subarachnoid neurolytics often fail to give as long a duration of relief in this region as they do lower down the cord (Swerdlow, 1981). This has been attributed to the relative shortness of the dural sheaths in which the neurolytic agent 'settles' in the cervical segments. Furthermore, the cervical nerve roots have a short intrathecal course and therefore are less exposed to the neurolytic than elsewhere. Moreover, the spinal canal is narrower with a stronger current of CSF which will tend to carry the neurolytic away from the target nerve roots. Bonica (1981) believes that better results can be obtained by inserting a needle through each of the interspinous spaces involved and injecting 0.2 ml absolute alcohol through each needle. Table 8.1 shows the results reported by various workers.

One possible alternative method is to use the extradural route (q.v.), which is safer but which unfortunately often fails to give an adequate duration of relief.

TABLE 8.1

Results of cervical intrathecal neurolysis

Author	Agent	No. of patients	Results	Duration	Comments
Churcher (1970)	Alcohol	9	4 good; 4 partial; 1 fail	1 month	
Stovner and Endresen (1972)	Phenol	5	2 good or moderate; 3 poor		
Papo (1976)	Phenol	19	Good relief 3; Partial relief 7; No relief 9		
Ventafridda and Martino (1976)	Alcohol or phenol	27	Good relief 56%	Mean of 18 days	Most had complications
Maher and Mehta (1977)	Phenol or chloro-cresol	38	Significant relief 12		
Swerdlow (1978, 1981)	Phenol or chloro-cresol	20	Little or no relief 9; Good or moderate relief 11	3 for 2 weeks; 4 for >2 weeks	4 survived less than 2 weeks
	Alcohol	4	Transient 2; Moderate or good 2	2 months	

Another method which has been advocated is *subdural* injection of phenol. The anatomy of the subdural space has been well described by Sechzer (1963). The injection is carried out with the aid of an image intensifier: preliminary injection of a small amount of iophendylate displays a typical honeycomb appearance when introduced subdurally. One to three ml of 5% phenol in glycerine is then injected, depending on the extent of analgesia required. The technique is not an easy one, and even when it is carried out successfully, it may fail to give a useful duration of relief. Not surprisingly, therefore, it is not achieving popularity.

A further alternative is *intracisternal neurolysis*. Injection of phenol into the cisterna magna was reported by Wilkinson et al. in 1964 and has more recently been advocated by Marini and Giunta (1975) for the treatment of head and neck pain. However, the radiofrequency electrode now probably offers safer and more effective therapy.

(2) Pain in the *perineal and rectal* area presents a very difficult problem, chiefly because of the serious risk of bladder and rectal involvement when neurolytic agents are applied to the lower lumbar and sacral segments. If incontinence is already present and the patient has an indwelling catheter, this problem does not arise. When the pain is situated in the perineum and the buttock or thigh on one side, a unilateral block will sometimes produce good relief without complications. At a later time, when required, the other side can be tackled to complete the analgesia. Even when the pain is midline and shows no bias to either side, the performance of two unilateral blocks at an interval of a day or two will sometimes produce a good result without bladder or rectal involvement. If the pain relief so obtained is inadequate, however, then, despite the risks, a further injection should be given with the patient sitting up without any attempt at lateral positioning. In cases where urinary complications would create excessive problems, an alternative means of relieving bladder and perineal pain is trans-sacral blockade (Simon et al., 1982; Robertson, 1985). The fourth sacral nerve is injected bilaterally with 2.5 ml 6% phenol; a repeat injection may be necessary 7–10 days later.

'LOWER END' INJECTION

The patient is sat up and bent forward in the lumbar puncture position, while a spinal needle is introduced intrathecally at the level of L_4–L_5. Maher (1963) believes that if the injection is made with the needle tip only just penetrating the arachnoid, then there is less risk of the sacral nerves and bladder being involved. If the block is being given for midline pain, the patient's shoulders and back are then lowered until at about 45° to the table and he is supported in this position by the nurse (Fig. 8.7) while the injection is being carried out.

If a unilateral block is being performed, the patient is lowered to 45° with the table and the upper part of his body is rotated towards the side to be blocked (Fig. 8.8).

Phenol or chlorocresol (0.5–0.7 ml) is now injected slowly (alcohol is not recommended for this purpose). The patient should soon report cutaneous sensations, analgesia and disappearance of pain as described above. The needle is removed when the injection is completed, the head end of the table is raised and pillows are placed behind the patient, so that he can lie comfortably in the injection position; he is retained thus for about 20 min.

When neurolytic block is successful, the duration of pain relief varies from weeks to many months and, of course, if the patient survives longer than the analgesia, the block may be repeated. When a good result is obtained and the pain has gone, the patient often sleeps a great deal. Patients have been reported to have died within a few days of a successful block – the stimulus has gone.

236

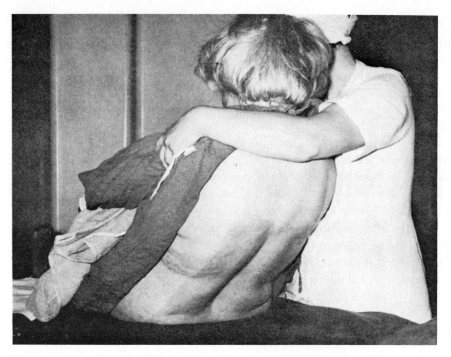

Fig. 8.7. Position for injection of hyperbaric solution for 'lower end' pain.

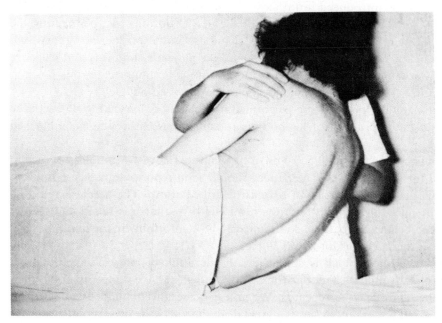

Fig. 8.8. Position for unilateral block of lower lumbar and sacral roots.

Failure

There are a number of reasons why intrathecal chemical neurolysis sometimes fails to provide pain relief. Inflammatory changes and cancerous infiltration may shelter the nerve roots from the injected agent and render a good result more difficult to obtain. Radiation therapy to the nerve roots also makes relief much more difficult to attain by intrathecal injections. On the other hand, Pellegrini et al. (1969) have found gross myelin and axon damage in patients in whom treatment failed to produce pain relief! Sometimes failure occurs because there is a large sympathetic nervous element in the pain aetiology. In patients suffering from pathological fracture of a vertebra or bone, intrathecal neurolytic injections will fail to relieve 'movement or incident pain' which appears to be transmitted by fibres which escape the intrathecal agent. In these patients, relief can be provided by appropriate splinting. The following case history is illustrative:

Mrs. S., aged 70, complained of severe pain in the right hip, buttock, thigh and leg following abdominoperineal resection of carcinoma recti. An intrathecal injection of 0.75 ml 7% phenol in glycerine was administered, after which she was quite free from pain when lying still, but movement of the right leg caused severe pain. X-Ray of the right hip demonstrated pathological fracture of the femoral neck. She was referred to an orthopaedic colleague and following surgical pinning she was able to move the hip painlessly.

Maher (personal communication, 1972) has shown that in cases with incident pain if the tumour can be made to regress by cytotoxic drugs or other means, then sufficient bone healing can occur to allow the patient once again to have reasonably free, painless movement (see also p. 332). Occasionally, a previous intrathecal injection will have caused some patchy meningitis which prevents a subsequent injection from gaining access to the nerve roots. The author had one patient who was given two intrathecal injections of chlorocresol at an interval of 2 days, the second of which produced no immediate effect. Four days later, there was a sudden onset of good and lasting analgesia.

Results of subarachnoid neurolysis

One of the difficulties in assessing and reporting results is that pain has three dimensions: degree, extent and duration. The patient's own degree of comfort varies from time to time, being influenced by innumerable physical and psychological factors. Patients often find it difficult to state the degree of relief, especially if they have other pains or physical disabilities. In assessing reported results, the actual duration and degree of relief which are adopted as being 'good' or 'fair' vary in different publications. Some patients require two, three or even more injections before a stable pain-free period is achieved, and this may give rise to some diffi-

238

culty in ascribing complications. Furthermore, new secondaries and pain may occur while the block for the previous pain is still perfectly effective. A technically 'good' result in only part of the pain area might score worse than a 'moderate result' in the whole pain area.

Bearing in mind that the following are composite tables and that there are the above differences in the statements of results, Tables 8.2 and 8.3 show the type of results obtained with phenol and with alcohol. Most workers find that the average duration of relief is about 2–4 months, but periods very much greater and shorter than this may be obtained (see below).

There is considerable divergence of opinion on the relative merits of alcohol and phenol as intrathecal agents. Few comparative trials of the two agents have as yet been reported.

Jacobs and Howland (1966) compared alcohol with 5% phenol in glycerine in 62 patients with advanced cancer; they found that alcohol impairs the sphincters significantly more than phenol, but otherwise the results were similar with the two agents. On the other hand, Cole (1965) considers that intrathecal phenol gives better results than alcohol, with fewer complications. After phenol, unlike alcohol, numbness may occur, but there will still be a sense of touch. Lourie and Vanasupa (1963) and Swerdlow (1963) consider that site localization and extent can be more easily controlled with phenol. A survey of recent publications suggests that phenol is now the more widely favoured agent. However, Gerbershagen has recently (1981) made a strong plea for the more frequent use of intrathecal alcohol.

There is as yet little information about the efficacy of chlorocresol. This agent was introduced in 1963 by Maher, who claimed it to be a better agent than phenol: more reliable, not so instantaneous in onset and affecting a greater length of nerve root. He also claimed that it affords better penetrability and causes no complications except occasional slight paresis.

For several years, the present author used phenol and chlorocresol more or less

TABLE 8.2

Results of subarachnoid phenol blocks

Authors	No. of cases	Percentage of patients obtaining relief		
		good	moderate	little or none
Maher (personal communication, 1972)	433	62	6	32
Swerdlow (1979)	320	57	19	24
Papo and Visca (1979)	290	40	35	25
Stovner and Endresen (1972)	151	77		23
Lifshitz et al. (1976)	117	77		23

TABLE 8.3

Results of subarachnoid alcohol block

Author(s)	No. of cases	Percentage of patients obtaining relief		
		good	fair	little or none
Kuzucu et al. (1966)	322	58	26	16
Hay (1962)	252	46	32	22
Bonica (1958)	182	53	29	18
Dogliotti (1931)	150	59	25	16
Greenhill (1947)	> 100	60	10	30

alternately in patients given intrathecal neurolysis. In many cases it was impossible to obtain a valid estimate of the duration and degree of effectiveness of the neurolytic applied. Complete results are available in 130 cases; all were suffering from cancer pain. Sixty nine had received phenol and 61 chlorocresol. Table 8.4 shows the results obtained in terms of degree and duration of relief. The table includes the duration of relief (or the time from the injection to death where this occurred before the block had worn off) in all single-dose cases and in patients who had had an injection on each side with a day or two interval for bilateral

TABLE 8.4

Analysis of duration of results – 130 patients

Duration of relief	Agent administered:	Phenol			Chlorocresol		
	Result of treatment:	good	moderate	poor	good	moderate	poor
Less than 1 month		11	5	6	14	6	3
1–2 months		6	3	2	7	4	2
2–3 months		7	1	3	3	2	1
3–4 months		3	1	2	2	2	1
4–5 months		8		1	1	0	1
6–8 months		6	1		8	1	
8–10 months		1			1		
10–12 months							
Over 1 year		1					
Over 2 years					1	1	
Total		44	11	14	37	16	8

pain. In patients who had received a succession of injections over a period of time, the duration of the first injection only has been inserted in the table. It can be seen that chlorocresol appears to have provided rather longer relief than phenol, although the great individual variation and the sparsity of numbers excludes a statistical approach. It may be that in some cases pain occurs late in the progress of the disease, but it is clear that many of the patients who survived for longer than 3 months obtained prolonged relief, and this underlines the importance of offering this form of treatment as early in the disease as pain becomes a serious factor.

Other intrathecal agents

A number of other neurolytic agents have been employed by the subarachnoid route to relieve intractable pain and are of historical interest.

Pantopaque (iophendylate, myodil) has been much used with phenol but this agent tends to protect the nerve roots and may interfere with subsequent injections (Maher, 1957). Pantopaque is advantageous when positioning neurolytic solution around nerve roots under X-ray control, but phenol in glycerine is generally agreed to be more neurolytic than phenol in Pantopaque (Khalili and Ditzler, 1968; White and Sweet, 1969), probably because the phenol diffuses more rapidly from glycerine than from Pantopaque. From a practical point of view, Pantopaque has the disadvantage that it has to be removed after the block and that its use may result in arachnoiditis (Howland et al., 1963).

Maher used a mixture of phenol and *silver nitrate* in cases resistant to phenol alone (1957). He thought that silver nitrate could be used safely at the lower thoracic level. Experience now shows that this agent is not safe at any level.

Alexander and Lewis (1963) employed ether as a (hypobaric) neurolytic agent. They found that it produced good analgesia but that it was difficult to control.

Bates and Judovich (1942) reported the use of intrathecal 6% *ammonium* sulphate or ammonium chloride for the relief of intractable pain in malignancy. They claimed that these agents produced good results, but other workers found the method unsatisfactory (Hand, 1944). In a later paper, Judovich et al. (1944) reported six cases of bowel and bladder paresis and recommended a lower dosage of the agent, greater dilution during injection and more accurate stabilization of the pH of the solution. Guttman and Pardee (1944) had a patient who developed persistent flaccid paraplegia with loss of sphincter control after intrathecal injection of ammonium sulphate. Post-mortem examination demonstrated necrosis of neural elements at the level of the injection. The use of ammonium salts intrathecally is not to be recommended.

In 1967, Hitchcock reported the production of pain relief following intrathecal injection of *cold saline*. More recently, hypertonic saline has been used at normal temperature with equal results; is would appear that the effects are due to the hypertonicity of the solution rather than its temperature. The original prognostications regarding the efficacy of this method have unfortunately proved inaccurate and moreover there are numerous reports of complications (Lucas et al., 1975). *Barbotage of CSF* is said to have first been used for pain relief by Speransky in 1935 in Moscow (Gillman, 1972). This method does not now appear to have any real clinical value.

Complications of intrathecal neurolysis

The intrathecal route provides easy and effective accessibility to the dorsal spinal nerve roots. Unfortunately, there are a number of complications which may ensue, some being due to the contact of the agent with unintended (e.g., motor and autonomic) nerve roots or with other structures (e.g., vascular supply of the CNS), while others are quite unrelated to the neurolytic drug (Swerdlow, 1980). The complications are usually transient or temporary but some persist and give rise to difficulties in patient management.

Table 8.5 shows the complications reported by a number of different authors. Tables 8.6 and 8.7 show the incidence and nature of the complications which have occurred in the present author's series of cases. Some of the patients had more than one complication but it can be seen that most of them were of a fairly minor nature. One hundred and seventy seven of the 300 patients had no complications at all.

In patients suffering from pain due to malignant disease, a number of factors may influence the incidence of complications, such as the size and situation of the tumour, whether the patient has had radiotherapy and whether there are pre-existing somatic or autonomic nervous deficits. However, the major factor depends on which part of the cord is being blocked and, to a lesser extent, how many nerve roots are involved.

It is convenient from a practical point of view to divide complications which may occur into 'common' (a) and 'uncommon' (b).

(a) *Common complications:* Retention of urine, often with overflow, is perhaps the most serious; it is very unlikely to occur, except after intrathecal injection in the lower lumbar and sacral regions, as is paralysis of the anal sphincter. A paper by Ischia et al. (1984) makes it clear that the use of higher concentrations of phenol in the lumbo-sacral theca is likely to increase the incidence of these complications.

In the 300 cases reported above, the author had only two patients who developed bladder paralysis after injection cephalad to the lumbar region: one occurred after a phenol block at T_7 in a patient who had had a great deal of radiotherapy to that portion of the spine, while the second followed phenol block at T_{11} after

TABLE 8.5

Complications of subarachnoid neurolysis

Author(s)	No. of patients	bladder paresis	bowel paresis	headache	muscle paresis	dysaesthesia	loss of proprioception	temporary paraplegia
Papo and Visca (1976)	270	15	–	–	24	–	–	–
Swerdlow (1975) (phenol or chlorocresol)	200	18	3	2	7	2	–	–
Stovner and Endresen (1972)	151	6	2	14	10	3	–	–
Mehta (1973) (phenol or chlorocresol)	55	8	8	2	10	27	–	–
Lifshitz et al. (1976)	133 blocks	22%	2.2%	5.3%	23%			1.5%

TABLE 8.6

Complications lasting longer than 7 days in 300 patients

Drug(s)	No. of patients	Bladder paresis	Bowel paresis	Muscle paresis	Headache	Paraesthesia	Numbness
Phenol	146	8	1	3	–	1	4
Chlorocresol	137	11	1	7	1	1	5
Phenol and chlorocresol	17	3	1	–	1	–	1

TABLE 8.7

Incidence and duration of complications

No. of patients with complication(s)		Duration of complication(s)
48		More than 3 days
28		More than 1 week
19		More than 2 weeks
10		More than 1 month
Total number of patients	300	
Total number of injections given	453	

three previous uncomplicated blocks at lower spinal levels. Retention was usually of only 1 or 2 days' duration, but in 22 of the author's patients, the paralysis lasted more than 1 week, in five it lasted more than 4 weeks, and in one patient it persisted until death some months later. Patients who develop retention of urine should be catheterized as necessary, a urinary antiseptic should be administered and carbachol should be given at intervals and may indicate returning bladder tone. Returning sensation in the perineum and penis may also signal the impending return of normal bladder function. It has recently been shown (Nathan, 1977), that a paralysed bladder can sometimes be made to empty by applying a vibrator to the lower anterior abdominal wall. In some patients, this initiates the micturition reflex and complete emptying follows: in others the vibration must be continued until the bladder is empty. Quite often, with the concurrence of the family doctor, the patient can be discharged with an indwelling catheter and bag. Subarachnoid neurolytic block sometimes aggravates latent bladder incompetence due, for example, to prostatism.

In Nathan's series (1967) of patients, 12% developed sphincter trouble. Jacobs and Howland (1966) report six cases of permanent urinary or rectal disability after intrathecal alcohol and two cases of permanent urinary disability after phenol. Alexander and Lewis (1963) had six cases of bladder paralysis severe enough to need catheterization for up to 6 weeks. In Stovner and Endresen's series (1972), six patients required catheterization for 1–10 days and two patients developed incontinence which lasted a day or two. Mathews (1969) had a 15% incidence of urinary and faecal incontinence after lumbosacral block with subarachnoid alcohol. Porges and Zdrahal (1985) report results in 47 patients with rectal carcinoma who received lower sacral root block with alcohol. Thirty-five of the patients did not need a catheter prior to treatment; of these, 11 required a permanent catheter after the block. Seven patients had intact rectal sphincter function before neurolysis and one of these became partly incontinent after treatment. Three patients developed lower limb paresis which disappeared within 3–14 days.

Persistent intense numbness is sometimes distressing, although obviously not as much so as the pain which it replaces. Paraesthesiae are sometimes complained of in the blocked area but are not usually persistent or troublesome. Paresis, when it occurs, usually diminishes rapidly and within a few days no longer restricts activity. In these cases, appropriate splinting, walking aid and physiotherapy are of great assistance in rehabilitating the patient. In the present series, ten patients developed weakness of more than 1 week's duration, in two patients the paresis lasted 3 weeks, and in one patient there was weakness of a leg which prevented the patient from walking for 6 weeks after the (intrathecal) injection. Derrick (1966) had two patients with permanent paralysis of both legs following intrathecal alcohol, and Alexander and Lewis (1963) reported two patients with leg paralysis which lasted 1 month. Bonica (1958) found that after subarachnoid neurolytic block, 25% of patients develop vesical paralysis, rectal dysfunction or limb paralysis. Headache is likely to occur when intrathecal injection is performed at a high thoracic level, but headache of the lumbar puncture type occurred here in two patients and persisted for several days. Two patients in the present series complained of nausea after the block. Intermittent vomiting has been reported after intrathecal block, especially upper- and midlumbar; this is thought to be due to diffuse sympathetic block. Severe headache can be relieved by epidural administration of normal saline or Hartman's solution, either by slow intermittent injection of 40–50 ml or by continuous catheter technique. Alexander and Lewis (1963) and Brown (1958) reported prolonged paraesthesia after intrathecal alcohol. Jacobs and Howland (1966) encountered persistent hyperaesthesia in two patients after phenol and in two after alcohol; persistent hypoaesthesia occurred in 12 cases. One patient in the present series complained of backache for a day or two after injection. Stovner and Endresen (1972) report the occurrence of undue pain and tenderness in the back in three out of 151 patients; they ascribe this to loss of phenol into the interspinous tissues.

(b) *Uncommon complications:* Tureen and Gitt (1936) and Sloane (1935) have reported cases of cauda equina lesion following intrathecal alcohol injection (although of course these date from the 'pre-autoclave' era). Stern (1937) points out that if the needle causes trauma to the cord or nerves of the cauda equina, then injection of even small amounts of alcohol will result in paralysis and severe sensory disturbances. He recommends that unless there is a free flow of CSF or if the CSF is persistently blood-stained, alcohol should not be injected.

Alcohol neuritis is an uncommon complication which has been reported by Gordon and Goel (1963) and by Katz (1970); however, the latter wondered whether some alcohol may have 'spilled' in the epidural space. Hay (1962) found that proprioceptive loss lasting 5–8 days occurred in four out of 252 cases.

Hughes (1970) reports a case of posterior spinal artery thrombosis following intrathecal injection of 1 ml 5% phenol in glycerine at T_3–T_4. The thrombosis syndrome appeared on the second post-injection day and lasted 8 days, and recovery occurred with only minor residual neurological signs. This syndrome may also occur in patients with cervical spondylosis when the neck is hyperextended.

Anterior spinal artery thrombosis is also a hazard; Totoki et al. (1979) have reported the development of anterior spinal artery occlusion syndrome following cervical subarachnoid injection of 0.3 ml 10% phenol in glycerine with disastrous consequences. Anecdotal and medico-legal evidence suggests that this syndrome occurs more frequently than would appear from the literature. The danger from the effects of neurolytic agents on the blood supply of the cord is perhaps not generally recognized. Nour-Eldin (1970) considered that phenol has a greater affinity for vascular than for brain tissue. More recently, Superville-Sovak and her colleagues (1975) have stressed the risks involved when phenol is introduced close to the vascular supply of the CNS. They describe a patient who received a cervical intrathecal injection of phenol and developed immediate respiratory difficulties which persisted until death 5 weeks later. A similar case has been reported more recently by Holland and Yousseff (1978). An earlier report by Wolman (1966) detailed a case with necrotic myelitis resulting from thrombosis of pial vessels near the injection site.

Meningismus is a rare complication which appears usually on the 3rd or 4th day after intrathecal injection (Stern, 1937; Bonica, 1953). The patient exhibits headache and neck rigidity and the CSF pressure is found to be raised.

Wilkinson and his colleagues (1964) describe a case in which cisternal injection of phenol for cervical root irritation was immediately followed by development of quadriplegia, which lasted 30 min and then gradually cleared.

Peyton et al. (1937) report a patient with pre-existing paresis due to a progressive cord lesion which was precipitated into complete paralysis by subarachnoid alcohol injection.

EPIDURAL NEUROLYTIC INJECTION

In 1901, Sicard reported the use of epidural cocaine, injected via the caudal route, for the relief of pain. Woodbridge (1930), in 1929, treated a patient suffering from cancer of the bladder with 8 ml 80% alcohol injected into the sacral foramina and obtained 9 months' pain relief. This method had, according to Woodbridge, already been used for a number of years by Labat and it subsequently achieved some popularity (Gilcreest and Mullen, 1931; Teevens, 1948). It is also of some historical interest that Kenny (1947), Teevens (1948) and Massey Dawkins (1963) employed 'Proctocaine' (procaine, 1.5% (w/v), butyl p-amino benzoate, 6% (w/v) with benzyl alcohol in arachis oil) epidurally in patients with cancer pain and sometimes obtained relief lasting for many months; repeat injections were often needed, but the method was claimed to be free from side effects. The solution was very oily and had to be warmed before use; this agent is no longer available. According to Dawkins (personal communication, 1972) cat nerve fibres of 1 mm section or less are completely destroyed by 10% benzyl alcohol. Theoretically, epidural injection of neurolytics offers distinct advantages over the intrathecal route. Meningeal irritation and the risk of spread within the cranial cavity are avoided and there is considerably less risk of bladder and rectal involvement and headache. It is somewhat surprising, therefore, that relatively little has been published on this method and that its value and indications cannot yet be authoritatively stated. Extradural injection has certainly found considerable usefulness as an interim measure in conditions due to peripheral vascular disorder and spasm and in autonomic nervous system disorders. In cases where an element of the pain is due to malignant involvement of blood vessels or viscera, phenol extradural block at the level of the coeliac plexus can be worthwhile. However, because it does not block vagal branches, this is not as effective as coeliac plexus block (see p. 268). The use of the epidural route for somatic nerve destruction in the relief of intractable pain, however, has been much less adequately documented.

The epidural route is also often preferred to subarachnoid injection when the painful dermatomes are cephalad to T_6, but alternative methods must be considered (see p. 234).

Technique

With the patient lying on the painful side in the lumbar puncture position, a 20 or 21 gauge spinal needle is introduced into the epidural space at the level corresponding to the middle of the painful area. After introducing the needle, the patient is tilted backwards into the 45° position as for intrathecal phenol (see p. 228). The position of the needle should be checked by the use of radio-opaque dye (Charlton, 1986). If an image intensifier is not available, a test dose of 0.2 ml phenol should be injected and after ensuring that the solution has not been deposited intrathecally, about 2 ml of 7% phenol in glycerine or of an 8–10% 'aqueous' solution of phenol are injected for each nerve root to be blocked; in the cervical region, the recommended dose is 1.5 ml per dermatome. The patient is retained in the tilted position for 40 min. Disappearance of pain occurs in about 10–15 min. With the small volume of solution required to block just a few segments of the cord, there should be little danger of hypotension. The technique is somewhat less precise than subarachnoid block, particularly in that the patient cannot immediately state where the solution is relative to the nerve roots. Because of the volume of neurolytic agent employed epidurally, it is more important than ever to take the greatest care to avoid accidental intrathecal injection. Furthermore, there is a large extradural plexus of veins and before injection it is important to ensure that the tip of the needle (or catheter) is not intravascular.

Some good results have been claimed with extradural alcohol (Patterson and Marcello, 1963; Spaetz and Wegner, 1963), and recently Korevaar and her colleagues have described the administration of alcohol via an epidural catheter on 3 successive days to 30 patients. Seventy percent of the patients obtained significant relief for an average duration of 5–8 months. The few reports of the use of phenol show some promising results. Lourie and Vanasupa (1963) employed 5% phenol extradurally for high thoracic and cervical pain, and claim more than 9 months relief, and Finer (1958) obtained good results with epidural 10% phenol in glycerine. Doughty (1972) advocates epidural injection of 5–10% phenol in glycerine at the level of T_{12}–L_1 for the relief of the attacks of tenesmus and burning pain which may occur with carcinoma of the rectum; in this condition, the somatic block produced by intrathecal phenol often fails to remove these distressing sensations. Madrid (1975) employed 7.5% phenol in glycerine for pain in the head and neck. Although this method was usually successful, relief was found to last for only 2–4 weeks.

Grunwald (1976) claims good results in 44.3% of 221 patients with cancer pain treated with 6–10% aqueous phenol administered epidurally. Raftery (1977) employs an indwelling epidural catheter and using intermittent 0.5–1 ml doses of 6% aqueous phenol he obtained good pain relief in 55% of 27 patients. If a catheter is inserted, a sterile microfilter should be used.

An interesting modification of the method has recently been proposed by Racz and his colleagues (1985), who employ doses of 2.5–5 ml 5.5% phenol in saline injected through an indwelling epidural catheter daily until complete or near-complete relief is attained for 24 h. The procedure is, however, terminated if signs of motor involvement appear. Further experience of the results of this technique must be awaited to confirm that it is indeed advantageous. Incidentally, Racz et al. have used the method successfully in six patients with upper limb spasticity.

NON-NEUROLYTIC EXTRADURAL BLOCK

Extradural medication as therapy in lumbo-sciatic syndrome

Historical

The epidural route was employed by Sicard as long ago as 1901 for the relief of lumbo-sciatic pain; he administered cocaine caudally to seven patients with lumbago or sciatica and obtained 2 weeks' relief of pain. Viner (1925) and Evans (1930) reported larger series of patients who were given a caudal epidural injection of 50–100 ml of procaine or normal saline with encouraging results. The injection of a large volume of fluid was thought perhaps to break down extradural adhesions or to stretch the sciatic nerve or its roots, while local anaesthetic might interrupt the vicious cycle of pain and muscle spasm. Coomes (1961) believed that a combination of anaesthetized nerve sheath plus hydrostatic effect plus painless lumbar movement resulted in improvement either by relieving pressure on the nerve root or by increasing pressure, either of which could relieve pain though by different mechanisms.

The extradural injection of a steroid for this purpose was first published by Lievere et al. (1953), and later Sehgal and Gardner (1960) reported the use of the subarachnoid route of injection. They subsequently showed that methylprednisolone suspension may persist in the lumbar subarachnoid space for 2 or 3 weeks after injection (Sehgal and Gardner, 1963). Steroid solutions probably assist healing of the inflamed nerve roots and reduce oedema by the anti-inflammatory effect of the steroid. Lindahl and Rexed (1951), who during laminectomy took biopsies of dorsal nerve roots affected by disc degeneration, found inflammatory changes in 70% of specimens.

The author has been using both types of agents since 1958 and has reported (Swerdlow and Sayle-Creer, 1970) a study in 325 patients suffering from lumbosciatic syndrome who received either saline, local anaesthetic or steroid by lumbar or sacral epidural routes.

Clinical

Extradural injection of local anaesthetic solution or more commonly of steroid has now become a widely used method in the treatment of lumbo-sciatic syndrome and wisely employed it can be both safe and valuable. It is best considered as one of a number of conservative measures (including bedrest, traction and postural advice) which might be helpful in acute and subacute episodes of back pain. Brown (1977) found that patients with discogenic disease of less than 3 months duration responded significantly better to epidural steroid than those with a longer duration of symptoms. It is important that before carrying out this form of treatment, the cause of the pain has been properly investigated to exclude the presence of spinal tumour or other space-occupying pathology and to ensure that a more appropriate form of treatment is not being neglected. The rationale should be explained simply to the patient and the possibility of complications enunciated.

The author prefers to perform the epidural injection into the lumbar (or cervical) epidural space at about the level of the painful dermatomes. The patient lies in the lateral lumbar puncture position with the painful side downwards and is maintained in this position for 5–10 min after the injection is completed. The dose given is 80 mg (2 ml) methylprednisolone acetate suspension in 4 ml 0.5% lignocaine. (The preparation should be shaken before injection.) The small volume results in the steroid being localized to the desired nerve roots and not widely dispersed in the epidural space, as would happen with a larger volume of solution. A further advantage of using such a small volume is that there is no appreciable motor or sympathetic block so that the procedure can safely be performed on an out-patient basis and the patient can be allowed to go home 1 h after treatment (provided accidental thecal puncture has not occurred).

Results

Immediate but transient pain relief occurs in most patients and is due to the local anaesthetic. A more long-lasting benefit does not usually become apparent until 2 or 3 days after the injection. Some patients are greatly helped, some experience partial or temporary relief and some do not benefit at all. If the injection produces only transient improvement, no further blocks are performed. If, however, improvement persists for 2 or 3 weeks and then starts to fade, a further epidural injection is then given.

There have now been a large number of clinical trials of the value of epidural injections for lumbo-sciatic pain relief. Miller et al. (1980) analysed the results obtained by ten different groups of workers and found that a mean of 62% (range 39–81%) of patients obtained complete or significant pain relief, that a large volume of local anaesthetic was no more effective than a large volume of saline and that steroid was more satisfactory than either. However, recent extensive reviews by Kepes and Duncalf (1985) and Benzon (1986) conclude that the value of the method has not been scientifically proved, although Benzon considers that the injection may be justified if there are signs and symptoms of nerve root irritation. Most studies have not included a control group. Of those that have, Dilke et al. (1973), Breivik et al. (1976) and Rogers et al. (1987) found that epidural local anaesthetic plus steroid gave significantly better results than local anaesthetic solution alone. However, Beliveau (1971), Snoek et al. (1977), Vent (1981) and Yates (1978) could find no significant difference.

Methylprednisolone acetate has been the steroid most commonly used but Delaney and his colleagues (1980) prefer to use triamcinalone as the steroid agent. They believe it remains in suspension longer than methylprednisolone and they administer 50 mg in 6 ml 1% lignocaine.

The results of a recent study (Delaney et al., 1980) suggest that local anaesthetic/steroid combinations do not cause significant damage to neural tissues when injected extradurally. A number of complications have been reported following subarachnoid injection, however, including conus medullaris syndrome, arachnoiditis and meningitis (Delaney et al., 1980). The subarachnoid route has been recommended for use if epidural injection is unsuccessful (Winnie et al., 1972). However, subarachnoid injection is thought to be no more successful than epidural (Abram, 1978). Intrathecal injection was also advocated by Goebert et al. (1961) and by Feldman and Behar (1961) for the relief of arachnoiditis, but intrathecal steroid has recently been indicted as a cause of arachnoiditis, probably due to the ethylene glycol used in depot steroid preparations. The subarachnoid route of administration of steroids is probably best avoided.

Other uses of extradural steroid

Epidural injection of steroid solution has recently been recommended for a number of conditions other than lumbo-sciatic syndrome.

Forrest (1980) reports the use of extradural injections of methylprednisolone in the treatment of 63 patients suffering from either chronic postherpetic or post-traumatic neuralgia. The patients were given three injections, at 1 week intervals, of 80 mg in 0.5–1 ml of 0.5% bupivacaine. One month after treatment, 56% of the postherpetic patients and 48% of the post-traumatic patients were pain-free. One year after treatment, 89% of postherpetics were pain-free, but only 59% of the post-traumatic patients. Lingenfelter (1981) advocates the use of extradural methylprednisolone for patients with pain due to degenerative arthritis of the spine and Dirksen et al. (1987) recommend its use in the treatment of reflex sympathetic dystrophy.

Intrathecal injection of methylprednisolone has been claimed to give relief of cancer pain for up to 3 months (Hatangdi et al., 1980) and extradural injection of local anaesthetic with long-acting steroid has also been found valuable (Melding, 1980).

INTRASPINAL NARCOTICS

A variety of narcotics have now been administered by both subarachnoid and extradural routes to provide pain relief, and in general, clinical reports have been favourable, at least in the short term, although the method is by no means uniformly successful, nor is it free from complications (Gustafsson et al., 1982). The subject is dealt with in Chapter 5.

Local anaesthetic epidural block

Bonica (1959) and Lund (1966) find that continuous epidural injection of local anaesthetic is especially useful in cases of postherpetic neuralgia, in post-toxic and neoplastic neuropathies, and in cases of severe peripheral nerve pain due to osteoarthritis, root sleeve fibrosis and other skeletal disorders. Bonica considers that continuous peridural block provides 'temporary relief, obviating the associated skeletal muscle spasm and sympathetic dysfunction, and permitting the use of traction and other physical therapeutic measures which otherwise would not be employed'. If, due to the condition of the patient or some other cause, the injection of a neurolytic agent is considered to be unwise, a temporary respite can be provided by repeated doses of a dilute solution of bupivacaine injected through a catheter. A polyvinyl catheter is inserted into the epidural space and efforts are made to get the tip of the catheter at about the middle of the painful segment. After ensuring that the catheter is extradural, 6–10 ml of dilute bupivacaine may be injected at intervals as required. It is advisable not to advance the catheter more than a few centimetres to avoid it becoming kinked and to avoid the possibility of tearing the peridural vessels which would result in haemorrhage, more rapid absorption, the possibility of toxic reactions, and the risk of failure of the block. Dogliotti and Ciocatto (1955) consider that by using continuous epidural injection of concentrated local anaesthetics for several days, a partial degeneration of sensory nerves is produced and a subsequent prolonged analgesia, even in patients with intractable pain from cancer. Bonica (1955) was unable to corroborate Dogliotti's and Ciocatto's results.

Finally, in terminal patients with widespread pain who are too ill for any other effective pain-relieving procedure, satisfactory analgesia can be achieved by intermittent injection of a dilute local anaesthetic solution through an epidural catheter. The use of a volumetric pump can be advantageous (Denson et al., 1982). The problems of tachyphylaxis may be reduced by the use of long-acting local anaesthetic agents.

COMPLICATIONS

The general complications of epidural injections have been fully detailed by Dawkins (1969) and Usubiaga (1975). Sequelae following specifically neurolytic epidural blocks are very unusual; backache is perhaps the commonest and is occasionally troublesome. Pitkin (1953) reported the occurrence of temporary paralysis of the bladder following injection of alcohol into the caudal epidural space and Grunwald (1975) noted that urinary incontinence occurred in about a quarter of the patients given epidural phenol. Muscular palsy has been described (Usubiaga, 1975) following lumbar epidural injection of both alcohol and phenol in the treatment of cancer pain; recovery began within 6 months. A more serious case has been reported recently where an epidural 'top-up' dose of local anaesthetic containing or contaminated by paraldehyde caused permanent tetraplegia (Swerdlow, 1982). Epidural injection of alcohol may also be followed by distressing neuritis. It is advisable not to perform extradural block in patients who are receiving anticoagulants because of the risk of extradural haematoma formation. Finally, the epidural administration of hypertonic saline has been the cause of permanent paraplegia (Usubiaga, 1975).

REFERENCES

Abram, S.E. (1978) Subarachnoid corticosteroid injection following inadequate response to epidural steroid for sciatica. *Anesth. Analg. Curr. Res.*, 57, 313–315.

Ahlgren, E.W., Stephen, C.R., Lloyd, E.A.C. and McCollum, D.E. (1966) Diagnosis of pain with a graduated spinal block technique. *J. Am. Med. Assoc.*, 195, 125–128.

Alexander, F.A.D. and Lewis, L.W. (1963) The control of pain. In: *Anesthesiology*. Editor: D.E. Hale. Blackwell, Oxford, p. 801.

Bates, E. and Judovich, B.D. (1942) Intractable pain. *Anesthesiology*, 3, 663.

Baxter, D.W. and Schacherl (1962) Experimental studies on the morphological changes produced by intrathecal phenol. *Can. Med. Assoc. J.*, 86, 1200.

Beliveau, P. (1971) A comparison between epidural anesthesia with and without corticosteroid in the treatment of sciatica. *Rheumatol. Phys. Med.*, 11, 40–43.

Benzon, H.T. (1986) Epidural steroid injections for low back pain and lumbosacral radiculopathy. *Pain*, 24, 277–295.

Berry, K. and Olszewski, J. (1963) Pathology of intrathecal phenol injection in man. *Neurology*, 13, 152.

Bonica, J.J. (1953) *Management of Pain*. Lea & Febiger, Philadelphia.

Bonica, J.J. (1955) Role of the anesthesiologist in the management of intractable pain. *Anesthesiology*, 16, 854.

Bonica, J.J. (1958) Diagnostic and therapeutic blocks: a reappraisal based on 15 years' experience. *Anesth. Analg. Curr. Res.*, 37, 58.

Bonica, J.J. (1959) *Clinical Applications of Diagnostic and Therapeutic Nerve Blocks*. Charles C. Thomas, Springfield.

Bonica, J.J. (1981) *Proc. International Seminar on Management of Superior Pulmonary Sulcus Syndrome, Stresa.*

Breivik, H., Hesla, P.E., Molnar, I. and Lind, B. (1976) Treatment of chronic low back pain and sciatica, comparison of caudal epidural injections of bupivacaine and methylprednisolone with bupivacaine followed by saline. *Advances in Pain Research Therapy, Vol. 1*. Editor: J.J. Bonica. Raven Press, New York, pp. 927–932.

Brown, F.W. (1977) Management of disogenic pain using epidural and intrathecal steroids. *Clin. Orthop.*, 129, 72–78.

Brown, A.S. (1958) Treatment of intractable pain by spinal carbolic acid. *Lancet*, 2, 975.

Charlton, J.E. (1986) Current views on the use of nerve blocking in the relief of chronic pain. In: *The Therapy of Pain*. Editor: M. Swerdlow. *2nd Edn.* pp. 133–164. M.T.P. Press, Lancaster.

Churcher, M. (1970) *Proc. Ann. Meeting Intractable Pain Society, Great Britain.*

Cole, R. (1965) The problem of pain in persistent cancer. *Med. J. Austr.*, 1, 682.

Coomes, E.N. (1961) A comparison between epidural anaesthesia and bed rest in sciatica. *Br. Med. J.*, 1, 20.

Corning, J.L. (1894) *Pain*. Lippincott, Philadelphia, p. 247.

Dawkins, M. (1963) Pain relief following the injection of oily solution of nupercaine and lignocaine into the peridural space. In: *Symposium on Treatment of Painful Syndrome by Nerve Block. Venice, 1963*. Editor: R. Rizzi. Consonni, Vicenza, p. 189.

Dawkins, C.J.M. (1969) An analysis of the complications of extradural and caudal block. *Anaesthesia*, 24, 554.

Delaney, T.J., Rowlingson, J.C., Carron, H. and Butler, A. (1980) Epidural steroid effects on nerves and meninges. *Anesth. Analg.*, 59, 610–614.

Denson, D.D., Thompson, G.A., Raj, P.P. et al. (1982) Continuous perineural infusions of bupivacaine for management of terminal cancer pain. *Anesthesiology*, 57, A215.

Derrick, W.S. (1966) Subarachnoid alcohol block for the control of intractable pain. *Acta Anaesth. Scand., Suppl.*, 24, 167.

Dilke, T.F.W., Burry, H.C. and Grahame, R. (1973) Extradural corticosteroid injection in management of lumbar nerve root compression. *Br. Med. J.*, 1, 635–637.

Dirksen, R., Rutgers, M.J. and Coolen, J.M.W. (1987) Cervical epidural steroids in reflex sympathetic dystrophy. *Anesthesiology*, 66, 71–73.

Dogliotti, A.M. (1931) Traitement des syndromes douloureux de la périphérie par l'alcoolisation subarachnoidienne. *Presse Med.*, 67, 11.

Dogliotti, A.M. and Ciocatto, E. (1955) Method of differential block in pain relief. *Anesthesiology*, 16, 623.

Doughty, A. (1972) In: *A Practice of Anaesthesia*. Editors: W.D. Wylie and H. Churchill Davidson. Lloyd Luke, London, p. 1099.

Evans, W. (1930) Intrasacral epidural injection in the treatment of sciatica. *Lancet*, 2, 1225.

Feldman, S. and Behar, A.J. (1961) Effect of intrathecal hydrocortisone on advanced adhesive arachnoiditis and C.S.F. pleocytosis. *Neurology*, 11, 251–256.

Finer, B. (1958) Epidural injection of carbolic acid in incurable cancer. *Lancet*, 2, 1179.

Flanigan, S. and Boop, W.C. (1974) Spinal intrathecal injection procedure in the management of pain. *Clin. Neurosurg.*, 21, 229.

Forrest, J.B. (1980) The response to epidural steroid injections in chronic dorsal root pain. *Can. Anaesth. Soc. J.*, 27, 40–46.

Gallagher, H.S., Yonezewa, T., Hay, R.C. and Derrick, W.S. (1961) Subarachnoid alcohol block. Histological changes in CNS. *Am. J. Pathol.*, 38, 679.

Gerbershagen, H.U. (1981) Subarachnoid neurolytic blockade. *Acta Anaesth. Belg.*, 1, 45–57.

Gilcreest, E.L. and Mullen, T.F. (1931) The epidural and trans-sacral injection of alcohol for the relief of pain. *Surg. Clin. North Am.*, 11, 989.

Gillman, J. (1972) Pain relief and other effects following barbotage. *Lancet*, 1, 746.

Goebert, H.W., Jallo, S.J., Gardner, W.J. and Wasmuth, C.E. (1961) Painful radiculopathy treated with epidural injections of procaine and hydrocortisone acetate: Results in 113 patients. *Anesth. Analg.*, 40, 130.

Gordon, R.A. and Goel, S.B. (1963) Intrathecal phenol block in treatment of intractable pain of malignant disease. *Can. Anaesth. Soc. J.*, 10, 357.

Greenhill, J.P. (1947) Sympathectomy and intraspinal alcohol injections for the relief of pelvic pain. *Br. Med. J.*, 2, 859.

Grunwald, I. (1976) Neurolise com fenol: Uso da via peridural no tratamento da dor de cancer. *Rev. Brasil de Anest.*, 26, 628.

Gustafsson, L.L., Schildt, B. and Jacobsen, K. (1982) Adverse effects of extradural and intrathecal opiates: Report of a nationwide survey in Sweden. *Br. J. Anaesth.*, 54, 479.

Guttman, S.A. and Pardee, I. (1944) Spinal cord level syndrome following intrathecal ammonium sulphate and procaine hydrochloride. A case report with autopsy findings. *Anesthesiology*, 5, 347.

Hand, L.V. (1944) Subarachnoid ammonium sulfate therapy for intractable pain. *Anesthesiology*, 5, 354.

Hansebout, R. and Cosgrove, J.B.R. (1966) Effects of intrathecal phenol in man – a histological study. *Neurology*, 16, 277.

Hatangdi, V.S., Melding, P.S., Boas, R.A. and Richards, E.G. (1980) Intrathecal methylprednisolone in relief of pain from the vertebral metastasis. *Anesth. Inten. Care*, 8, 370.

Hay, R.C. (1962) Subarachnoid alcohol block in the control of intractable pain. *Anesth. Analg. Curr. Res.*, 41, 12.

Hitchcock, E.R. (1967) Hypothermic subarachnoid irrigation for intractable pain. *Lancet*, 1, 1133.

Hitchcock, E.R. and Prandini, M.N. (1973) Hypertonic saline in management of intractable pain. *Lancet*, 1, 310.

Holland, A.J.C. and Yousseff, M. (1978) A complication of subarachnoid phenol blockade. *Anaesthesia*, 34, 260.

Howland, W.J., Curry, J.L. and Butler, A.K. (1963) Pantopaque arachnoiditis. Experimental study of blood as a potentiating agent. *Radiology*, 80, 489.

Hughes, J.T. (1966) Pathological findings following intrathecal injection of ethyl alcohol in man. *Paraplegia*, 4, 1671.

Hughes, J.T. (1970) Thrombosis of the posterior spinal arteries. *Neurology*, 20, 659.

Ichiyanagi, K., Matsuku, M., Kinefuchi, S. and Kato, Y. (1975) Progressive changes in the concentrations of phenol and glycerine in the human subarachnoid space. *Anesthesiology*, 42, 622.

Ischia, S., Luzzani, A., Ischia, A., Magon, F. and Toscano, D. (1984) Subarachnoid neurolytic block (L5-S1) and unilateral percutaneous cervical cordotomy in the treatment of pain secondary to pelvic malignant disease. *Pain*, 20, 139–147.

Jacobs, R.G. and Howland, W.S. (1966) A comparison of intrathecal alcohol and phenol. *J. Ky. Med. Assoc.*, 64, 408.

Judovich, B.D., Bates, W. and Bischop, K. (1944) Intraspinal ammonium salts for the intractable pain of malignancy. *Anesthesiology*, 5, 341.

Katz, J. (1970) Pain. Theory and management. In: *Scientific Foundations of Anaesthesia*. Editors: C. Scurr and S. Feldman. Heinemann, London.

Kenny, M. (1947) Relief of pain in intractable cancer of the pelvis. *Br. Med. J.*, 2, 862.

Kepes, E.R. and Duncalf, D. (1985) Treatment of backache with spinal injection of local anaesthetics. Spinal and systemic steroids; a review. *Pain*, 22, 33–47.

Khalili, A.A. and Ditzler, J.W. (1968) Neurolytic substances in the relief of pain. *Med. Clin. North Am.*, 52, 161.

Korevaar, W.C., Kline, M.T. and Donelly, C.C. (1987) Thoracic epidural neurolysis using alcohol. *Proc. 5th World Congress on Pain, Pain*, Suppl. 4, 133.

Kuzucu, E.Y., Derrick, W.S. and Wilber, S.A. (1966) Control of intractable pain with subarachnoid alcohol block. *J. Am. Med. Assoc.*, 195, 133.

Lievere, J.A., Block-Michel, H., Peas, G. and Uro, J. (1953) L'hydrocortisone en injection locale. *Rev. Rheum. Mal. Osteoartic.*, 20, 310.

Lifshitz, S., Debacker, L.J. and Buchsbaum, H.J. (1976) Subarachnoid phenol block for pain relief in gynecological malignancy. *Obstet. Gynecol.*, 48, 316.

Lindahl, O. and Rexed, B. (1951) Histologic changes in spinal root of operated cases of sciatica. *Acta Orthop. Scand.*, 20, 215.

Lingenfelter, R.W. (1981) Use of epidural steroids for treatment of arthritic pain. *Third World Pain Congress Abstracts, Pain*, Suppl. 1, 227.

Lipton, S. (1981) Intractable pain – the present position. *Ann. R. Coll. Surg.*, 63, 157.

Lourie, H. and Vanasupa, P. (1963) Comments on the use of intraspinal phenol-pantopaque for relief of pain and spasticity. *J. Neurosurg.*, 20, 60.

Lucas, J.T., Ducker, T.B. and Perot, P.L. (1975) Adverse reactions to intrathecal saline injection for control of pain. *J. Neurosurg.*, 42, 557.

Lund, P.C. (1966) *Peridural Analgesia and Anesthesia*. Charles C. Thomas, Springfield.

Madrid, J. (1975) In: *Proceedings of the First World Congress on Pain, Florence*.

Maher, R.M. (1955) Relief of pain in incurable cancer. *Lancet*, 1, 18.

Maher, R.M. (1957) Neurone selection in relief of pain. Further experiences with intrathecal injections. *Lancet*, 1, 16.

Maher, R.M. (1960) Further experiences with intrathecal and subdural phenol. Observations on two forms of pain. *Lancet*, 1, 895.

Maher, R.M. (1963) Intrathecal chlorocresol in the treatment of pain in cancer. *Lancet*, 1, 965.

Maher, R.M. and Mehta, M. (1977) Spinal and extradural analgesia. In: *Persistent Pain, Vol. 1.* Academic Press, London.

Marini, G. and Giunta, F. (1975) Phenol into posterior fossa for the treatment of facial and oral pain. In: *Proceedings of the First World Congress on Pain, Florence.*

Mathews, W.A. (1969) Neurolytic blocks in the management of pain. *Ariz. Med.*, 1050.

Matsuki, M., Kato, Y. and Ichiyanagi, K. (1971) Progressive changes in concentration of ethyl alcohol in the human and canine subarachnoid spaces. *Anesthesiology*, 36, 617.

Matthews, G.J., Ambruso, V.T. and Osterholm, J.L. (1970) Hypothermic hyperosmolar saline irrigation of cisterna magna: a new method for the relief of pain. *Surg. Forum*, 21, 445.

Mehta, M. (1973) *Intractable Pain.* Saunders, London.

Melding, P. (1980) The management of pelvic cancer pain. In: *Problems in Pain.* Editors: C. Beck and M. Wallace. Pergamon Press, Oxford, p. 253.

Miller, R.D., Munger, W.L. and Powell, P.E. (1980) Chronic pain and local anaesthetic neural blockade. In: *Neural Blockade.* Editors: M.J. Cousins and P.O. Bridenbaugh. Lippincott, Philadelphia, pp. 616–636.

Nathan, P.W. (1967) Control of pain. *Ann. R. Coll. Surg. Engl., Suppl.*, 82, 41.

Nathan, P.W. (1977) Emptying the paralysed bladder. *Lancet*, 1, 377.

Nathan, P.W. and Scott, T.G. (1958) Intrathecal phenol for intractable pain: safety and dangers of the method. *Lancet*, 1, 76.

Nathan, P.W., Sears, T.A. and Smith, M.C. (1965) Effects of phenol solutions on the nerve roots of the cat: an electrophysiological and histological study. *J. Neurol. Sci.*, 2, 7.

Nour-Eldin, F. (1970) Preliminary report: uptake of phenol by vascular and brain tissue. *Microvasc. Res.*, 2, 224.

Papo, I. and Visca, A. (1976) Intrathecal phenol in the treatment of pain and spasticity. *Prog. Neurol. Surg.*, 1, 56.

Papo, I. and Visca, A. (1979) Phenol subarachnoid rhizotomy for the treatment of cancer pain: A personal account of 290 cases. In: *Advances in Pain Research Therapy, Vol. 2.* Editors: J.J. Bonica and V. Ventafridda. pp. 339–346, Raven Press, New York.

Patterson and Marcello (1963) Quoted by Alexander and Lewis. In: *Anesthesiology.* Editor: D.E. Hale. Blackwell, Oxford, p. 801.

Pellegrini, G., Visca, A. and Papo, I. (1969) Considerazioni sul meccanismo di azione antalgico delle soluzione de fenolo intratecali. *Acta Neurol.*, 24, 85.

Peyton, W.T., Semansky, E.J. and Baker, A.B. (1937) Subarachnoid injection of alcohol for relief of intractable pain with discussion of cord changes found at autopsy. *Am. J. Cancer*, 30, 709.

Pitkin, G.P. (1953) *Conduction Anesthesia. 2nd Edn.* Lippincott, Philadelphia.

Porges, P. and Zdrahal, F. (1985) Die intrathekale Alkoholneurolyse der unteren sakralen Wurzeln beim inoperabelen Rectumkarzinom. *Anaesthesist*, 34, 627–629.

Racz, G.B., Heavner, J. and Haynsworth, R. (1985) Repeat epidural phenol injections in chronic pain and spasticity. In: *Persistent Pain, Vol. 5.* Editors: S. Lipton and J. Miles. Grune & Stratton, London.

Raftery, H. (1977) *Proceedings of Intractable Pain Society of Great Britain Annual Meeting, 1977.*

Robertson, D.H. (1985) Transsacral neurolytic nerve block. *Br. J. Anaesth.*, 55, 873–874.

Rogers, P., Schiller, D. and Nash, T.P. (1987) Personal Communication.

Schaumburg, H.H., Byck, R. and Weller, R.O. (1970) The effect of phenol on peripheral nerve. A histological and electrophysiological study. *J. Neuropath. Exp. Neurol.*, 29, 615.

Sechzer, P.H. (1963) Subdural space in spinal anesthesia. *Anesthesiology*, 24, 869.

Sehgal, A.D. and Gardner, W.J. (1960) Corticosteroids administered intradurally for relief of sciatica. *Cleveland Clin. Quart.*, 27, 198.

Sehgal, A.D. and Gardner, W.J. (1963) *Transact. Am. Neurolog. Assoc.*, 88, 275.

Sicard, M.A. (1901) Les injections médicamenteuses extradurales par voie sacro-coccygienne. *C.R. Soc. Biol. (Paris)*, 63, 396.

Simon. D.I., Carron, H. and Rowlingson, J.C. (1982) Treatment of bladder pain with transsacral nerve block. *Anesth. Analg.*, 61, 46.

Sloane, P. (1935) Syndrome referrable to the cauda equina following the intraspinal injection of alcohol for relief from pain. *Arch. Neurol. Psychiatry (Chicago)*, 34, 1120.

Smith, M.C. (1964) Histological findings following intrathecal injections of phenol solutions for relief of pain. *Br. J. Anaesth.*, 36, 387.

Snoek, W., Webber, H. and Jorgensen, B. (1977) Double blind evaluation of extradural corticosteroid methylprednisolone for herniated lumbar discs. *Acta Orthop. Scand.*, 48, 635–641.

Spaetz and Wegner (1963) Quoted by Alexander and Lewis. In: *Anesthesiology*. Editor: D.E. Hale. Blackwell, Oxford, p. 801.

Stern, E.L. (1937) Dangers of intraspinal (subarachnoid) injection of alcohol. Their avoidance and contra-indications. *Am. J. Surg.*, 45, 99.

Stovner, J. and Endresen, R. (1972) Intrathecal phenol for cancer pain. *Acta Anaesth. Scand.*, 16, 17.

Superville-Sovak, B., Rasminsky, M. and Finlayson, M.H. (1975) Complications of phenol neurolysis. *Arch. Neurol. (Chicago)*, 32, 226.

Swerdlow, M. (1963) In: *Symposium on Treatment of Painful Syndromes by Nerve Block. Venice, 1963*. Editor: R. Rizzi. Consonni, Vicencza, p. 174.

Swerdlow, M. (1967) Four years' pain clinic experience. *Anaesthesia*, 22, 568.

Swerdlow, M. (1968) The relief of intractable pain. In: *Proceedings of the Fourth World Congress Anaesthesiologists*. ICS No. 200. Excerpta Medica, Amsterdam, p. 270.

Swerdlow, M. (1975) In: *Proceedings of the First World Congress International Association Study of Pain, Florence*.

Swerdlow, M. (1978) In: *Complications of Neurolytic Blocks in Neural Blockade*. Editors: M.J. Cousins and P.O. Bridenbaugh. Lippincott, Philadelphia.

Swerdlow, M. (1979) Subarachnoid and extradural neurolytic blocks. In: *Advances in Pain Research and Therapy, Vol. 2*. Editors: J.J. Bonica and V. Ventafridda. Raven Press, New York, pp. 325–339.

Swerdlow, M. (1981) Spinal and peripheral neurolysis in relief of Pancoast Syndrome. *Proceedings of the International Seminar on Management of Superior Pulmonary Stress Syndrome, Stresa*.

Swerdlow, M. (1982) Medico-legal aspects of complications following pain relieving blocks. *Pain*, 13, 321.

Swerdlow, M. (1988) The history of neurolytic block. In: *Techniques of Neurolysis*. Editor: G.B. Racz. Nijhoff Publishing, New York.

Swerdlow, M. and Cockings, E.C. (1958) Pethidine and promazine supplementation of regional analgesia. *Br. J. Anaesth.*, 30, 375.

Swerdlow, M. and Sayle-Creer, W. (1970) The use of extradural injections in the relief of lumbosciatic pain. *Anaesthesia*, 25, 128.

Teevens, W.P. (1948) Relief of sciatica, in carcinoma of the prostate, by proctocaine. *Can. Med. J.*, 58, 384.

Totoki, T., Kato, T., Nomoto, Y., Kurakazu, M. and Kanaseki, T. (1979) Anterior spinal artery syndrome – a complication of cervical intrathecal phenol injection. *Pain*, 6, 99.

Tuffier, M.P. (1899) Analgésie chirurgicale par l'injection sous-arachnoidienne lombaire de cocaine. *C.R. Soc. Biol. (Paris)*, 51, 882.

Tureen, L.L. and Gitt, J.J. (1936) Cauda equina syndrome following subarachnoid injection of alcohol. *J. Am. Med. Assoc.*, 106, 18.

Usubiaga, J.E. (1975) *Neurological Complications Following Epidural Anesthesia*. Little, Brown, Boston.

Vent, J. (1981) Prospective randomized study on influencing complaints, following discotomy by intraoperative application of cortisone via intrathecal and peridural injection. *Z. Orthop.*, 119, 284–286.

Ventafridda, V. and Martino, G. (1976) Observations on the relationships between plasma concentration and analgesic activity of a soluble acetylsalicylic acid derivative after intravenous administration in man. In: *Advances in Pain Research and Therapy, Vol. 1*. Editors: J.J. Bonica and D. Albe-Fessard, pp. 529–536. Raven Press, New York.

Viner, N. (1925) Intractable sciatica – the sacral epidural injection – an effective method of giving relief. *Can. Med. Assoc. J.*, 15, 630.

White, J.C. and Sweet, W.H. (1969) *Pain and the Neurosurgeon*. Charles C. Thomas, Springfield.

Wilkinson, H.A., Mark, V.H. and White, J.C. (1964) Further experiences with intrathecal phenol for the relief of pain. *J. Chron. Dis.*, 17, 1055.

Winnie, A.P. and Collins, V.J. (1968) Differential neural blockade in pain syndromes of questionable etiology. *Med. Clin. N. Am.*, 52, 123.

Winnie, A.P., Hartman, J.T. and Myers, H.L. (1972) Pain Clinic II. Intradural and extradural corticosteroids for sciatica. *Anesth. Analg. (Cleveland)*, 51, 990.

Wolman, L. (1966) The neuropathological effects resulting from the intrathecal injection of chemical substances. *Paraplegia*, 4, 97.

Woodbridge, P.D. (1930) Therapeutic nerve block with procaine and alcohol. *Am. J. Surg.*, 9, 278.

Yates, D.W. (1978) A comparison of the types of epidural injection commonly used in the treatment of low back pain and sciatica. *Rheumatol. Rehab.*, 17, 181–186.

M. Swerdlow and J.E. Charlton (eds.) Relief of Intractable Pain
© 1989, Elsevier Science Publishers B.V. (Biomedical Division)

9

The sympathetic nervous system and pain relief

Robert A. Boas

There exists, both in the literature and in established clinics, a well-founded basis for the use of sympathetic blocks in the treatment of many specific pain disorders. Authoritative texts are available covering applied anatomy of the sympathetic system (Pick, 1970); excellent clinical descriptions of disease states and how blocks should be applied to their treatment (Bonica, 1953) and specialist procedure monographs (Moore, 1954, 1965) now serve as classics in the subject. Many subsequent publications have added new methods and given results of extensive case studies (Reid et al., 1970; Hannington-Kiff, 1974; Cousins et al., 1979), while a spate of recent review chapters in special texts or monographs (Challenger, 1978; Boas, 1978; Bonica, 1980, 1981; Löfström et al., 1980) have rapidly disseminated and consolidated advances in techniques and our understanding of sympathetic dysfunction. This chapter assumes that the history and detail of these papers are accepted and seeks to extend discussion into areas of current advances in neurophysiology, neurochemistry, technical precision and case series, with particular application in management of the commoner chronic pain problems. There is little doubt that further rapid strides will be made, especially in areas of neurochemical change related to specific disorders.

Despite many recent developments, it is perhaps surprising to note the restraint still evident in extending well established procedures such as chemical sympathectomies into more widespread use. In part, this may be due to a failure of our teaching system in offering only limited didactic instruction and opportunity for special training, as well as reflecting carry over attitudes of speciality boundaries and levels of responsibility. Some centres have limitations on medical staff, so that those already committed to ongoing service needs are not logistically able to undertake long-term clinical pain service care as an additional responsibility. There is no doubt as to the daunting challenge of providing a full spectrum of treatment options for the care of chronic pain patients if a proper facility is to be maintained and recognized. Without well-integrated therapeutic options, the complexity and diversity of disease presentations would inevitably reduce a singular block service to an empirical, technical, subservient role from which patients receive only limited benefit and for which staff committment and continuity is difficult to sustain. While there seems little need to still justify the establishment of a pain service for the general hospital and community, there is little doubt that the application of sympathetic blocks provides one of the major benefits accruing from such a service. These techniques offer great benefit to the patient at minimal cost and negligible risk. Sympathetic blockade is effectively directed to relief of vasospastic and post-traumatic pain syndromes of upper and lower limbs and provides the definitive treatment of visceral pain of malignancy in the upper abdomen, while chemical lumbar sympathetic block has improved to such an extent that it now provides the best approach to permanent sympathectomy.

PAIN AND THE SYMPATHETIC NERVOUS SYSTEM

Autonomic function is served by sympathetic preganglionic fibres extending from the thoracolumbar sympathetic outflow with wide visceral and somatic ramifications. Parasympathetic neurones with long preganglionic fibres extend to synapse at visceral end organs, but common to all classes of these nerve fibres is the manner by which they exert their effector actions through release of catecholamines or acetylcholine. Afferent transmission of nociceptive impulses giving dull, aching, diffuse pains is via unmyelinated fibres travelling with splanchnic or somatic nerves from vessels and viscera. Pick (1970) has provided extensive anatomical detail on this system though only recently has information been forthcoming from Cervero (1982) on the receptor system involved in the visceral transmission of stimuli. The neurochemistry of activation and central transmission of this visceral nociception is eagerly awaited as this is likely to provide a key to further understanding and treatment of sympathetic pain. Visceral afferent termination in the spinal cord and the phenomenon of viscerosomatic convergence has detailed the processes of referred pain phenomena (Milne et al., 1981), while also offering models for further investigation. Convergence is probably at lamina VII and VIII levels in the spinal cord (Bowsher, 1978) in immediate proximity to the lateral horn subserving sympathetic neurones. Dysfunctional states of hyperactivity derived from activity at this dorsal horn level may be the origin of many of the bizarre changes observed from dissemination of neuronal hyperactivity in central pain states. As presented by Loh et al. (1981), the peripheral sympathetic manifestations of these pains can be ameliorated by chemical or pharmacological block of the peripheral fibres giving short-term clinical relief, even though the lesion remains in the central nervous system. However, the overwhelming failure of peripheral neuroablative measures to yield permanent relief after initial good results with block procedures in 100 consecutive cases reported by Tasker et al. (1980) is stark testimony to the failure of measures directed solely to conduction mechanisms in dealing with processes having a major central nervous component. Whatever the central component in pains of thalamic syndrome, phantom limb, etc., with major sympathetic dysfunction as part of the presentation, whether it be a primary local discharge focus in the CNS, or derived from reentry type phenomena or internal reverberating circuits or aberrations of neurotransmitters, it cannot be 'cut out' or 'blocked out' with peripheral procedures. On the other hand, disorders of tissue injury involving peripheral nerves or joints with sustained nociceptive input are a critical element as reviewed by Bonica (1979) in the development of all sympathetic dystrophies such as causalgia or Sudeck's atrophy, etc. These disorders respond quickly and dramatically to peripheral interruption of the efferent sympathetic response but to remain effective treatment must also be directed to resolution of the somatic disorder as well, or the pain syndrome will again return. The neurochemical abnormality mediating the hyperaesthetic peripheral response was shown by Wall and Gutnick (1974) to be an increased release of noradrenaline, which lowered the threshold to nociceptive stimulation in damaged nerves or neuroma sprouts. Further support for this is derived from the relief of pain and sympathetic hyperactivity obtained by block of noradrenaline with regional guanethine, reserpine or prazosin (Hannington-Kiff, 1974, 1979; Benzon et al., 1980; Abram and Lightfoot, 1981).

It would seem from these findings that sympathetic pain, bearing the stigmata of burning dysaesthetic pain and hyperaesthesia, plus trophic and vasomotor disturbances, requires the following sequence. Initially, there needs to be a somatic or centrally derived nociceptive input to a spinal level, a hyperactivity state to be activated at this level, then an efferent response derived from this level which leads to increased noradrenaline release at the periphery. This noradrenergic activity is diffuse, affecting the entire limb or body quadrant because of the diffuse segmental derivation of this response. However, the critical element in sustaining or aggravating the syndrome is the action of peripheral somatic disease to lower the threshold to stimulation in damaged nerve fibres, such that benign stimuli are perceived as being noxious. When vasospastic responses and motor dysfunction produce regional ischaemia and nutritional losses leading to further somatic damage, a sequence of changes is activated to sustain and extend a vicious cycle thus producing the full syndrome of a sympathetic dystrophy. Advances in understanding these processes have improved the rationality and methodology of treatment for such disorders, providing several clinical objectives for sympathetic blockade, as shown in Table 9.1. The common therapeutic aim of these treatments is both to block the peripheral efferent noradrenaline-mediated responses and to stop affe-

TABLE 9.1

Clinical objectives of sympathetic blockade

---

1. Sympathetic dystrophy
   (a) diagnostic confirmation
   (b) treatment

2. Blood flow improvement
   (a) vasospastic disorders
   (b) acute cold, trauma, thromboembolic ischaemia
   (c) post-surgical vasodilation
   (d) arteriosclerotic disease

3. Visceral pain
   (a) diagnosis
   (b) long-term treatment

4. Differential diagnosis
   (a) sympathetic pain vs. peripheral neuralgia
   (b) somatic vs. visceral pain

5. Hyperhydrosis and herpes zoster – treatment

---

rent nociceptive entry to the spinal cord. Future treatments are likely to be directed at inhibition of the central spinal mediation of both these processes as well.

CONDITIONS AMENABLE TO TREATMENT

Peripheral vascular disease

Permanent neurolytic sympathectomy is the treatment of choice when ischaemic arteriosclerotic disease of the legs is not amenable to surgery. In a local experience of 600 patients who received lumbar sympathetic block, 500 (80%) were suffering from some form of arteriosclerotic induced ischaemia. Foot rest pain was the dominant clinical presentation in 68% of these cases. Intermittent claudication was present in 40% of all cases as an added component to their symptomatic presentation, but was not accepted as a primary disorder for treatment. Ulceration was present in 39% of referrals, gangrene in 15% and pregangrenous changes in 7% of the patient group, with many patients having more than one complaint. This distribution does not accurately represent the spectrum of peripheral arterial disease as the selection is biased in favour of conditions caused by superficial vessel disease, this group being more likely to respond to sympathectomy. At follow-up, two-thirds of this group had resolution of their ischaemic changes, rest pain showing the best improvement, while small vessel disease from diabetic arteriosclerosis showed poor improvement compared to those with proximal vessel involvement. Patients with deep vessel disease causing claudication showed improvement in only 30% of cases. This benefit may have come not from sympathectomy but from the slow improvement evident in the natural history of the disease as collateral circulation is developed (Fyfe and Quinn, 1975). In this group, no clinical evidence was found for a steal response, whereby blood flow is diverted from deep to more dilated superficial vessels. However, crossover response was observed in many patients with a moderate contralateral temperature rise on the side opposite to that blocked.

The response to sympathetic block for treatment of other small vessel diseases such as thromboangiitis obliterans and Raynaud's phenomenon was initially good but not sustained beyond a few weeks or months at most. Erythromyalgia must be considered a contraindication based on our results, with over half (five of nine cases) having increased burning pain after sympathectomy.

The benefits of improved blood flow (100% mean increase overall in the 500 arteriosclerotic group) decline rapidly to a 50% increase from pretreatment flows over the next month and are lost completely at 6 months. Fortunately, this is usually sufficient to resolve local ischaemic changes and allow collaterals to develop, so sustaining clinical improvement. In some cases, sympathectomy block was used as an adjunct to subsequent arterial graft surgery 1 or 2 days before operation to improve runoff, giving better graft patency and clinical resolution as described by Cousins and Wright (1971).

Sympathetic dystrophies and vasospastic ischaemic disease

All of the sympathetic dystrophies, vasospastic disorders, cold injury, thromboembolic disease (without gangrene) and post-traumatic ischaemic states, affecting the upper or lower limbs, respond dramatically to sympathetic block or pharmacological sympathectomy. Blood flows of up to 3-times pretreatment levels can be obtained in some cases and one block sometimes produces an immediate and total clinical resolution. This same group also responds to repeat TNS or acupuncture stimulation, while the Raynaud's patients may improve to a lesser extent with temperature biofeedback therapy. While these disorders make up only 5% of our current clinic case load for sympathetic block, they provide a formidable challenge in both diagnosis and management. The diagnosis of sympathetic dystrophy is dependent on the identification of a specific precipitating factor plus a minimum of three features, additional to the burning dysaesthetic pains and hyperaesthesia, these being temperature, colour, swelling, sweating, trophic, bony, sensory or motor change in the involved limb. Many of these responses may accompany central neuralgic disorders which may manifest with features mimicking a sympathetic dystrophy. In these cases, when the abnormal efferent response is derived from a central neuralgic syndrome, sympathectomy almost never provides sustained benefit. In fact, these are the patients who have shown some of the more intractable forms of post-sympathectomy dysaesthesia. Tabetic pain, thalamic pain, phantom pains and post-denervation neuralgias are examples of central neuralgias which do not respond on a lasting basis to neurolytic sympathectomies as primary treatment, though temporary symptomatic relief is obtained.

Distinction of central pain from peripheral neuralgic disorders as the underlying disorder can be gained from the response to intravenous lignocaine. A dose of 1.5 mg/kg will suppress the pain of central origin, yet cause little suppression of peripheral pain (Boas et al., 1982).

The treatment of patients with sympathetic dystrophies and vasospastic ischaemias is more difficult than treating those with arteriosclerotic disease. Not only is the diagnosis less absolute but in addition the treatment frequently demands continuing use of temporary blocks or pharmacological interruption rather than permanent sympathectomy. Preference to intravenous guanethidine block on a once to twice weekly basis has greatly simplified this aspect of care. The out-patient visits for these injections are further used to promote increasing exercise therapy and functional activity of the involved limb, together with treatment directed to management of any underlying musculoskeletal or neurological disorder which has almost invariably initiated the dystrophic response. The benefits of sympathetic block may be as great in allowing these other treatments to proceed expeditiously and effectively as in breaking the efferent response in itself. Where neither local anaesthetic nor pharmacological sympathetic block can be employed or where logistical problems reduce the opportunity for out-patient visits, patients can direct their own care with transcutaneous electrical stimulation therapy and physiotherapy, given a good set of instructions and followed by telephone contact. Somewhat empirically four electrodes are applied, two proximally at the appropriate paravertebral level, one at the axilla or groin and one distally about the foot or hand, using low frequency stimulation for 0.5–1 h periods three or four times daily together with exercises and anti-inflammatory or other analgesics.

Recurrent seasonal ischaemic conditions such as those seen with Raynaud's disease are best treated with intravenous regional guanethidine on a demand basis while acute ischaemic lesions such as frostbite, thrombo embolic disease or traumatic/surgical insufficiency may be best treated with sympathetic ganglion block. This, too, is likely to change as drugs such as Ketanserin, a 5HT peripheral blocker, are applied in wider practice giving increasing specificity to treatment of the aetiological processes.

Malignancy

When analgesic drugs fail to provide adequate relief or cause profound side effects in the treatment of visceral cancer pain, the use of neurolytic blocks is an effective alternative to treatment. Tumours of the upper abdomen frequently cause severe pain and are readily managed with splanchnic/coeliac block giving good results with minimal morbidity. The separation of somatic from sympathetic fibres within the abdomen is a critical anatomical distinction. Selective block at this level confers major advantages over intrathecal neurolytic injection, which carries risks of sensory, sphincter and motor block. Carcinoma of the pancreas in particular is probably best managed with splanchnic block giving upwards of 80% relief, though tumour extension into the posterior abdominal wall is a limiting factor in this response. When tumour of other organs or paravertebral lymphatic spread invades vessels or the coeliac plexus, or causes obstruction to a hollow viscus, visceral deafferentation will again give relief of much of the pain. Breakthrough arises when parasympathetic vagal fibres provide an alternative nociceptive pathway or when somatic structures are also involved. Pelvic pain not relieved with sacral block can be helped with coeliac and L_1 lumbar sympathetic block as these levels contribute to the hypogastric plexus. Elsewhere, sympathetic blocks are of little benefit in treatment of the pain of malignancy unless a major sympathetic component is present, such as occurs when tumour invades peripheral nerves.

At best, these blocks confer relief for weeks to a few months duration, often requiring both supplementary analgesics and repeat blocks, so that they are not advocated for long-term or non-malignant conditions.

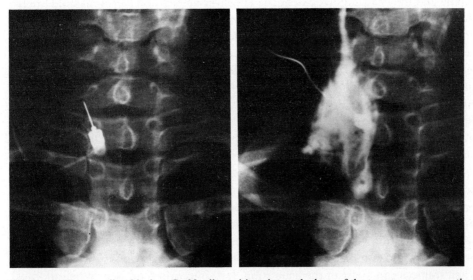

Fig. 9.1. Stellate ganglion block at C_7. Needle positioned over the base of the transverse process, then withdrawn 3–4 mm to lie in the prevertebral fascia, using an extension line to aid needle stability. Solution spread with 10 ml of contrast medium (Conray 420) shows a typical pre-fascial compartment spread from C_6 to T_2 with the rounded inferolateral border formed by the pleural dome.

Other disorders

Historically, sympathetic block has been used in a wide variety of visceral and so-matic pain complaints. However, its use in the treatment of common problems such as ischaemic cardiac pain has now been superseded by drug treatment and surgery. Sympathetic block for acute Herpes Zoster pain has been advocated by many, though it has not yet been proved to reduce the incidence of postherpetic neuralgia. Neither is sympathetic block effective in long-term treatment of post-herpetic or other neuralgias, where antiepileptic and psychotropic drugs are the treatment of choice. Hyperhydrosis without pain or trophic changes does respond well to sympathetic block and has been treated effectively with chemical lumbar sympathectomy. This has not been extended to the stellate ganglion, where a sur-gical ablation is recommended because of greater risk at this site with neurolytic solutions.

TECHNIQUES

Stellate ganglion block

The best approach to the stellate ganglion is the anterior one with the patient lying supine and the head slightly extended. The large vessels and sternomastoid are re-tracted slightly laterally by firm downward pressure with the index and middle fingers of the left hand alongside the trachea, with the lower finger just above the head of the clavicle. A 5–6 cm 22G needle is inserted through a local anaesthetic infiltration in the skin between the index and middle fingers about 3 cm from the clavicle. While maintaining pressure with the left hand the needle is advanced at 90° to the skin surface alongside the trachea until the needle tip touches the trans-verse process of the 7th cervical vertebra close to its junction with the body, as shown in Fig. 9.1. The needle is then withdrawn about 3 mm to lie in the preverte-bral fascia and after a negative aspiration a dose of about 10 ml of 1% lignocaine or 0.25% bupivacaine is ready to be injected. Two manoeuvres can stabilize the needle at this point to maintain correct positioning. One is to hold the needle hub between thumb and index fingers of the left hand, the other is to attach an in-travenous extension line between needle and syringe as described by Winnie (1969). In addition to added needle stability, these measures allow for easy aspira-tion testing and use of test doses, as well as serving as an aid during teaching when trainees can assist in the aspiration, test, injection sequence. When thoracic ganglia are sought to provide greater block to the arm, doses of 10 ml are needed, and while most texts advocate sitting the patient up immediately after injection, dye studies do not demonstrate any facilitation of downward spread with this move. The distribution of 10 ml of radio opaque dye correctly placed using this method is also shown in Fig. 9.1.

The classical monograph by Moore (1954) suggests the stellate approach at a C_6 level is the easier landmark with lesser risk of pneumothorax and vertebral artery puncture. However, with this method, the block of thoracic components to sympathetic supply of the arm is more frequently missed unless large volumes are used. This increases the risk of inadvertent spread to include the opposite side or the recurrent laryngeal nerve. When assessing the response to the block it should be recognized that Horner's syndrome merely indicates block of cervical sympathetics, while changes of warming, vasodilation, loss of sweating and subjective change in the hand more accurately denote block of sympathetics to the arm. As nearly all stellate blocks are performed for disorders of the upper limb, it is recommended that one or more pre- and post-block measurements of either skin temperature, blood flow, cold pressor responses, sweating tests, electrical skin resistance or sympathogalvanic reflex responses be used to confirm an appropriate block. This adds qualitative and quantitative response data to the procedure giving valuable measures of prognostic, therapeutic and comparative worth.

Minimizing complications with careful technique is the basis of good practice. Accurate needle placement, pre-injection aspiration and use of test doses will ensure that the incidence of complications will be so low as to be negligible. Vasovagal attacks can occur directly consequent to needle insertion, complemented to an extent by block of cardiac sympathetics, but these responses are readily treated with atropine and should pose no serious hazard. Recurrent laryngeal nerve block is the most frequent inadvertent response resulting from solution spread to a more superficial plane. A hoarse voice and some loss of laryngeal protection occurs so this block is not advised as a concurrent bilateral procedure. Patients should be forewarned of possible hoarseness and the need to avoid food and drink until the effect wanes. Less frequently, lateral spread to the brachial plexus or medial spread in the pre-vertebral fascia to the opposite side will result in anaesthesia to the arm or bilateral sympathetic block. Neither carries risk when consequent to injection with local anaesthetic drugs. Bleeding causing a major haematoma is always possible, especially if coagulation defects are present. More serious complications unfortunately do occur, if only rarely, and may follow inadvertent vertebral artery injection (Korevaar et al., 1979), accidental spinal anaesthesia after injection into a root sleeve extension of the dural sac, pneumothorax following needling through the dome of the pleura or even a pneumochylothorax (Thompson et al., 1981) when the thoracic duct and pleura have been perforated during needling. Each of these potential emergencies demands the availability of full resuscitative measures immediately on hand whenever a stellate or other sympathetic block is performed, no matter how quickly or easily the block may be performed. The simplicity of the technique belies its hazardous potential.

Splanchnic nerve/coeliac plexus block

In recent years, the techniques for performing coeliac plexus block have been called to question. The points at issue are the anatomical variability of the coeliac plexus (Ward, 1979), the lack of precision of needle placement (Singler, 1982) and unpredictable radio opaque solution spread (Boas, 1978), when using the classical techniques of Bonica (1953) and Moore (1965). Moore et al. (1981) subsequently verified these findings supported further by Singler (1982) using C.T. scanning to give three-dimensional visualization of contrast media dispersement. An approach to overcome this limitation was the development of a splanchnic block technique which sought to place solution dorsal rather than ventral to the diaphragmatic crura. This distinction has major advantages of true compartmental spread giving precision, safety and greater comfort during injection. It is now our preferential technique for neurolytic block, especially when tumour or previous surgery has caused loss of anatomical integrity. Critical to the safety of this approach is the use of direct visualization under fluoroscopic control, for both needle placement and solution spread. However, where needling is done using landmarks and needle depths without radiological control, the safest technique remains the classical approach.

The anatomy for splanchnic nerve block is depicted in Fig. 9.2. The retrocrural compartment is well confined, lying in a narrow plane formed between the pleura and vertebra, bounded anteriorly by each crus of the diaphragm and posteriorly by the fibrous pleural attachment to the posteromedial aspect of each vertebral body and annulus fibrosis. Needle entry is made on either side just lateral to the tip of the L_1 transverse process just beneath the twelfth rib margin with only a slight medial and cephalad angulation during insertion until the lateral edge of

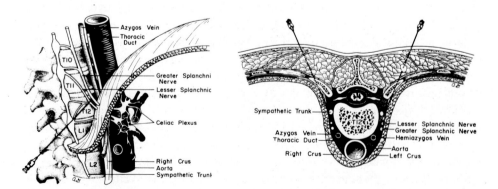

Fig. 9.2. Splanchnic nerve blocks showing anatomy of the splanchnic nerves in the retrocrural compartment where they lie in close proximity alongside the body of T_{12}. Note symmetrical needle placement and critical position abutting the vertebral body at its anterolateral edge.

the body of T_{12} is contacted, as in Figs. 9.2 and 9.3. At this level, the needle is 0.5 cm dorsal to the edge of the vertebra behind the diaphragm and two segments below the lower limits of the lung. Asymmetry of entry is not required with this method, the two or three splanchnic nerves being together and symmetrical at this point as they convene behind the crura just before piercing them to enter the retroperitoneal tissues and form the coeliac plexus as depicted in Fig. 9.2. The confinement of dye spread within the retrocrural compartment is shown in Fig. 9.4. following bilateral injection of 10 ml of 7% phenol in Conray 420. There are no other vital structures within this compartment, though needle insertion shallower by 1–1.5 cm could readily cause segmental somatic nerve block or spinal/epidural injection producing paraplegia. In a total of 20 such injections, we have seen no neurological sequelae, but have achieved about 75% success in relieving pain of pancreatic carcinoma. The failures may be due to tumour erosion into the dorsal retroperitoneal tissues or afferent nociceptive transmission in vagal fibres.

The asymmetrical approach to coeliac plexus block as described by Singler (1982) is shown in Fig. 9.5, with the left needle more vertically placed, but using the same landmarks as for a classical approach or a splanchnic nerve block. This more vertical inclination avoids penetration of the aorta and gives improved solution spread.

Whatever the approach, hypotension is the invariable consequence of these blocks, requiring 1000–1500 ml of crystalloid infusion as a precautionary antecedent to the block. Blood pressures can usually be maintained with the patient lying flat, but full supportive measures must be at hand. Hiccoughs or pleuritic irritation have occurred temporarily with splanchnic or coeliac injection, and although neurolytic solution about the great vessels might seem a risk factor with potential for erosion of a vessel wall, no cases of haemorrhage or thrombosis have been

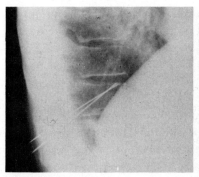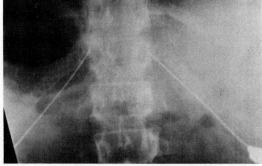

Fig. 9.3. Splanchnic nerve block radiographs showing lateral and A-P projections of needle positions. Note the diaphragm forming an anterior dome and the absence of lung tissue in the vicinity of the retrocrural compartment.

270

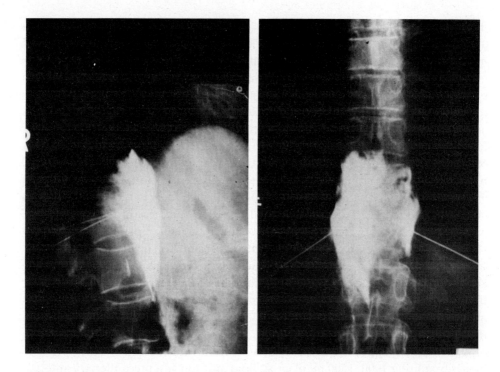

Fig. 9.4. Splanchnic nerve block radiographs showing the compartmental spread of bilateral 10 ml injections of phenol 7% in Conray 420. Spread is limited ventrally and inferiorly by the diaphragmatic crura with free movement rostrally. Solution does not spread dorsally beyond the mid portion of the vertebral body.

observed. As with lumbar sympathectomy, somatic nerve block or spinal injection are possibilities but the utilization of direct fluoroscopy virtually precludes this happening in practice. Splanchnic block provides a further example of the specificity and safety of ablative sympathetic block at compartmental sites where there is well-defined anatomical separation of the somatic and sympathetic nerve fibres.

Lumbar sympathetic block

Neurolytic lumbar sympathectomy for occlusive vascular disease is an under-utilized procedure in most medical centres. Though many reports attest to its safety (no mortality and little morbidity), simplicity, efficacy and outstanding cost benefits when compared with a surgical alternative, only a few centres have established lumbar sympathectomy via the percutaneous chemical approach as a routine procedure. The studies of Löfström (1969) and Reid et al. (1970), with further important contributions by Cousins and Wright (1971), Cousins et al. (1979) and Löf-

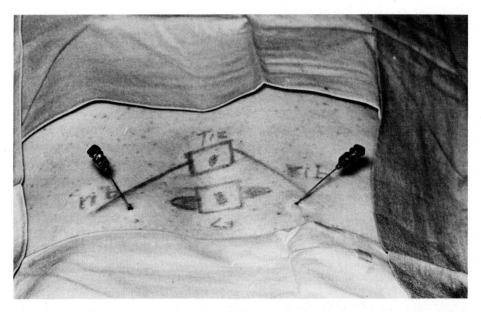

Fig. 9.5. Coeliac plexus block showing entry levels at the lateral edge of the L_1 transverse processes beneath the lower edge of the twelfth rib. The left needle is slightly more vertical than the right so that it will glance by the side of the aorta to lie just ventral to it in the retroperitoneal space at the level of the coeliac axis.

ström et al. (1980), have consolidated the place of chemical lumbar sympathectomy in the treatment of ischaemic disease of the legs. Using phenol in x-ray contrast solutions, we reported an improved direct visualization of needle placement and solution dispersement under fluoroscopic control, using a two-needle technique at L_3 and L_4 levels (Boas et al., 1976). After 600 cases, the technique has again been modified to a single needle fluoroscopic approach. Consideration of the lumbar sympathetic chain anatomy suggested that since all lumbar sympathetic fibres pass through or synapse at the L_2 ganglion level and most pass through L_3, a block of the chain at either of these levels should abolish nearly all sympathetic supply to and from the lower limb. An analysis of almost 200 cases having singular injections at either L_2 or L_3 showed no difference in short- or long-term responses when compared with two- or three-needle techniques for the same procedure. On this basis, a single-needle neurolytic block is now recommended for all but those patients with extensive degenerative bony changes or locally destructive lesions, where accurate needle placement and solution spread is hard to attain.

The approach as depicted in Fig. 9.6 employs a one-needle insertion 8–10 cm lateral to the midline, advancing the needle medially to glance off the anteromedial

CHEMICAL LUMBAR SYMPATHECTOMY

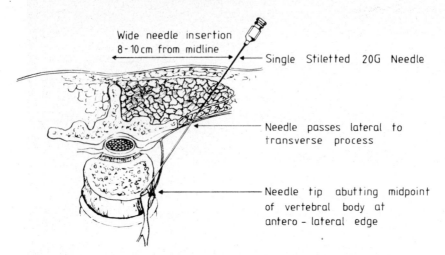

Wide needle insertion
8 - 10 cm from midline

Single Stiletted 20G Needle

Needle passes lateral to
transverse process

Needle tip abutting midpoint
of vertebral body at
antero - lateral edge

Fig. 9.6. Lumbar sympathetic block anatomy. The single needle wide entry approach at the L_2 or L_3 level avoids the transverse process, usually missing the segmental nerve, to bring the needle point to the mid-front level of the vertebral body.

edge of the midpoint of the vertebral body. This critical medial position of the needle tip should be 0.5 cm within the lateral edge of the vertebra when viewed in the A.P. projection and at the anterior edge of the body in a lateral view. The one-needle method usually requires 10 ml of 7% phenol in Conray 420 solutions to give a longitudinal spread to adjacent vertebra in a narrow prevertebral plane containing the sympathetic ganglia and fibres in the anterolateral quadrant of the prevertebral fascia (Fig. 9.7). Direct visualization under fluoroscopic control is quick with a cumulative 1.5–2 min of screening time, which above all, ensures that the solution is correctly dispersed in the appropriate anatomical plane. Even with seemingly correct needle placement, perhaps 10% of cases require repositioning of the needle when the solution is seen to be in a vessel or incorrect plane. With this control, there has not been a single case of inadvertent somatic block or functional morbidity of any note in the 600 sympathectomies performed to date. Failure to employ fluoroscopic control would seem to invite misplaced solution spread in a significant proportion of cases leading to a failure of therapeutic outcome and exposing the patient to potential risk from inadvertent spread to other nerves or structures.

The immediate post-block measurements of sympathetic block in 500 patients with arteriosclerotic disease is shown in Table 9.2 derived from a study which also included detailed flow responses on 25 of these cases.

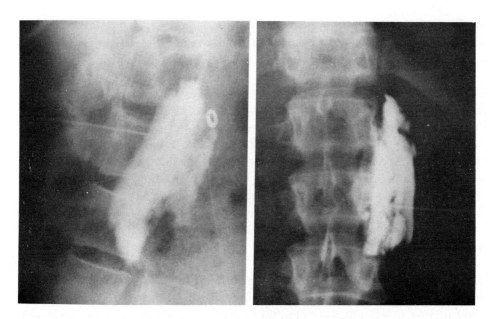

Fig. 9.7. Single needle sympathetic block showing solution spread of 10 ml 7% phenol in Conray 420 extending from L_1 to L_3 with injection at L_2. Although the needle lies slightly too laterally giving some dorsolateral spread into the psoas groove, the sympathetic chain is well covered and the intervertebral foramina clearly spared of any solution encroachment near the somatic lumbar nerve.

As many patients presented with more than one symptom, the results are expressed as a total of all complaints. Rest pain clearly responds best in terms of immediate improvement in calf blood flow as well as giving higher ankle systolic blood pressure to Doppler measurement and gives a greater rise in venous oxygen tension taken from the dorsum of the foot. Rest pain showed the best outcome, approaching 70% resolution of pain at 1 month follow-up. The worst responses

TABLE 9.2

Arteriovascular disease: 1 h post-sympathectomy changes from preblock control

	% Incidence in 500 cases	Ankle Pr. (ΔmmHg)	PvO_2 (ΔmmHg)	Calf blood flow (% Δ)	Foot temp. (Δ °C)
Rest pain	68	22 $\pm$ 31	20 $\pm$ 13	120 $\pm$ 130	4 $\pm$ 2.9
Ulcers	40	9 $\pm$ 14	15 $\pm$ 16	92 $\pm$ 104	4 $\pm$ 2.8
Claudication	39	1.8 $\pm$ 13	15 $\pm$ 16	61 $\pm$ 58	3.8 $\pm$ 3.0
Pregang./gangr.	22	insufficient data	insufficient data	insufficient data	3.9 $\pm$ 3.0

occurred in those with intermittent claudication, though detailed results from only six patients of the pregangrene/gangrene group suggest these might fare worst of all, with only half the response improvement as seen in the already poor claudication group. Similarly, the long-term response to claudication shows little change from a non-treatment control. Temperature changes of approximately 4°C rise at the level of the dorsum of the forefoot were non-discriminatory, indicating only that some flow improvement in cutaneous vessels had occurred as a result of a functional sympathectomy. As a test of prognostic value, the improvement in Doppler-measured posterior tibial artery systolic pressure is the most sensitive as well as being simple, relatively cheap and non-invasive. Its discriminative capacity appears better than that of direct flow measures, which are difficult, expensive and time-consuming, while the venous oxygen levels gave too wide a scatter of responses to be of value in projecting the outcome in any individual case if the value was low.

Further breakdown of variables as to injection site showed no difference between outcomes, whether the block was provided as a single injection at L_2 or L_3 or whether a two-needle technique was done at L_2 and L_3 or L_3 and L_4 levels. The data base was insufficient to test three-needle sympathectomies, this approach being abandoned soon after initiating the service.

The only untoward consequence of this technique is the occurrence of a post-sympathetic dysaesthesia, which has fallen to less than 5% with the single-needle approach. The pain is usually sharp, burning or dysaesthetic, situated about the inner thigh and groin, which may arise intermittently or with hot or cold stimulation or develop spontaneously, but usually subsides over several weeks without treatment. In severe cases, intravenous lignocaine, about 1.5 mg/kg (Boas et al., 1982), gives dramatic and sometimes sustained resolution, while refractory cases benefit from electrical stimulation therapy, carbamazepine and tricyclics. The presentation and treatment responses suggest a deafferentation-type neuralgia (Kerr et al., 1982), perhaps as a result of the loss of sympathetic afferent input, causing referred pain in a somatic distribution at the same segmental level as the destroyed sympathetic fibres. In any event, there is no cutaneous sensory or motor deficit in these patients, indicating the absence of peripheral somatic nerve damage as the cause of these complaints.

Bilateral injection performed in 112 patients has not caused any sexual dysfunction, nor has any case of renal penetration been seen in this group, though needles at the L_2 level must be close to the medial border of the kidney. At this level, an 8 cm entry point from the midline is considered the lateral limit, while immediate medial direction of needle insertion to the side of the vertebral body ensures sufficient latitude is provided for safety. However, until studies are undertaken with contrast media within the kidney parenchyma at the time of block, no definitive statement can be made on this point of potential renal damage. Hypotension has not been a problem, even in patients with poorly controlled heart failure, but major haemorrhage has been seen in two cases on anticoagulation therapy, where the blocks were undertaken in other centres. Minor and transient radicular pains have been seen in a few patients following traumatic needling of a somatic nerve, mostly with injection techniques closer to the midline. As a general statement, lumbar sympathectomy can be regarded as an effective and safe procedure when undertaken with fluoroscopic control. How one assesses the response to block depends to a great extent on the facilities available. Skin temperature changes, sweat testing, sympathogalvanic or skin resistance changes give an indication as to whether a functional block has been accomplished, but more quantitative testing will give better information. In particular, the measures of systolic pressure change at the ankle as shown in these results or direct flow measurements are recommended. Doppler techniques with small pencil probes are both simple and cheap and will aid in more accurate forecasting of those patients likely to yield a good response (Yao and Bergan, 1973).

Pharmacological sympathectomy

Depletion of noradrenaline stores or receptor block by regional injections of guanethidine, reserpine or prazosin offer a simple alternative to regional blocks, giving excellent results, as reported by Hannington-Kiff (1974, 1979), Loh and Nathan (1978), Loh et al. (1980), Benzon (1980), Abram and Lightfoot (1981). The duration of action is longer than with local anaesthetic blocks, the full repletion of noradrenaline taking approximately 10 days. Eriksen (1981) showed guanethidine to give complete block for 3 days compared to 10 h with a bupivacaine stellate ganglion block, while our own experience suggests that weekly injections are usually adequate for most chronic dystrophies. A dose of 10 mg guanethidine + 500 I.U. of heparin in 25 ml normal saline is used for the arm and 20 mg guanethidine + 1000 I.U. heparin in 50 ml saline is injected for the leg; the limb is occluded for 20 min. Patient discomfort is confined to that arising from cuff occlusion and morbidity is virtually nil, a point of merit when considered as an alternative to stellate blocks. Data are not yet available regarding flow changes, but clinical circulatory improvement is marked once the initial stimulatory action of increased noradrenaline release is past. In the treatment of Raynaud's disease or cold ischaemia, intravenous regional blocks with guanethidine would appear to offer the best available treatment. This can be instituted at short notice with the minimum of equipment and without special training.

For those patients who fear even these simple procedures, occasional benefit has been obtained with temperature biofeedback training to control vasospastic states but does not seem effective in sympathetic pain states. Acupuncture has been reported to give sustained relief in 70% of sympathetic dystrophies in a study of Chan and Chow (1981), while transcutaneous electrical stimulation has given benefit in some of our cases where regular clinic attendance was not possible. Carron and his group (Stilz et al., 1977) report a successful outcome using TNS in a child with sympathetic dystrophy. The mode of this action for both TNS and acupuncture is conjectural, though it possibly involves combinations of small fibre fatigue, central gating and neurochemical changes.

CHOICE OF AGENTS

Local anaesthetic block

There is no major distinction between the various drugs in respect of their merits for sympathetic blocks. Bupivacaine, 0.25%, possesses potency, duration and dosage toxicity limits sufficient to provide block at any level for several hours duration. When only short-lived or diagnostic testing is undertaken, 0.5–1% lignocaine is a better choice. Where vasodilation is to be sustained, bupivacaine or continuous or repeat injections will be needed, but for most pain states, the interruption of the so-called vicious cycle seems sufficient to institute active exercise therapy and overcome pain and dystrophy for days or weeks with one treatment, that is, the clinical response far out-lasts the pharmacological one – a dramatic feature of sympathetic dystrophy treatment.

Adrenergic block

Guanethidine works by being preferentially absorbed into the nerve terminal where it blocks noradrenaline release and brings about a depletion of stores in the nerve terminal. This potent binding action ensures that most of the administered drug is held in the tissues after a 20 min occlusion and thus diminishes the systemic action of the drug. While this is not a full sympathetic block, the reduction of vasoconstriction, hyperaesthesia and hyperpathia is sufficient to resolve the peripheral efferent component of sympathetic responses and bring about a clinical resolution of symptoms. Definitive treatment of any underlying lesion and an exercise programme can then be effectively instituted. Where guanethidine is not available, reserpine can be substituted in doses of 1–2 mg given intra-arterially or by ischaemic intravenous block type injection in 20 ml of solution. Reserpine is not bound to the same extent but prevents noradrenaline uptake into terminal vesicles and so leads to depletion from nerve endings and brings about a similar though less complete adrenergic block. The use of phentolamine or phenoxybenzamine is not reported in this manner, but the latter would appear to have theoretical merit because of its potent α-adrenergic binding and receptor-blocking action.

Neurolytic block

Alcohol has been widely employed as a standard neurolytic solution, but its action is accompanied by a burning, which, in procedures such as sympathectomy or coeliac block, is very painful. This is so severe with coeliac block that an anaesthetic must be given at the same time or a prior local anaesthetic block administered to counter this response. Phenol in water is soluble to a limit of 7% giving destruction of small nerves and fine fibres as in sympathetic nerves and ganglia, without causing pain. To facilitate correct placement of phenol, a mixture with the iodinated contrast solution Conray 420 was made, which showed far higher solubility limits of phenol in this solution without alteration of the chemical structure for either compound. Ultraviolet spectrophotometry of the separate solutions and a combined phenol/Conray mixture show that each appeared at the same wavelength alone and in combined form, indicating their chemical stability (Fig. 9.8). In particular, no free iodine is released and phenol is not degraded. Further studies on the long-term stability of 10% phenol solutions showed no changes after 3 months, apart from the formation of very small amounts of phenol oxidation products called phenoxides, which gave a slight darkening of the solutions when exposed to light.

Since first describing the use of this solution (Boas et al., 1976), over 1000 peripheral neurolytic blocks have been undertaken locally with phenol/Conray 420 or phenol/Renografin-76 solutions without report of adverse responses. These

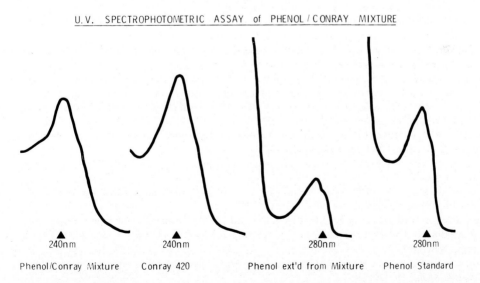

U.V. SPECTROPHOTOMETRIC ASSAY of PHENOL / CONRAY MIXTURE

240nm   240nm   280nm   280nm

Phenol/Conray Mixture   Conray 420   Phenol ext'd from Mixture   Phenol Standard

Fig. 9.8. 10% Phenol in Conray 420: spectrophotometric analysis showing stability of each of the components when in solution.

278

phenol solutions are easily prepared in any hospital pharmacy and are strongly recommended as the standard preparation for all neurolytic blocks.

REFERENCES

Abram, S.E. and Lightfoot, R.W. (1981) Treatment of long standing causalgia with prazosin. *Reg. Anesth.*, 6, 79–81.

Benzon, H.T., Chomka, C.M. and Brunner, E.A. (1980) Treatment of reflex sympathetic dystrophy with regional intravenous reserpine. *Anesth. Analg.*, 59, 500–502.

Boas, R.A. (1978) Sympathetic blocks in clinical practice. *Int. Anesthesiol. Clin.*, 16, 4, 149–182.

Boas, R.A., Hatangdi, V.S. and Richards, E.G. (1976) Lumbar sympathectomy, a percutaneous chemical technique. In: *Advances in Pain Research and Therapy, Vol. 1.* Editors: J.J. Bonica and D. Albe-Fessard. Raven Press, New York, pp. 685–689.

Boas, R.A., Covino, B.G. and Shahnarian, A. (1982) Analgesic responses to intravenous lignocaine. *Br. J. Anaesth.*, 54, 501–505.

Bonica, J.J. (1953) *Management of Pain.* Lea and Febiger, Philadelphia.

Bonica, J.J. (1979) Causalgia and other reflex sympathetic dystrophies. In: *Advances in Pain Research and Therapy, Vol. 3.* Editors: J.J. Bonica, J.C. Liebeskind and D. Albe-Fessard. Raven Press, New York.

Bonica, J.J. (1980–1981) *Sympathetic Blocks for Pain Diagnosis and Therapy, Vols. I and II.* Breon Laboratories Inc.

Bowsher, D. (1978) Pain pathways and mechanisms. *Anaesthesia*, 33, 935–944.

Cervero, F. (1982) Afferent activity evoked by natural stimulation of the biliary system in the ferret. *Pain*, 13, 137–151.

Challenger, J.H. (1978) Sympathetic nervous system blocking and pain relief. In: *Relief of Intractable Pain.* Editor: M. Swerdlow. Excerpta Medica, Amsterdam.

Chan, C.S. and Chow, S.P. (1981) Electroacupuncture in the treatment of post traumatic sympathetic dystrophy (Sudeck's Atrophy). *Br. J. Anaesth.*, 53, 899–901.

Cousins, M.J. and Wright, C.J. (1971) Graft, muscle, skin blood flow after epidural block in vascular surgical procedures. *Surg. Gynec. Obstet.*, 133, 59–64.

Cousins, M.J., Reeve, T.S., Glynn, C.J., Walsh, J.A. and Cherry, D.A. (1979) Neurolytic lumbar sympathetic blockade: duration of denervation and relief of rest pain. *Anaesth. Intens. Care*, 7, 121–135.

Eriksen, S. (1981) Duration of sympathetic blockade. Stellate ganglion versus intravenous regional guanethidine block. *Anaesthesia*, 36, 768–771.

Fyfe, T. and Quin, R.O. (1975) Phenol sympathectomy in the treatment of intermittent claudication: a controlled clinical trial. *Br. J. Surg.*, 62, 68–71.

Hannington-Kiff, J.G. (1974) Intravenous regional sympathetic block with guanethidine. *Lancet*, i, 1019–1020.

Hannington-Kiff, J.G. (1979) Relief of causalgia in limbs by regional intravenous guanethidine. *Br. Med. J.*, 279, 367–368.

Kerr, F.W.L., Wall, P.D., Loeser, J.D. and Tasker, R.R. (1982) Deafferentation pain – Papers from Proceedings 3rd World Congress IASP. In: *Advances in Pain Research and Therapy, Vol. 4.* Raven Press, New York.

Korevaar, W.C., Burney, R.G. and Moore, P.A. (1979) Convulsions during stellate ganglion block. *Anesth. Analg.*, 58, 329–330.

Löfström, J.B. (1969) Lumbar sympathetic blocks in the treatment of patients with obliterative arterial disease of the lower limb. *Int. Anesthesiol. Clinc.*, 7, 423.

Löfström, J.B., Lloyd, J.W. and Cousins, M.J. (1980) Sympathetic neural blockade of upper and lower extremity. In: *Neural Blockade in Clinical Anesthesia and Management of Pain*. Editors: M.J. Cousins and P.O. Bridenbaugh. Lippincott, Philadelphia, pp. 355–382.

Loh, L. and Nathan, P.W. (1978) Painful peripheral states and sympathetic blocks. *J. Neurol. Neurosurg. Psych.*, 41, 664–671.

Loh, L., Nathan, P.W., Schott, G.D. and Wilson, P.G. (1980) Effects of regional guanethidine infusion in certain painful states. *J. Neurol. Neurosurg. Psych.*, 43, 446–451.

Loh, L., Nathan, P.W. and Schott, G.D. (1981) Pain due to lesions of central nervous system removed by sympathetic block. *Br. Med. J.*, 282, 1026–1028.

Milne, R.J., Foreman, R.D., Giesler, G.J. and Willis, W.D. (1981) Convergence of cutaneous and pelvic visceral nociceptive inputs onto primate spinothalamic neurones. *Pain*, 11, 163–183.

Moore, D.C. (1954) *Stellate Ganglion Block*. Thomas, Springfield.

Moore, D.C. (1965) *Regional Block*. Thomas, Springfield.

Moore, D.C., Bush, W.H. and Burnett, L.L. (1981) Celiac plexus block: A roentgenographic, anatomic study of technique and spread of solution in patients and corpses. *Anesth. Analg.*, 60, 369–379.

Pick, J. (1970) *The Autonomic Nervous System*. Lippincott, Philadelphia.

Reid, W., Watt, J.K. and Gray, T.G. (1970) Phenol injection of the sympathetic chain. *Br. J. Surg.*, 57, 45–50.

Singler, R.C. (1982) An improved technique for alcohol neurolysis of the celiac plexus. *Anesthesiology*, 56, 137–141.

Stilz, R.J., Carron, H. and Saunders, D.B. (1977) Reflex sympathetic dystrophy in a 6 year old: Successful treatment by transcutaneous nerve stimulation. *Anesth. Analg.*, 56, 438–443.

Tasker, R.R., Orgon, L.W. and Hawrylyshyn, P. (1980) Deafferentation and causalgia. In: *Pain*. Editor: J.J. Bonica. Raven Press, New York.

Thompson, K.J., Melding, P. and Hatangdi, V.S. (1981) Pneumochylothorax: a rare complication of stellate ganglion block. *Anesthesiology*, 55, 589–591.

Wall, P.D. and Gutnick, M. (1974) Ongoing activity in peripheral nerves: the physiology and pharmacology of impulses originating from a neuroma. *Exp. Neurol.*, 43, 580–593.

Ward, E.M., Rorie, D.K., Nauss, L.A. and Bahn, R.C. (1979) The celiac ganglia in man: normal anatomic variations. *Anesth. Analg.*, 58, 461–465.

Winnie, A.P. (1969) An immobile needle for nerve blocks. *Anesthesiology*, 31, 577–578.

Yao, J.S.T. and Bergan, J.J. (1973) Predictability of vascular reactivity relative to sympathetic ablation. *Arch. Surg.*, 107, 676–680.

M. Swerdlow and J.E. Charlton (eds.) Relief of Intractable Pain
©1989, Elsevier Science Publishers B.V. (Biomedical Division)

10

Electrical stimulation for pain relief: transcutaneous, peripheral nerve, spinal cord and deep brain stimulation

Richard B. North

INTRODUCTION

Over the past two decades, electrical stimulation for the relief of intractable pain has become well established in medical practice. Many thousands of peripheral nerve, spinal cord and deep brain stimulation devices have been implanted, and a much larger patient population has been treated with transcutaneous electrical nerve stimulation. The physiological mechanisms of stimulation analgesia remain the subject of controversy, but the efficacy of these techniques in properly selected patients has been well established in clinical experience.

It has been known since antiquity that electrical stimulation has analgesic effects. A bioelectric generator, the torpedo fish, was used in the first century B.C., as described by Scribonius Largus (Stillings, 1975). As methods for artificial generation of electricity were developed in the 17th and 18th centuries, medical applications, among them the management of pain, were reported by a number of investigators, including Benjamin Franklin. In 1859, Althaus described the occurrence of analgesia and anaesthesia following stimulation of the ulnar nerve.

In 1965, the publication of the so-called 'gate theory' (Melzack and Wall, 1965) provided a rationale for, and engendered new interest in, this form of treatment. Melzack and Wall postulated that neural activity encoding pain is transmitted centrally via a 'gate' at the level of the spinal cord, which opens and closes as a function of the relative activity of small and large fibre activity in the mixed population of fibres in peripheral nerve. The differential susceptibility to recruitment by electrical stimulation of large (low threshold) and small (high threshold) fibres in a mixed population might be exploited, therefore, to close the 'gate'. Electrical stimulation for this purpose could be delivered not only orthodromically, from a mixed peripheral nerve, but also antidromically, via ascending collaterals of primary afferents in the dorsal columns of the spinal cord.

Concurrent with the publication of the 'gate theory', and with the empirical demonstration of pain relief by electrical stimulation with implanted electrodes (Wall and Sweet, 1967), the technology necessary to implement treatment, with chronically implanted devices, was under development for other purposes, notably cardiac pacing. Among the most important developments were solid-state circuitry, sufficiently compact and efficient for portable and implantable systems; methods for encapsulating and packaging implanted electronics; implantable power sources; and techniques of transcutaneous radiofrequency power transmission and telemetry.

Physiological mechanisms of stimulation analgesia

Always the subject of controversy (Nathan, 1976), the gate theory provided a theoretical rationale for development of a new technique: neural stimulation with implanted devices. Peripheral nerve and spinal cord stimulation for pain have succeeded empirically, and have become standard techniques, even as evidence countering certain aspects of the gate theory continues to emerge.

There is, for example, evidence that hyperalgesia is mediated by large fibres (Campbell and Meyer, 1986). Selective recruitment by electrical stimulation of large fibres should not, therefore, be effective in relieving hyperalgesia by the simple mechanism originally suggested by the gate theory. Frequency-related conduction block, rather than a central gating mechanism, may explain this effect (Campbell, 1981). Clinically, peripheral nerve stimulation achieves its analgesic effect at pulse repetition rates and intensities which may produce frequency-related conduction block (Campbell and Taub, 1973; Ignelzi and Nyquist, 1976), but this is controversial (Swett and Law, 1983). Branch points are especially sensitive to this effect; this may explain the relief of pain by spinal cord ('dorsal column') stimulation, by virtue of blockade at branch points of primary afferents which ascend in the dorsal columns after giving off collaterals to dorsal horn.

The analgesic affects of spinal cord stimulation, in clinical practice, usually persist for many minutes, and even hours, following stimulation; the latency of the effect is similar (North et al., 1977). This observation is not readily explained by frequency-related conduction block as the sole mechanism of stimulation analgesia.

Transcutaneous electrical nerve stimulation at typical 'high frequency' parameters (50–100 pulses per second) reportedly is not reversible in man by narcotic antagonists, such as naloxone (Abram et al., 1981; Woolf et al., 1978; Freeman et al., 1983). 'Acupuncture-like' TENS at low frequencies (two pulses per second) (Chapman and Benedetti, 1977) or at high pulse repetition rates, in pulse trains of low frequency (Sjolund and Eriksson, 1979) is reportedly reversible by naloxone. The latter regimes, therefore, would appear to involve a central mechanism, mediated by or under the influence of endogenous opioid systems, rather than an effect on primary afferents.

As detailed below, stimulation at higher levels of the nervous system with implanted intracerebral electrodes has a similar basis, in that successful clinical application continues empirically, in parallel with investigations of its mechanism(s) of action.

The effects of electrical stimulation at any level of the nervous system are not necessarily excitatory (Ranck, 1975). Inhibition, conduction block and even unidirectional action potential propagation (Van den Honert and Mortimer, 1979) may be achieved with appropriate stimulation waveforms and electrode configurations. In a mixed peripheral nerve, subpopulations of specific fibres may be selected on the basis of diameter (Accornero et al., 1977). Experimental observations and mathematical models of these effects have been limited to idealized electrode geometries (in some cases circumferential) applied to peripheral nerve. Limited inferences may be drawn for spinal cord stimulation, delivered via electrodes which are not only not circumferential, but also are separated from neural tissue by anisotropic media of variable thickness. Finite element modelling has been applied to this situation (Coburn and Sin, 1985); for standard spinal electrode geometries, voltage and current profiles predicted by the model approximate to those obtained by probe measurements in primate and cadaver spinal cord preparations (Sances et al., 1975).

Peripheral nerve stimulation

In 1967, Wall and Sweet reported the first clinical application of the 'gate theory', involving electrical stimulation of mixed peripheral nerves for the treatment of pain. They described eight patients in whom temporary peripheral nerve stimulating electrodes were implanted. A larger series of eighteen patients was reported in 1968 by Sweet and Wepsic. In 1976, long-term follow-up data were published for thirty-one patients treated by this group, with chronically implanted devices: nineteen patients (61%) had experienced lasting relief of pain. In other series of patients, followed as long as 10 years, success has been reported in 45–79% of patients (Campbell and Long, 1976; Law et al., 1980; Long et al., 1981; Picaza et al., 1978; Waisbrod et al., 1985). Peripheral nerve stimulation has, in fact, been among the most successful applications of implanted electrical stimulation devices for the relief of pain at long-term follow-up (Long et al., 1981). In general, treatment with implanted peripheral nerve electrodes has been most successful in documented cases of nerve injury peripheral to the site of electrode placement. Patients with, for example, sciatica due to lumbosacral radiculopathy have not responded favourably to peripheral, sciatic nerve stimulation (Meyer and Fields, 1972; Campbell and Long, 1976). Diagnostic peripheral nerve blocks, at a proposed implanted stimulating electrode site, have been helpful in patient screening (Nashold and Goldner, 1975). Diagnostic electrophysiological testing may also have predictive value (Waisbrod et al., 1985).

Before treatment with an implanted peripheral nerve stimulator is considered, a trial of transcutaneous electrical nerve stimulation (TENS) is useful; in fact, this alone may prove to be adequate treatment. If selective stimulation coverage of appropriate topography cannot be achieved by this method, then a trial with a temporary, percutaneous electrode is appropriate. Stable, chronic delivery of peripheral nerve stimulation requires electrode implantation and fixation, under direct vision. An electrode array supported by a circumferential sleeve of silicone rubber, which may include fabric reinforcement, has been used most commonly. This achieves stable fixation, although at some risk of compromising the nerve, which may swell postoperatively. Extensive testing of combinations of electrodes from the array to achieve appropriate, selective stimulation coverage is necessary to optimize therapeutic effect. The first generation of radiofrequency coupled devices, which were limited to a single, hard-wired configuration, involved lengthy intraoperative testing. More recently, non-invasive selection of anodes and cathodes from an array has been made possible by programmable, multi-contact implanted devices.

Transcutaneous electrical nerve stimulation (TENS)

Transcutaneous electrical nerve stimulation for the relief of pain and other maladies was among the first applications of artificially generated electricity, in the 18th and 19th centuries (Stillings, 1975). The development of contemporary devices shares the theoretical rationale and technical foundations of implantable devices. TENS was, in fact, reintroduced as a screening technique for potential candidates for peripheral nerve and spinal cord implants (Long, 1976). Many patients, however, found TENS alone to be adequate therapy (Long and Hagfors, 1975). As a benign, noninvasive procedure, TENS lends itself to blind, controlled studies to a far greater extent than techniques involving implanted devices. Placebo-controlled trials have, in fact, demonstrated therapeutic benefit and have defined the extent of the placebo response, which is similar to that observed with drugs during the first few days of treatment (Long, 1977; Thorsteinsson et al., 1978).

In routine clinical use, TENS requires empirical determination, in each patient, of optimal electrode placement sites, following a few basic principles (electrodes over or proximal to the distribution of pain, dipole parallel to major nerve trunks, avoiding motor points) (Mannheimer and Lampe, 1984). The applications of TENS have become far broader than those of implanted devices, and include postoperative pain (Vanderark and McGrath, 1975), visceral pain and acute and chronic pain of musculoskeletal and neurological origin (Mannheimer and

Lampe, 1984). Among patients with chronic pain syndromes, in particular lumbar post-laminectomy syndrome, few will report satisfactory analgesia with simple TENS (Loeser et al., 1975). This does not, however, preclude a favourable response to treatment with an implanted stimulator. TENS is useful in this group, however, as a form of initial, conservative management and as an introduction to the concept of pain management with an electronic device.

Transcutaneous electrical nerve stimulation is an especially benign form of treatment, with few reported adverse effects and few contraindications:

TENS: Contraindications

(1) Cardiac pacemakers: Although most contemporary R wave sensing schemes are immune to this effect, some demand cardiac pacemakers may be inhibited by externally applied electrical fields such as TENS. Early cardiac pacemaker designs, which were fixed-rate, precluded this effect; but these are uncommon today, because of the advantages of demand pacing for the great majority of patients. The presence of an implanted cardiac pacemaker, therefore, is generally a contraindication to the use of TENS, and for that matter, of an implanted stimulator.
(2) Pregnancy: The safety of transcutaneous electrical nerve stimulation in pregnancy, as well as in labour and delivery, has not been demonstrated; the available information on this subject is rather limited (Mannheimer and Lampe, 1984).
(3) Psychiatric disease, dementia or mental retardation, to a degree rendering the patient incompetent to use the device.

TENS: Precautions

(1) Hypersensitivity reactions to topical conductive gels and adhesives are common; hypoallergenic materials (such as karaya, combining adhesive and conductive properties in a single medium) are available. Careful attention to ordinary principles of skin hygiene is of obvious importance.
(2) Precordial application should be avoided in a patient with a history of cardiac arrhythmia; no adverse effect has been reported in this circumstance, but prudence dictates caution. Likewise, cephalic application should be avoided in patients with seizures and cerebrovascular disease.
(3) Application near the eyes, or in close proximity to mucous membranes, should be avoided.
(4) Application over the carotid sinus may induce bradycardia or hypotension, and should be avoided, especially in cerebrovascular or cardiac disease.

Spinal cord stimulation

In more than two decades of experience with implanted neural stimulation devices, the most common application has been spinal cord stimulation. The first electrodes developed for this purpose were planar, with silicone rubber backing to insulate and support the electrode or electrode array. Implantation over the dorsal surface of the spinal cord required a laminectomy for epidural (or in some cases, subdural or endodural) placement under direct vision (Shealy et al., 1967; Nashold and Friedman, 1972; Sweet and Wepsic, 1974). Electrodes were implanted at high thoracic levels in the usual patient with 'post-laminectomy syndrome'; this was intended to provide stimulation paraesthesias involving all segments caudal to the electrode. Excessive thoracic radicular stimulation, however, often predominated over the desired low back and sciatic coverage. Electrode placement at more caudal levels proved superior in this sense. The optimal level of placement was found to vary, however, from patient to patient. Under local anaesthesia, a patient could provide useful feedback, but extensive longitudinal mapping of the epidural space by stimulation via laminectomy remained cumbersome.

Electrodes amenable to percutaneous introduction into the epidural space were developed, therefore, to determine the optimal level of placement in individual patients, as well as to screen for analgesic efficacy before implantation of a permanent device (Erickson, 1975). Such electrodes, could, in fact, be implanted permanently, avoiding the need for laminectomy (Fig. 10.1). These electrodes often migrated, however, and required surgical revision (North et al., 1977); this was particularly problematic when electrodes were implanted in pairs, to achieve bipolar stimulation. Linear arrays of electrodes which could be introduced via a Tuohy needle were developed to ameliorate this (Leclercq, 1984) (Fig. 10.2). Concurrently, implantable multichannel pulse generators were introduced to permit noninvasive selection of electrode combinations from these arrays. The active electrodes along an array could then be varied postoperatively by noninvasive adjustments to the system. Artifacts introduced by electrode placement with the patient in the prone position, and minor postoperative changes in the position of the electrode itself, may be overcome by these versatile systems.

The following specific indications for treatment with an implanted spinal cord stimulator have been developed over two decades of experience.

Spinal cord stimulation for intractable pain: specific indications

(1) Lumbosacral spinal fibrosis (lumbar arachnoiditis). Among patients with post-laminectomy syndrome, those with radicular symptoms and signs are more amenable to therapy than those with predominantly axial or mechanical pain.

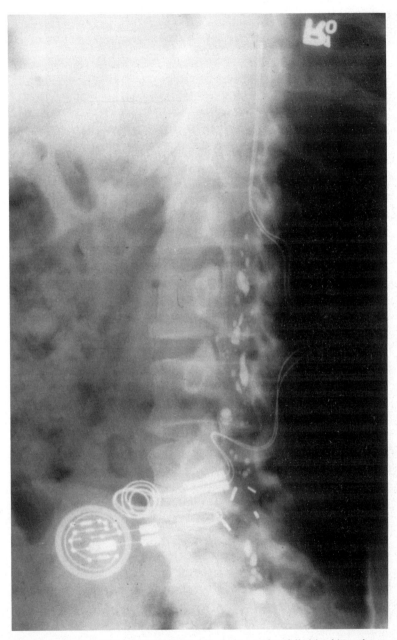

Fig. 10.1. Typical dorsal epidural electrode placement for 'failed back' syndrome, with arachnoid fibrosis. (Note myelographic contrast residue and post-surgical changes.) Independently inserted, individual epidural electrodes, as shown here, have been particularly vulnerable to spontaneous migration. In this bipolar configuration, the electrodes are hardwired to a single-channel, radiofrequency-coupled subcutaneous receiver.

288

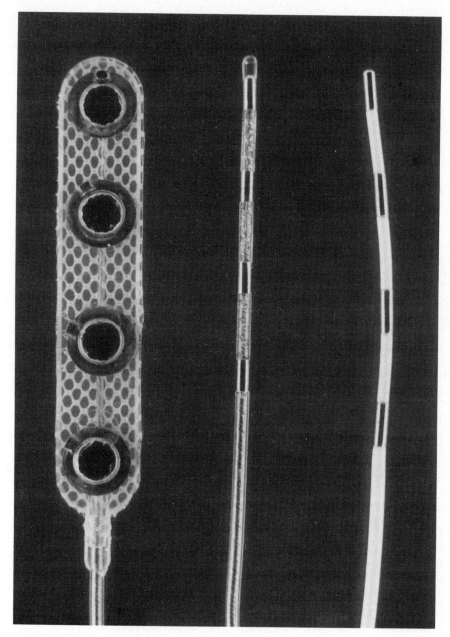

Fig. 10.2. Representative, contemporary spinal cord stimulating electrode arrays. On the left, an array requiring a laminectomy, or laminotomy, for introduction into the dorsal epidural space. In the centre and on the right, arrays designed for introduction into the dorsal epidural space via a percutaneous 15 or 16 gauge Tuohy needle. To facilitate steering the electrode in the epidural space, the array in the centre permits introduction of a central, malleable stylet. Percutaneous arrays of up to eight electrodes, and laminectomy arrays of up to 64 electrodes are available.

(2) Lower extremity ischaemic pain due to occlusive aorto-femoral or peripheral vascular disease (Broseta et al., 1986).

(3) Peripheral nerve injury, phantom limb or stump pain.

(4) Painful peripheral neuropathy.

(5) Pain following spinal cord injury, particularly when confined to a radicular distribution at the level of injury, as opposed to a more diffuse distribution, below the level of injury.

The results of treatment of lumbosacral spinal fibrosis (arachnoiditis) have been 'good' or 'excellent' in the majority of patients in reported series in the literature (De la Porte and Siegfried, 1983). Outcome measures used in these series have varied widely.

The experience at Johns Hopkins with a cohort of patients, followed for 8 years, is representative. At 6 month mean follow-up (North et al., 1977), 12 of 24 patients reported 70–100% relief and 6 reported 40–70% relief. Eighteen of 24 judged the procedure to be 'much more effective' than any prior treatment and 20 of 24 indicated that they would go through the procedure again, given the result obtained. Concurrently, patients described improvement in ability to perform various everyday activities, and usage of analgesics and benzodiazepines was reduced or eliminated. At 8-year follow-up (North and Long, 1984), 7 of 20 maintained an excellent result, reporting 75% relief or better.

Patients in this series were treated with percutaneously inserted electrodes, implanted in pairs to deliver bipolar stimulation, and adapted to chronic use with a single-channel implant (Fig. 10.1). This configuration proved to be vulnerable to spontaneous electrode migration and other technical problems requiring surgical revision. At 21-month follow-up of our first 31 patients, there had been 47 instances of electrode migration or malposition, 9 lead wire fractures, 5 failures of lead insulation and 1 receiver failure (North and Long, 1984). Because of this experience, we reverted for a time to implanting fixed arrays, via laminectomy, precluding delayed electrode migration (Fig. 10.2). A trial period with temporary, percutaneous leads addressed the problem of postural effects, which can lead to inappropriate electrode placement based upon a patient's responses while in the prone position during surgery. This issue was, ultimately, addressed more elegantly by the development of implantable systems with multiple channels, which may be selected noninvasively, effectively moving the active electrodes. At the same time, arrays of electrodes amenable to insertion through a Tuohy needle were developed. These preclude migration of one electrode with respect to another, and migration of the entire array has, with improvements in its design and in anchoring techniques, become a rare occurrence. We now reserve the laminectomy technique for patients in whom extensive epidural scarring precludes percutaneous electrode placement (North, 1988).

Deep brain stimulation (DBS)

Over 30 years ago, the analgesic effects of electrical stimulation of subcortical structures, via stereotactically implanted electrodes, were reported by Pool (1956) and by Heath and Mickle (1960). Deafferentation pain was first treated in this fashion by Mazars, who in 1960 reported the analgesic effects of stimulating the somatosensory system via the spinothalamic fasciculus (Mazars et al., 1960). Electrical stimulation of specific thalamic sensory nuclei (Mazars, 1975; Hosobuchi et al., 1975), as well as of the internal capsule (Adams et al., 1974; Fields and Adams, 1974; Hosobuchi et al., 1975) was employed for the same purpose in later series.

Even before the demonstration of opiate receptors in nervous tissue (Pert and Snyder, 1973) and their regional localization, the analgesic effects of electrical stimulation of periaqueductal grey (PAG) had been described (Reynolds, 1969). The periaqueductal grey was later demonstrated to be an area rich in opiate receptors (Kuhar et al., 1973). Subsequent animal studies have shown a descending inhibitory pathway, in the dorsal lateral quadrant of the spinal cord, mediating this effect, which is reversible by naloxone, the narcotic antagonist, and cross-tolerant with opiate analgesia (Basbaum and Fields, 1978; Liebeskind et al., 1973; Mayer et al., 1971; Mayer and Liebeskind, 1974; Mayer and Hayes, 1975; Mayer and Price, 1976). Periaqueductal grey stimulation in humans may (Adams, 1976, Hosobuchi et al., 1977) or may not (Young and Chambi, 1987) be naloxone-reversible. It has been reported that cerebrospinal fluid levels of beta-endorphin are elevated by PAG stimulation (Akil et al., 1978; Hosobuchi et al., 1979). Subsequent studies have, however, suggested that this is in fact an effect of ventriculography with iodinated contrast (Dionne et al., 1980; Fessler et al., 1984). There is mounting evidence that the analgesic effects of PAG stimulation are independent of endogenous opiate release (Young and Chambi, 1987). In clinical practice, however, this method has succeeded empirically, not only in the management of chronic benign pain, but also of cancer pain (Richardson and Akil, 1977; Young et al., 1985; Hosobuchi, 1986).

Periaqueductal grey stimulation has been most effective in the management of nociceptive, as opposed to deafferentation, pain syndromes (Levy et al., 1987). A morphine infusion test has been advocated as a screening procedure (Hosobuchi, 1986), but this is controversial (Young and Chambi, 1987). Among the specific conditions treated have been:
1. Lumbar post-laminectomy or 'failed back': syndrome (although this may include a component of deafferentation pain).
2. Cancer pain (on the basis of neoplastic infiltration causing nociception, as opposed to deafferentation).
3. Abdominal, pelvic and perineal pain of non-neoplastic origin.

4. Atypical facial pain.

Deafferentation pain syndromes, on the other hand, are more responsive to electrical stimulation of specific thalamic relay nuclei:

1. Thalamic syndrome (Dejerine-Roussy syndrome), on the basis of thalamic infarct or injury, in cases in which an anatomical substrate for stimulation remains.
2. Anaesthesia dolorosa.
3. Postherpetic neuralgia.
4. Phantom limb pain.
5. Post-cordotomy dysaesthesias.
6. Brachial or lumbosacral plexus lesions.
7. Lumbosacral polyradiculopathy.
8. Pain following spinal cord injury.

DBS electrodes are implanted by standard stereotactic techniques using either contrast ventriculography or computed tomography (transmission X-ray or magnetic resonance). Two electrode arrays commonly are implanted simultaneously: in patients with axial or bilateral pain of nociceptive origin, bilateral PAG electrodes are placed. In patients with unilateral pain with a deafferentation component, one array may be placed in contralateral sensory thalamus, in ventral posterolateral lateral or ventral posteromedial medial nucleus (VPL or VPM), as appropriate for the anatomical location of the patient's pain, and a second contralateral PAG electrode may be placed through the same burr hole (Fig. 10.3). As for other implanted stimulator procedures, percutaneous test leads are employed for a trial period, prior to pulse generator implantation.

Stimulation of specific thalamic sensory nuclei, like peripheral nerve or spinal cord stimulation, produces paraesthesias; empirically, overlap of these paraesthesias with the patient's topography of pain is a necessary condition for stimulation analgesia. PAG stimulation, on the other hand, may not produce any distinct subjective sensation at parameters adequate to produce pain relief. (At excessive stimulation amplitude, or with electrode placement caudal to the iter of the aqueduct of Sylvius, it may produce eye movement abnormalities.) The analgesic effects of PAG stimulation may persist for many hours; this makes exhaustive assessment of electrode combinations and stimulation parameters difficult. As soon as stimulation analgesia has been achieved, the implanted electrodes are adapted to long-term use by connecting lead wires and an implanted pulse generator, usually in an infraclavicular subcutaneous pocket. This phase of the procedure does not require patient participation and may be performed under general anaesthesia. If stimulation analgesia is not achieved and the intracerebral electrodes are to be removed, this may be accomplished under local or general anaesthesia.

The potential complications of intracerebral electrode implantation are more serious than those of other implanted stimulator procedures. As reported in the

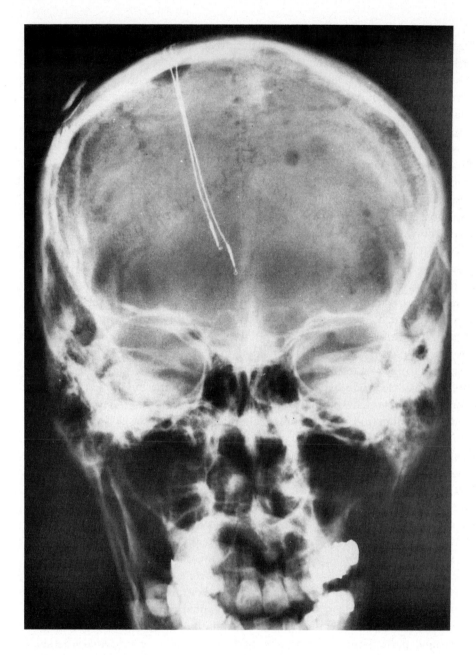

Fig. 10.3. Intracerebral stimulating electrode placement for intractable pain due to metastatic cancer, involving the forequarter and the upper thoracic spine. On the left, specific thalamic sensory (VPL) electrodes for deafferentation pain; in paramedian position, periaqueductal grey electrodes for nociceptive and axial components of the patient's pain.

largest series of patients (Hosobuchi, 1986; Plotkin, 1982; Young et al., 1985), they are: (1) Intracranial haemorrhage in 2–4% of cases, with a mortality of between 0–2%. Candidates for the procedure, particularly patients with cancer pain, should be screened carefully for coagulopathy. (2) Wound infection, which may necessitate removal of some or all implanted hardware, has occurred in 3–6% of patients. One risk factor, the duration of the percutaneous test phase, can be minimized by using multichannel, programmable implants, which permit noninvasive, postoperative selection of optimal electrode combinations, so that they need not be identified and hardwired at the time of pulse generator implantation. (3) For electrode tip positions rostral to the iter of the aqueduct of Sylvius, eye movement abnormalities occur less frequently; overall, the reported frequency is from 2–4%. (4) Failures of implanted hardware have been reported in 2–12% of cases. Migration of electrodes and various electronic and electromechanical failures have been reported. Based upon the limited available pathological material, no deleterious effect of stimulation or of electrode implantation has been identified; gliosis or reaction around implanted electrodes has been minimal (Baskin et al., 1986).

A number of outcome measures have been used to assess the results of pain management with intracerebral stimulating electrodes. They range from direct patient assessments of pain relief to indirect measures such as stimulator usage, concurrent analgesic intake, functional capacity, and employment. As reviewed by Levy (Levy et al., 1987), PAG stimulation for nociceptive pain and thalamic stimulation for deafferentation pain have been successful in 60% of patients. A 1985 review by Young (Young et al., 1985) reported success in 57% overall; between 50% (Plotkin, 1982) and 80% (Siegfried, 1982) of patients responded to thalamic stimulation, and between 0% (Amano et al., 1980) and 90% (Boivie and Meyerson, 1982) responded to PAG stimulation. Between 70 and 76% of patients with cancer pain have been treated successfully by these techniques (Hosobuchi, 1986; Young and Brechner, 1986).

Although its risks exceed those of other implanted stimulator techniques for intractable pain, intracerebral electrode implantation may succeed in patients refractory to other techniques. In central deafferentation pain states, it is the only available reversible, non-ablative neurosurgical procedure.

Chronic pain management: general considerations

Over the past two decades, concurrent with the development and refinement of electrical stimulation techniques, the overall management of chronic pain syndromes has evolved as a multidisciplinary subspecialty (Bonica, 1977). Psychological issues in the management of chronic pain in general and in patient selection for invasive procedures, in particular implanted stimulators (Daniel et al., 1985), are now widely appreciated. Many of the disappointing results in early series of patients with implanted stimulators may be explained on this basis. Contemporary patient selection criteria for treatment with an implanted stimulator address this explicitly.

Implanted stimulation devices for pain: general indications

(1) An objective basis for the patient's complaint of pain has been demonstrated (e.g., arachnoid fibrosis, documented myelographically, in lumbar post-laminectomy or 'failed back' syndrome).

(2) Alternative treatments have been exhausted, or are unacceptable (because of low yield or potential morbidity). Lysis of arachnoid scar by microsurgical techniques, for example, is associated with a high incidence of neurological complications, with limited analgesic benefit. Ablative neurosurgical procedures, such as cordotomy, share these problems, and delayed failures, including post-cordotomy dysaesthesias, are common. Stimulator implantation has the obvious advantage of reversibility, as a non-ablative technique.

(3) Psychological or psychiatric evaluation, as part of a multidisciplinary assessment, reveals no primary psychiatric illness, major drug habituation or drug-seeking behaviour, or serious issues of secondary gain. Long-term treatment with an implanted stimulator requires a well-motivated patient, capable of commitment to and involvement with a comprehensive treatment program.

(4) The pathophysiological basis and the anatomical distribution of pain are amenable to stimulation therapy. Sciatica, for example, is typically more amenable to coverage by spinal stimulation than is axial low back pain. Periaqueductal grey stimulation, on the other hand, is applicable to axial and to diffuse distributions of pain. Pain which responds to opiates, it has been reported, is more responsive to periaqueductal grey stimulation (Hosobuchi, 1986), but this remains controversial (Young and Chambi, 1987).

A patient chosen by these criteria as an appropriate candidate for an implanted stimulator must meet yet another criterion if the procedure is to be reimbursed by Medicare and, following their example, third party insurers: 'Demonstration of pain relief with a temporary implanted electrode precedes permanent implantation.' This condition might be fulfilled, in a limited sense, if a patient reported pain relief intraoperatively, during implantation of a complete system in a single-stage procedure. This would be expected, however, to result in a higher incidence of failures of treatment, and even of explants. A more prolonged trial of stimulation, via temporary, percutaneous leads, not only improves patient selection, but also, in the case of spinal electrodes, offers several technical advantages: (1) A temporary spinal electrode may be placed in a fluoroscopy suite, away from the time constraints of the operating room, affording the physician and the patient the opportunity to inventory a large number of potential electrode placement sites. (2)

When, after a period of trial stimulation, the temporary electrode has been removed (to reduce the risk of infection) and the patient is taken to the operating room for implantation of a permanent electrode, this earlier experience facilitates the rapid implantation of the permanent electrode, which in turn further reduces the risk of infection. (3) If implantation of a totally implanted device, powered by a primary cell, is contemplated, measurements of stimulation pulse parameters required by a particular patient may be made with the temporary electrode. This permits, in turn, an estimate of the time to battery depletion in a particular patient and an informed judgement as to whether such a device is appropriate. (4) The patient can assess the analgesic effects of stimulation at leisure, while engaging in everyday activities and in postions other than the prone position assumed during electrode placement.

Candidates for an implanted peripheral nerve stimulator benefit in the same ways from a trial with a temporary, percutaneously placed electrode. A peripheral nerve cuff, however, whose placement requires an open surgical procedure, should be tested with temporary percutaneous lead extensions; only the latter are removed if, after a stimulation trial, a permanent pulse generator is implanted. Intracerebral stimulating electrodes, like peripheral cuff electrodes, are best left in place and adapted for chronic implantation because of the potential technical problems and the morbidity involved in removal and replacement of the entire array following percutaneous testing. Programmable, multi-contact implants, which permit the selection of electrodes from an array by noninvasive means, even after implantation of the permanent device, permit selection of the optimal electrode combination or combinations after the fact. Formerly, with single channel devices hard-wired to a single electrode combination, extended intraoperative or percutaneous testing was necessary.

During the percutaneous test phase, the analgesic effects of stimulation should be assessed under a variety of conditions. Ideally, treatment should be evaluated by an individual other than the primary surgeon. A crossover protocol, including periods of time without any stimulation, helps to establish that relief reported by the patient is indeed an effect of stimulation. Among the outcome measures which are useful in determining a patient's candidacy for a permanent implant, and in assessing long-term results, are not only estimates of analgesic effect per se by analogue rating scales, but also indirect indices such as intake of medications, ability to engage in everyday activities and (at extended follow-up) disability status and ongoing use of other health care resources.

Implanted neurological stimulation systems

The earliest systems developed for chronic neural stimulation via implanted electrodes consisted of an external radiofrequency transmitter and a passive, implanted receiver. Major refinements have been added over the past two decades, but this scheme remains the most common in clinical use (Fig. 10.4). The battery-powered external transmitter emits radiofrequency (455 kHz–2 MHz) bursts via a circular antenna, which is applied to the intact skin over the implanted receiver. A matching antenna in the receiver, coupled to the external antenna, feeds this signal to a simple AM demodulator, which rectifies and integrates the radiofrequency bursts into rectangular stimulation pulses. The output of the implant is capacitatively coupled to the electrodes so that no potentially injurious direct current flows through the circuit. The amplitude, duration and repetition rate of the radiofrequency bursts emitted by the transmitter determine the stimulation parameters delivered to the electrodes. The implanted receiver is entirely passive; it contains no battery, whose longevity might limit its useful life span.

Contemporary radiofrequency-coupled systems are capable of supporting multiple (4–8) electrodes, permitting the selection of stimulating anodes and cathodes from an array. This may be accomplished noninvasively, by simple adjustments to switch settings on the external radiofrequency transmitter (Fig. 10.4). Formerly, with single channel systems, this could be accomplished only by surgical revision of hardwired connections or of electrode position. This in turn minimizes the duration of the percutaneous test phase to determine the optimal electrode combination and permits postoperative adjustments to compensate for any changes which may occur between intraoperative and postoperative trials, or during the postoperative period. This reduces the need for subsequent surgical revisions of the implanted hardware.

In parallel with the development of cardiac pacing technology, totally implantable pulse generators have been developed for neural stimulation. The design requirements for these two applications differ in many respects. Whereas cardiac pacing is a critical, life-supporting function, which may not tolerate even momentary interruption, neural stimulation for pain is less demanding in this regard. A totally implanted pulse generator, containing its own power source and capable of functioning autonomously, is quite appropriate for such purposes as cardiac pacing and diaphragmatic pacing (phrenic nerve stimulation). Applied to neurostimulation for pain, on the other hand, the major advantage of a total implant is convenience to the patient, who need not be encumbered by an external power supply. Patient control over the function of the implant, however, is a requirement of this application. In order to turn the implant on and off, and to control certain parameters of stimulation (e.g., amplitude, within preprogrammed ranges), an external device is still necessary. Whether this takes the form of a magnet or of a battery-powered transmitter, the patient remains encumbered by external hardware.

The major disadvantage of an implanted primary cell or expendable power source is its limited useful life span: replacement of a depleted unit involves a sur-

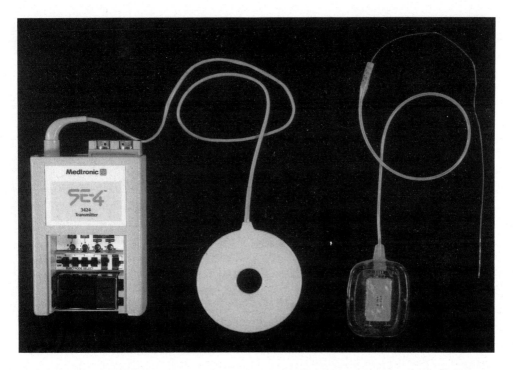

Fig. 10.4. A typical contemporary radiofrequency-coupled, multi-contact neurostimulation system. On the left, a battery-powered radiofrequency transmitter, whose switch settings determine the configuration of anodes and cathodes selected from an array of four electrodes. A circular antenna, connected by a flexible lead to the transmitter, is placed over the radiofrequency receiver, on the right. The passive, implanted receiver supports an array of four intraspinal electrodes, seen on the far right.

gical procedure. As neural stimulation applications may require from 1–3 orders of magnitude more power than cardiac pacing, a typical pacemaker primary cell may not yield acceptable longevity. A typical 1–2 ampere hour lithium primary cell, powering an implanted cardiac pacemaker, may last a decade or more; but in certain neural stimulation applications, it may last only a few weeks. Implantable, rechargeable systems, originally developed for cardiac pacing, have been applied successfully for neural stimulation (Fischell et al., 1978), but these have been implemented only in prototype form. Another approach to this problem is a hybrid system, powered by a primary cell, but capable of accepting power from an external radiofrequency transmitter to maximize battery life (Fig. 10.5). This system also permits noninvasive selection of electrodes from an array, like contemporary radiofrequency-coupled devices.

New design features and improved reliability have enhanced the clinical efficacy of implanted neural stimulation devices for the many reasons enumerated above.

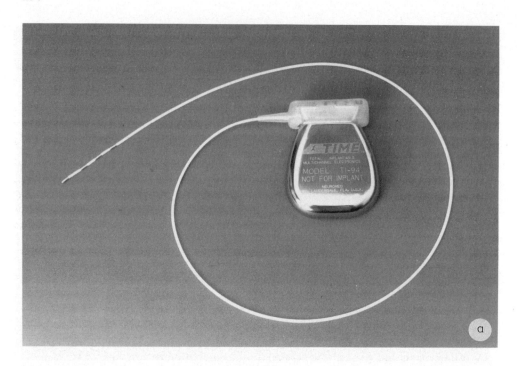

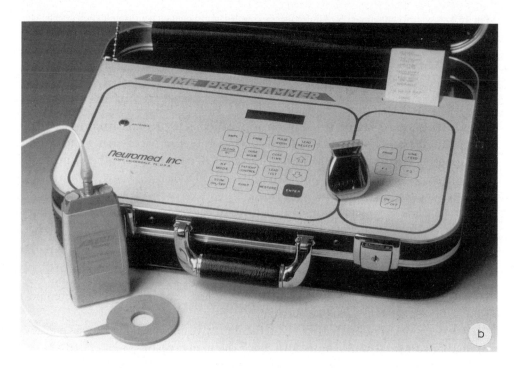

As the number of available stimulation channels and stimulation parameters increases, however, the number of possible settings increases disproportionately. Whereas, for a single channel system, only stimulation amplitude, pulse width and pulse repetition rate required adjustment to optimize effect, contemporary devices permit selection from among many possible combinations of electrodes. If these are to be tested exhaustively, to optimize therapeutic effect, the task may grow beyond the capabilities of the physician or his assistant to perform in a reasonable time.

As the number of available stimulation channels increases, the number of available electrode combinations grows disproportionately, in a nonlinear fashion. This may be expressed by the following formulae:

An array of n electrodes, where $n \geqslant 2$, allows combinations of m active and $n-m$ inactive electrodes numbering:

$$C(n,m) = n!/(n-m)!m!$$

Each combination of m active electrodes permits 2^m choices of stimulation anodes and cathodes. Two of these combinations (all electrodes anodes, or all cathodes) are open-circuit; $2^m - 2$ configurations, therefore, are useful. The total number of unique, useful electrode combinations, therefore, is given by:

$$\sum_{m=2}^{n} n!(2^m - 2)/(n-m)!m!$$

For an array of four electrodes, which is the most common contemporary configuration, this yields $12 + 24 + 14 = 50$ combinations. Eight electrodes, on the other hand, allow $56 + 336 + 980 + 1680 + 1736 + 1008 + 254 = 6050$ combinations of electrodes.

In practice, many of these electrode combinations will be equivalent physiologically or psychophysically. A more manageable subset of electrode combinations,

---

Fig. 10.5 (a). A totally implantable, multichannel, programmable device. Note the array of four electrodes, from which combinations of stimulating anodes and cathodes may be selected noninvasively. (b) Although powered by a lithium primary cell and able to operate autonomously, the implant is also capable of operating in a passive, radiofrequency-coupled mode, to prolong battery longevity. The radiofrequency transmitter is shown on the left. Also shown is the portable, external programming unit, which the physician uses to control the implant's stimulation parameters and electrode settings. Note printout emerging (upper right). The patient controls the implant with either the external transmitter or a hand-held magnet with which the unit may be turned on and off and the stimulation amplitude adjusted within programmed limits.

assumed a priori to be representative and most appropriate, may be developed to reduce the magnitude of the task. It remains, however, a major undertaking for patient and staff alike.

Given means of controlling appropriate stimulation parameters, within defined limits, the patient himself is best able to manage the task of stimulator adjustment for optimal pain management. The roles of the physician or his assistant (supervision, data acquisition and expert advice), may, to a large degree, be automated.

We have developed, to this end, a personal computer-controlled stimulation system with 'user-friendly' software for direct patient interaction, which supports standard, commercially available radiofrequency-coupled devices (Fowler and North, 1986; North and Fowler, 1987). The system is designed for greater ease of operation by the patient than the standard radiofrequency transmitter. In routine clinical use, the system will test, in random or pseudorandom order, subsets of the available electrode combinations and stimulation parameters. The patient records the topography of stimulation via a graphics tablet and psychophysical thresholds via potentiometer settings. For research purposes, the system is capable of delivering stimulation pulse sequences which are not available from the standard, commercial transmitter. Electrode combinations and stimulation pulse parameters may be reprogrammed in as little as 1 ms between pulses. This would permit, for example, interleaving two stimulation pulse sequences involving different electrodes, to determine whether their effects are additive. Modulation of the interpulse interval, reportedly a useful strategy for TENS (Mannheimer and Carlsson, 1979), is another potential application.

CONCLUSION

Electrical stimulation by invasive and noninvasive techniques has been increasingly successful in the management of pain, in particular of chronic, intractable pain. The exact mechanisms of stimulation analgesia remain controversial. Contemporary devices permit increasingly complex, programmable stimulation regimes and electrode geometries, enhancing clinical efficacy and opening new research opportunities.

REFERENCES

Abram, S. Reynolds, A. and Cusick, J. (1981) Failure of naloxone to reverse analgesia from transcutaneous electrical stimulation in patients with chronic pain. *Anesth. Analg.* 60(2), 81–84.
Accornero, N., Bini, G., Lenzi, G. and Manfredi, M. (1977) Selective activation of peripheral nerve fibre groups of different diameter by triangular shaped stimulus pulses. *J. Physiol.* 273, 539–560.

Adams, J.E., Hosobuchi, Y. and Fields, H.L. (1974) Stimulation of the internal capsule for relief of chronic pain. *J. Neurosurg.* 41, 740–744.

Adams, J.E. (1976) Naloxone reversal of analgesia produced by brain stimulation in the human. *Pain*, 2, 161–166.

Akil, H., Richardson, D.E. and Hughes, J. (1978) Enkephalin-like material elevated in ventricular cerebrospinal fluid of pain patients after analgetic focal stimulation. *Science*, 201, 463–465.

Amano, K., Kitamura, K. and Kawamura, H. (1980) Alterations of immunoreactive β-endorphin in the third ventricular fluid in response to electrical stimulation of the human periaqueductal gray matter. *Appl. Neurophysiol.*, 43, 150–158.

Basbaum, A.I. and Fields H.L. (1978) Endogenous pain control mechanisms: Review and hypothesis. *Ann. Neurol.*, 4, 451–462.

Baskin, D.S., Mehler, W.R., Hosobuchi, Y., Richardson, D., Adams, J. and Flitter, M. (1986) Autopsy analysis of the safety, efficacy and cartography of electrical stimulation of the central gray in humans. *Brain Res.*, 371, 231–236.

Boivie, J. and Meyerson, B.A. (1982) A correlative anatomical and clinical study of pain suppression by deep brain stimulation. *Pain*, 13, 113–126.

Bonica, J.J. (1977) Basic principles in managing chronic pain. *Arch. Surg.*, 112; 783–788.

Broseta, J., Barbera, J., DeVera, J., Barcia-Salorio, J., March, G., Gonzalez-Darder, J., Rovaina, F. and Joanes, V. (1986) Spinal cord stimulation in peripheral arterial disease. *J. Neurosurg.*, 64, 71–80.

Campbell, J. and Taub, A. (1973) Local analgesia from percutaneous electrical stimulation. *Arch. Neurol.*, 28, 347–350.

Campbell, J.N., Long, D.M. (1976) Peripheral nerve stimulation in the treatment of intractable pain. *J. Neurosurg.*, 45, 692–699.

Campbell, J.N. (1981) Examination of possible mechanisms by which stimulation of the spinal cord in man relieves pain. *Appl. Neurophys.*, 44, 181–186.

Campbell, J.N. and Meyer, R.A. (1986) Primary afferents and hyperalgesia, In: *Spinal Afferent Processing*. Editor: T.L. Yaksh. Plenum, New York, pp. 59–81.

Chapman, C. and Benedetti, C. (1977) Analgesia following transcutaneous electrical stimulation and its partial reversal by a narcotic antagonist. *Life Sci.*, 21, 1645–1648.

Coburn, B. and Sin, W. (1985) A theoretical study of epidural electrical stimulation of the spinal cord. Part I: Finite element analysis of stimulus fields. *Biomed. Eng.*, 32(11), 971–977.

Daniel, M., Long, C., Hutcherson, M. and Hunter, S. (1985) Psychological factors and outcome of electrode implantation for chronic pain. *Neurosurgery*, 17 (5), 773–777.

De la Porte, C. and Siegfried, J. (1983) Lumbosacral spinal fibrosis (spinal arachnoiditis): Its diagnosis and treatment by spinal cord stimulation. *Spine*, 8 (6), 593–603.

Dionne, R.A., Muller, G.P., Young, R.F., Greenberg, P. Hargreaves, K.M. Gracely, R. and Dubner, R. (1980) Contrast medium causes the apparent increase in β-endorphin levels in human cerebrospinal fluid following brain stimulation. *Pain*, 20, 313–321.

Erickson, D.L. (1975) Percutaneous trial of stimulation for patient selection for implantable stimulating devices. *J. Neurosurg.*, 43, 440–444.

Fessler, R.G., Brown, F.D., Rachlin, J.R. and Mullan, S. (1984) Elevated β-endorphin in cerebrospinal fluid after electrical brain stimulation: Artifact of contrast infusion. *Science*, 224, 1017–1019.

Fields, H.L. and Adams, J.E. (1974) Pain after cortical injury relieved by electrical stimulation of the internal capsule. *Brain*, 97, 169–178.

Fischell, R.E., Schulman, J.H. and Cooper, I.S. (1978) An intracorporeal system for cerebellar stimulation. In: *Cerebellar Stimulation in Man*. Editor: I.S. Cooper. Raven Press, New York, pp. 195–206.

Fowler, K. and North, R. (1986) Patient-interactive PC interface to implanted, multichannel stimulators. *Proceedings of the 39th ACEMB*, Baltimore, Maryland, p. 380.

302

Freeman, T.B., Campbell, J.N. and Long, D.M. (1983) Naloxone does not affect pain relief induced by electrical stimulation in man. *Pain*, 17, 189–195.

Heath, R. and Mickle, W.A. (1960) Evaluation of seven years experience with depth electrode studies in human patients. In: *Electrical Studies on the Unanesthetized Brain*. Editor: E.R. Ramey. Hoeber, Inc., New York, pp. 214–247.

Hosobuchi, Y., Adams, J.E. and Rutkin, B. (1975) Chronic thalamic and internal capsule stimulation for the control of central pain. *Surg. Neurol.*, 4, 91–92.

Hosobuchi, Y., Adams, J.E. and Linchitz, R. (1977) Pain relief by electrical stimulation of the central gray matter in humans and its reversal by naloxone. *Science*, 197, 183–186.

Hosobuchi, Y., Rossier, J., Bloom, F.E. and Guilleman, R. (1979) Stimulation of human periaqueductal gray for pain relief increases immunoreactive β-endorphin in ventricular fluid. *Science*, 203, 279–281.

Hosobuchi, Y. (1986) Subcortical electrical stimulation for control of intractable pain in humans. Report of 122 cases (1970–1984). *J. Neurosurg.*, 64, 543–553.

Ignelzi, R.J. and Nyquist, J.K. (1976) Excitability changes in peripheral nerve fibers after repetitive electrical stimulation. *J. Neurosurg.*, 45, 159–165.

Kuhar, M., Pert, C. and Snyder, S. (1973) Regional distribution of opiate receptor binding in monkey and human brain. *Brain*, 245, 447.

Law, J.D., Swett, J. and Kirsch, W.M. (1980) Retrospective analysis of 22 patients with chronic pain treated by peripheral nerve stimulation. *J. Neurosurg.*, 52, 482–485.

Leclercq, T.A. (1984) Electrode migration in epidural stimulation: Comparison between single electrode and four electrode programmable leads. *Pain*, 20 (Suppl. 2), 78.

Levy, R.M., Lamb, S. and Adams, J.E. (1987) Treatment of chronic pain by deep brain stimulation: Long term follow-up and review of the literature. *Neurosurgery*, 21 (6), 885–893.

Liebeskind, J.C., Guilbaud, G., Besson, J.M. et al. (1973) Analgesia from electrical stimulation of the periaqueductal gray matter in the cat: Behavioral observations and inhibitory effects on spinal cord interneurons. *Brain Res.*, 40, 441–446.

Loeser, J.D., Black, R.G. and Christman, A. (1975) Relief of pain by transcutaneous stimulation. *J. Neurosurg.*, 42, 308–314.

Long, D.M. and Hagfors, N. (1975) Electrical stimulation in the nervous system: The current status of electrical stimulation of the nervous system for relief of pain. *Pain*, 1, 109–123.

Long, D.M. (1976) Cutaneous afferent stimulation for relief of chronic pain. *Clin. Neurosurg.*, 21, 257–268.

Long, D. (1977) Electrical stimulation for the control of pain. *Arch. Surg.*, 112, 884–888.

Long, D.M., Erickson, D., Campbell, J. and North, R. (1981) Electrical stimulation of the spinal cord and peripheral nerves for pain control. *Appl. Neurophysiol.*, 44, 207–217.

Mannheimer, C. and Carlsson, C.A. (1979) The analgesic effect of transcutaneous electrical nerve stimulation (TNS) in patients with rheumatoid arthritis: A comparative study of different pulse patterns. *Pain*, 6, 329–334.

Mannheimer, J.S. and Lampe, G.N. (1984) *Clinical Transcutaneous Electrical Nerve Stimulation*, F.A. Davis, Philadelphia.

Mayer, D.J., Wolfe, T.L., Akil, H. et al (1971) Analgesia from electrical stimulation in the brainstem of the rat. *Science*, 174, 1351–1354.

Mayer, D.J. and Liebeskind, J.C. (1974) Pain reduction by focal electrical stimulation of the brain: An anatomical and behavioral analysis. *Brain Res.*, 68, 73–93.

Mayer, D.J. and Hayes, R.L. (1975) Stimulation-produced analgesia: Development of tolerance and cross-tolerance to morphine. *Science*, 188, 941–943.

Mayer, D.J. and Price, D.D. (1976) Central nervous system mechanisms of analgesia. *Pain*, 2, 379–404.

Mazars, G., Roge, R. and Mazars, Y. (1960) Results of the stimulation of the spinothalamic fasciculus and their bearing on the physiopathology of pain. *Rev. Neurol.*, 103, 136–138.

Mazars, G.J. (1975) Intermittent stimulation of nucleus ventralis posterolateralis for intractable pain. *Surg. Neurol.*, 4, 93–95.

Melzack, P. and Wall, P.D. (1965) Pain mechanisms: A new theory. *Science*, 150 (3699), 971–979.

Meyer, G.A. and Fields, H.L. (1972) Causalgia treated by selective large fiber stimulation of peripheral nerve. *Brain*, 95, 163–168.

Nashold, B.S. Jr. and Friedman, H. (1972) Dorsal column stimulation for control of pain, preliminary report on 30 patients. *J. Neurosurg.*, 36, 590–597.

Nashold, B.S. and Goldner, J.L. (1975) Electrical stimulation of peripheral nerves for relief of intractable chronic pain. *Med. Instrum.*, 9 (5), 224–225.

Nathan, P.W. (1976) The gate-control theory of pain: A critical review. *Brain*, 99, 123–158.

North, R.B., Fischell, T.A. and Long, D.M. (1977) Chronic stimulation via percutaneously inserted epidural electrodes. *Neurosurgery*, 1, 215–218.

North, R.B., and Long, D.M. (1984) Spinal cord stimulation for intractable pain: Eight-year followup. *Pain*, 20 (Suppl. 2), 79.

North, R.B. and Fowler, K.F. (1987) Computer-controlled, patient-interactive, multichannel, implanted neurological stimulators. *Appl. Neurophys.*, 50, 39–41.

North, R.B. (1988) Spinal cord stimulation for intractable pain: Indications and technique. In: *Current Therapy in Neurological Surgery*. Editor: D.M. Long, B.C. Decker, Philadelphia.

Pert, C.B. and Snyder, S.H. (1973) Opiate receptor: Demonstration in nervous tissue. *Science*, 179, 405–423.

Picaza, J.A., Hunter, S.E. and Cannon, B.W. (1978) Pain suppression by peripheral nerve stimulation. *Appl. Neurophysiol.*, 40, 223–234.

Plotkin, R. (1982) Results in 60 cases of deep brain stimulation for chronic intractable pain. *Appl. Neurophysiol.*, 45, 173–178.

Pool, J.L. (1956) Psychosurgery in elderly people. *J. Am. Geriatr. Soc.*, 2, 456–465.

Ranck, J. (1975) Which elements are excited in electrical stimulation of mammalian central nervous system: A review. *Brain Res.*, 98, 417–440.

Reynolds, D.V. (1969) Surgery in the rat during electrical analgesia induced by focal brain stimulation. *Science*, 164, 444–445.

Richardson, D.E. and Akil, H. (1977) Pain reduction by electrical stimulation in man (Part I). *J. Neurosurg.*, 47, 178–183.

Sances, A., Swiontek, T.J., Larson, S.J., Cusick, J.F., Meyer, G.A., Millar, E.A., Hemmy, D.C. and Myklebust, J. (1975) Innovations in neurologic implant systems. *Med. Instrum.*, 9 (5), 213–216.

Shealy, C., Mortimer, J. and Reswick, J. (1967) Electrical inhibition of pain by stimulation of the dorsal columns: A preliminary report. *Anesth. Analg.*, 46, 489–491.

Siegfried, J. (1982) Monopolar electrical stimulation of nucleus ventroposteromedialis thalami for postherpetic facial pain. *Appl. Neurophysiol.*, 45, 179–184.

Sjolund, B. and Eriksson, M. (1979) The influence of naloxone on analgesia produced by peripheral conditioning stimulation. *Brain Res.*, 173, 295–301.

Stillings, D. (1975) A survey of the history of electrical stimulation for pain to 1900. *Medical Instrum.*, 9 (6), 255–259.

Sweet, W.H. and Wepsic, J.G. (1968) Treatment of chronic pain by stimulation of fibers of primary afferent neuron. *Trans. Am. Neurol. Assoc.*, 93, 103–107.

Sweet, W.H. and Wepsic, J.G. (1974) Stimulation of the posterior columns of the spinal cord for pain control. *Clin. Neurosurg.*, 21, 278–310.

Swett, J. and Law, J. (1983) Analgesia with peripheral nerve stimulation: absence of a peripheral mechanism. *Pain*, 15, 55–70.

Thorsteinsson, G. Stonnington, H.H., Stilwell, G.K. and Elveback, L.R. (1978) The placebo effect of transcutaneous electrical stimulation. *Pain*, 5, 31–41.

Van den Honert, C. and Mortimer, J. (1979) Generation of unidirectionally propagated action potentials in a peripheral nerve by brief stimuli. *Science*, 206, 1311–1312.

Vanderark, G. and McGrath, K.A. (1975) Transcutaneous electrical stimulation in treatment of postoperative pain. *Am. J. Surg.*, 130, 338–340.

Waisbrod, H., Panhans, C., Hansen, D. and Gerbershagen, H.U. (1985) Direct nerve stimulation for painful peripheral neuropathies. *J. Bone Joint Surg.*, 67 (3), 470–473.

Wall, P.D. and Sweet, W.H. (1967) Temporary abolition of pain in man. *Science*, 155, 108–109.

Woolf, C.J., Mitchell, D., Myers, R.A. and Barrett, G.D. (1978) Failure of naloxone to reverse peripheral transcutaneous electro-analgesia in patients suffering from acute trauma. *SA Med. J.*, 53, 179–180.

Young, R.F., Kroening, R., Fulton, W., Feldman, R. and Chambi, I. (1985) Electrical stimulation of the brain in treatment of chronic pain: experience over 5 years. *J. Neurosurg.*, 62, 389–396.

Young, R.F. and Brechner, T. (1986) Electrical stimulation of the brain for relief of intractable pain due to cancer. *Cancer*, 57, 1266–1272.

Young, R.F. and Chambi, V.I. (1987) Pain relief by electrical stimulation of the periaqueductal and periventricular gray matter: Evidence for a non-opioid mechanism. *J. Neurosurg.*, 66, 364–371.

M. Swerdlow and J.E. Charlton (eds.) Relief of Intractable Pain
© 1989, Elsevier Science Publishers B.V. (Biomedical Division)

11

The place of neurosurgery in the treatment of intractable pain

Blaine S. Nashold, Jr., Elizabeth Bullitt and Allan Friedman

'Not everyone has a soul of fire, and in actual human life even in the case of the great mystics, the struggle against pain exacts a high price.'

Leriche

The neurosurgical treatment of intractable pain should be based on a precise knowledge of the aetiology of the pain along with neuroanatomical, neurophysiological and pharmacological information which would give a complete understanding of the patient's pain problem. Unfortunately this is not the ideal and one might think of mechanisms of pain as an ancient mosaic where the vague outlines are visible, but closer inspection gives us only a fragmentary picture of the entire problem. Certainly neuroanatomical information has improved so that the neurosurgeon can direct surgical treatment to specific pain pathways or areas of central integration in the midbrain and thalamus. As soon as the anatomists could agree on the function of the dorsal and ventral spinal roots, the logical consequence for the surgeon to was section surgically the dorsal roots (rhizotomy) and this was done in 1888 by Bennett for relief of pain (Bennett, 1889). Thirty years later, the neurologist Spiller made an astute clinical observation when examining a patient with a spinal cord tumour, which enabled him to define the function of the lateral spinothalamic tract as a pain pathway. Spiller encouraged Martin, a surgeon, to perform the first spinothalamic tractotomy (1912). Surgical access to deeper regions of the central nervous system such as the thalamus and upper midbrain was not possible until the development of the human stereotactic instrument (Spiegel and Wycis, 1947). Since that time, both spinal and central brain targets have been readily accessible to the neurosurgeon.

Long-term chronic pain in man results in physical, mental, social and economic breakdown. Why does one person suffering from paraplegia due to spinal cord trauma develop pain whereas an identical paraplegic with the same type of trauma remains pain-free? At the present time there is no answer to this dilemma. How does the surgeon explain to a patient the cause of phantom limb pain, a perplexing problem to say the least. Neurosurgical treatment of intractable pain has evolved from two main sources: (1) a better understanding of neuroanatomical pain pathways in the CNS; (2) the development of neurosurgical techniques that can safely reach deeper regions of the central nervous system (stereotactic neurosurgery) together with the ability of the neurosurgeon to produce precise therapeutic lesions destroying the appropriate pain pathways or central pain centre.

THE NEUROSURGICAL RELIEF OF PAIN

Non-cancerous pain

This type of pain is usually the result of a specific insult to peripheral nerves or structures in the central nervous system, trauma, infection or metabolic disturbance as such. The aetiological causes of the pain are often not difficult to determine; for example, traumatic avulsion of the brachial or sacral plexus, postherpetic pain (shingles) or thalamic syndrome due to a thalamic infarct. The onset of the pain may begin immediately after the insult to the CNS and the pain can plague the patient for his entire lifetime. Treatment that will give long-term or permanent pain relief should be planned. This is a difficult task, as we shall see. Medical and other active therapy should always be used in the first 6 months after the onset of the pain, but if there is no clinical response, then neurosurgical treatment should be considered. The longer a person suffers unremitting pain the more difficult it is to institute any treatment that will be completely successful. The neurosurgical treatment discussed here is destructive in nature and requires a specific understanding of the neuroanatomy of the region to be lesioned. The specific target structures include the spinal dorsal roots, the dorsal root entry zone (DREZ), and the nucleus caudalis of the trigeminal nerve at the medullary spinal junction. In the central nervous system lesions may be made in the midbrain, thalamus or fibres of the cingulum of the frontal lobes.

Dorsal rhizotomy

With the discovery that the ventral spinal roots were motor and the dorsal roots sensory, it was logical that surgical section of the dorsal roots would be involved in any operation for pain relief (Fig. 11.1). Abbe (1896) carried out the first dorsal rhizotomy for 'neuralgia'. For many years, this was a standard neurosurgical operation, but its efficacy has recently become doubtful. Loeser (1974) concluded that rhizotomy for postherpetic, post-thoracotomy and coccygeal pain is generally

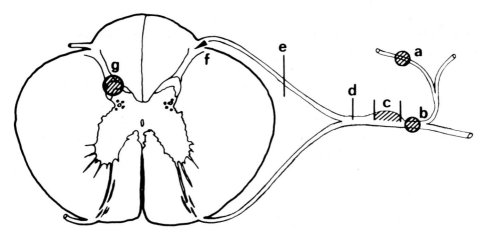

Fig. 11.1. Targets of root surgery: (a) coagulation of medial branch of posterior primary ramus; (b) coagulation of spinal nerve trunk; (c) excision of dorsal root ganglion; (d) extradural section of dorsal root; (e) intradural section of dorsal root; (f) selective dorsal rhizidotomy (partial section of rootlets); (g) coagulation of dorsal root entry zone.

unsuccessful for long-term relief. Another problem following dorsal rhizotomy is the occurrence of a deafferentation pain syndrome which may be more serious than the original neuralgia. The second reason for possible failure of dorsal root rhizotomy is the anatomical evidence that the ventral root contains some afferent fibres. This point is contested by the clinical observations, where no sensory responses were elicited on stimulating the ventral roots in an awake person. (Sweet, personal communication).

An exception to the poor results of dorsal rhizotomy for pain relief is the surgery for relief of spontaneous tic pain of the trigeminal and the glossopharyngeal nerves. Glossopharyngeal tic is characterized by severe explosive pains occurring in the throat and posterior pharynx triggered by talking, eating, swallowing or touching the area. Cocainization of the posterior pharyngeal wall often results in temporary relief and an intracranial section of the glossopharyngeal nerve along with section of the upper rootlets of the adjacent vagus nerve will give long-term relief. Recently, percutaneous techniques have been introduced in which radiofrequency (RF) lesions are produced by the percutaneous method. Both techniques seem equally successful and their use depends upon the expertise and experience of the neurosurgeon.

Trigeminal neuralgia (tic douloureux)

Painful facial tic is a severe, spontaneous pain involving one or more divisions of the trigeminal nerve. The pain commonly occurs in the lower cheek and chin (third division) with sudden bursts of electrical shock-like pains which immobilize the person during a painful episode. Each episode may last only seconds, but they can occur in continuous bursts so that the patient experiences a continuous type of pain. The painful paroxysm may spread into other regions of the face, oral cavity, throat or inner ear. Occasionally the pain may involve the teeth, but extraction of the teeth does not produce relief. Tic occurs more frequently in men and the patient is usually over 50 years of age, with a median of about 60 years. The age of the patient may be important in selecting the appropriate neurosurgical treatment. The diagnosis is not difficult, since the history is quite typical. On physical examination there may be little or no sensory change over the face, but the pain can often be triggered by touching the skin at sensitive spots located in the various divisions of the trigeminal nerve. Normal activities, such as talking and eating, may set off the pain. The pain can spread beyond the territory of the trigeminal nerve, such as into the pharynx (9th cranial nerve) or inner ear (7th cranial nerve – nervus intermedius). The aetiology of tic douloureux is still unknown. Recently, Jannetta (1967) has emphasized the role of vascular compression of the nerve and the dorsal root entry zone in the pons as a possible cause (an idea originally suggested by Dandy). Based on this, Jannetta introduced the vascular decompressive operation for relief of trigeminal pain.

Most of the time, the initial treatment should be medical. Two exceptions are the development of acute drug toxicity and the elderly patient with severe pain that is triggered by talking, chewing or swallowing, so that he may be unable to eat and rapidly becomes debilitated. The best treatment in this patient is to carry out an immediate percutaneous RF lesion, which will immediately relieve the pain and allow him to resume normal activity.

Neurosurgical treatment

Vascular decompression

Jannetta (1967) reported the surgical decompression of the trigeminal nerve for the relief of tic pain. He postulated that the trigeminal nerve was compressed by either an artery or a vein, resulting in an irritation of the nerve at its exit from the pons. There has been some debate as to the significance of vascular compression, but the improvement in pain following this surgery has been impressive with long-term relief in 85% of patients (Apfelbaum, 1977). An important advantage of this operation over the destructive operation has been the preservation of sensation over the face, plus the occasional discovery of a small tumour or AV aneurysm compressing the nerve which had escaped detection. The operation is best suited to the younger patient with tic or to one who does not want postoperative numbness of the face.

The surgical operation is major in contrast with the simpler percutaneous treatment. The morbidity is 3% with loss of hearing as an undesirable side effect and with 1% mortality. (Recently, I have seen patients with post-traumatic facial pain and anaesthesia dolorosa who underwent vascular decompression, which makes no sense in these two conditions. This stresses the importance of correct diagnosis.)

Percutaneous techniques

Sweet and Wepsic (1974) introduced selective RF lesions of the Gasserian ganglion. This procedure is the one of choice for elderly persons who need quick and certain pain relief; a disadvantage is the production of varying degrees of hypaesthesia over the face, but this is tolerable if the pain has gone. Loeser (1977) reports that in a large series of patients who had received percutaneous treatment, pain relief lasted for one year in 80% and for five years in 50% of the patients; the complication rate was 0.5%. The most serious consequence of the RF lesions of the trigeminal nerve is the development of a trigeminal dysaesthesia or anaesthesia dolorosa whose treatment is discussed later.

Atypical facial pain

The use of the word 'atypical' to describe certain types of cranial pain is somewhat misleading. Whatever definition one prefers, there is general agreement that surgical treatment in this group of patients is not as successful. The pains usually originate from varying degrees of involvement of the peripheral branches of the trigeminal nerve caused by facial trauma, either accidental, surgical or after dental operations, sinus or plastic surgery on the face. Percutaneous RF lesions have been used in treatment of this condition, but are usually unsuccessful, often leaving the patient with the dreaded 'anaesthesia dolorosa'.

Deafferentation pain – the DREZ operation

Deafferentation pain can be defined in several ways. It is pain following total or near total disconnection of the afferent input to the central nervous system. Clinical examples are traumatic avulsions of the dorsal roots most commonly in the brachial and lumbosacral regions. Phantom limb pain is another example where the missing limb continues to be perceived by the person as painful. When central pain pathways are involved, such as the lateral spinothalamic, trigeminal or spinoreticular pathway, pain syndromes may develop such as the pain of paraplegia, thalamic syndrome, or anaesthesia dolorosa.

Tasker et al. (1980) define the term 'deafferentation pain' as discomfort arising in any part of the body once the flow of afferent impulses has been partially or completely interrupted. They also say that it can theoretically also result "from injury to receptors caused by lesions of nerves, dorsal roots, spinal cord, brain stem or cerebral cortex."

Interruption of the ascending pain pathways at any anatomical level is capable of producing deafferentation pain. Wall (1980), describing it from the neurophysiologist's point of view, states that dysaesthetic pain is due to 'not only a loss of pain input but actual degeneration so that spinal cells were free to act in a pathological way'. The exact pathological origin of deafferentation pain is still an unsolved question. There are complex pharmacological changes in the deafferented CNS and these changes can occur at various levels, either upstream or downstream, involving the sensory system. The pathological process may be expressed as a hyperactivity of the secondary neurons probably due to deafferentation hypersensitivity. In animals with experimental avulsion injuries, deafferentation hypersensitivity of the secondary sensory neurons in the CNS may also be the origin of the pain.

Although the exact nature of deafferentation syndrome still eludes us, it is possible to reduce this pain by producing lesions in the secondary neurons of the afferent system. The DREZ operation has successfully relieved pain in this group of patients. In the early 1970s, we decided to produce localized lesions in the deafferented dorsal horn of persons with intractable pain due to brachial plexus avulsion (Fig. 11.2). Since then, we have performed over 500 DREZ operations in patients with deafferentation pain including paraplegia with pain, postherpetic pain and phantom pain (Fig. 11.3). The specific details of the DREZ operation and the relief of pain have been published (Nashold, 1984). This report gives the general details of patient selection, the surgical results of DREZ as well as the risks and benefits of the DREZ operation (Table 11.1).

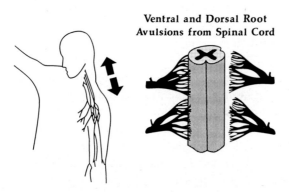

**Ventral and Dorsal Root
Avulsions from Spinal Cord**

Fig. 11.2. Brachial plexus root avulsion.

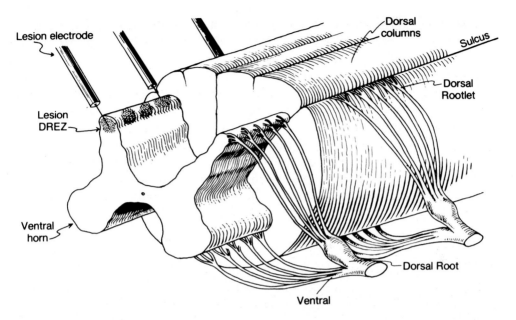

Fig. 11.3. Schematic drawing of spinal cord showing location of dorsal root entry zone (DREZ) lesions.

Brachial and lumbosacral avulsion injuries with deafferentation pain

These injuries are the result of high speed accidents; the motorcycle is the worst offender, followed by automobiles, snowmobiles and speedboats (Nashold and Ostdahl, 1979). The dorsal and ventral roots are torn from their connection on the spinal cord. The patient is left with a paralyzed arm or leg with a complete loss of sensation. Fortunately, only 10% of patients develop a severe chronic deaf-

Table 11.1. Results of the DREZ operation

	Average incidence of complications after cordotomy (%)	
	Unilateral	Bilateral
Death	5	8
Lack of initial pain relief	10	25
Dysaesthesias	7	–
Weakness	7	25
Urinary incontinence	5	25
Respiratory insufficiency	2	15

ferentation pain syndrome. The pain occurs immediately after the injury and if it does not respond to medical treatment within 6 months, the DREZ operation is recommended. The diagnosis is not difficult with a history of trauma and the neurological deficit in the involved limb. A myelogram or magnetic resonance imaging study of the involved segment of the spinal cord often reveals multiple traumatic myeloceles at the spinal level of the trauma, confirming the diagnosis. Avulsion injuries involving the lower extremity, although less frequent, can be confused with injuries to the peripheral nerves in the pelvis. These individuals suffer from severe trauma to the pelvis and lower extremity with extensive pelvic and/ or sacral fractures. Radiographic studies reveal traumatic myeloceles and the DREZ procedure in the conus medullaris relieves this pain in 80% of patients (Moossy, 1987).

Paraplegia with chronic pain

Ten percent of paraplegics suffer from chronic pain as a long-term problem. Trauma to the spinal cord, especially when caused by gunshot wounds, has the highest incidence of chronic pain. The pain may be experienced almost immediately after the injury. If the pain is described as 'burning or shock-like' and localized to the cutaneous dermatomes just above the level of the trauma, the DREZ operation will relieve 60% of these paraplegics (Nashold and Bullitt, 1981). If the pain is more diffuse in nature and localized to the legs and sacral region, surgery is of no value. Some paraplegics do not develop pain immediately after their injury but months or years later. In our experience, when delayed onset of pain occurs, a high percentage of these paraplegics will suffer from an intraspinal cyst. The cyst may occur in the segments of the spinal cord either above or below the level of the trauma. In the past, surgical drainage of the cyst alone was thought to be sufficient to relieve the pain, but in our experience surgical drainage combined with DREZ lesions has the best chance of reducing the pain, as found in 90% of our patients. All paraplegics with intractable pain should either have myelography combined with CT scanning or magnetic imaging scans of the involved segments of the spinal cord to rule out cysts (Nashold and Vieira, 1988).

Phantom limb pain due to avulsion or amputation

The development of a phantom sensation of a missing part of the body is especially troublesome to a patient and the physician is often at a loss to explain its cause and suggest a treatment. It should be remembered that the loss of a part of the body that extends beyond the surface, such as nose, ear, breast, arm, leg, penis, etc. will be followed by a temporary phantom sensation of the missing part that gradually fades away. The phantom phenomenon is probably the normal consequence of disturbing the CNS schema of the body image; however, the locus of this complex body image in the nervous system is not known, although some have implicated the cerebral cortex. The awareness of our body image requires some learning and imprinting of the body image engrams in the central nervous system. When this occurs and how long this takes in human development is unknown. However, it is interesting that children born without a limb usually do not experience phantom sensation, so that it seems that a learning process is necessary before one can experience a phantom. When pain and phantom occur together, the problem is especially difficult to treat. It is important for a surgeon carrying out an amputation to explain in detail to his patient before operating about the appearance of the phantom. The surgeon should reassure the person that the phantom will fade away. The continued presence of pain in the involved extremity tends to perpetuate both the phantom and the painful sensation. We have studied 22 patients with amputation due to trauma and surgical amputation who were suffering from painful phantom (Saris et al., 1985). Overall, only 36% of the patients with amputation and stump pain alone were relieved by the DREZ operation. In contrast, 67% of patients with phantom pain alone were relieved, as were five out of six patients with traumatic amputations associated with traumatic dorsal root avulsions. Poor results were noted in those patients with a combination of phantom and stump pain or stump pain alone.

Chronic sciatica following multiple lumbar disc operations

A most difficult pain problem is the individual who has been operated on many times for spondylitic or lumbar disc herniation and then suffers continued pain in the distribution of the sciatic nerve. Examination of these patients often reveals reduced or absent sensation in the painful areas of the leg, usually in the distribution of the L_5 or S_1 dermatome or both. In other words, the patient experiences pain in an analgesic limb (a deafferentation pain). In some patients, in an effort to relieve the pain, a dorsal rhizotomy was done; this did not relieve the pain, but may have converted the painful sensation into a burning dysaesthesia which is probably of central origin. We have carried out the DREZ operation on selected lumbosacral dorsal roots in 12 people after multiple disc operations and dorsal rhizotomies, but the results after DREZ were disappointing, with only 18% relieved (Saris et al., 1987) and even medical treatment was of little value. The same dismal results were obtained in patients with post-thoracotomy or post-surgical inguinal pain.

Postherpetic pain

Chronic postherpetic pain has been resistant to most medical and surgical treatment. The virus initially involves the dorsal root ganglion, then the peripheral nerve and in some patients may invade the dorsal and ventral horns of the spinal cord. The postherpetic pain that results is a form of deafferentation dysaesthesia. Elderly persons are more often involved with pain over the dermatomes of the chest or abdominal region. When the pain persists for more than 6 months, surgical treatment should be considered. Two types of pain are described. One is an intense burning with shooting characteristics; the skin is scarred and there is dysaesthesia in the involved dermatomes. This type of pain can be reduced with a DREZ operation carried out on the involved dorsal root entry zone regions. (However, if the pain has a deep aching quality, surgical relief is difficult. The use of transcutaneous electrical stimulation in the early phases of the disorder may be helpful, but after 6 months the difficulties mount.) We have studied 32 patients with chronic postherpetic pain and carried out dorsal root entry zone lesions on the involved dorsal roots (Friedman et al., 1984). The pain in these people had been present for 7 months – 11 years. There were two patients who were under 60 years of age while the oldest was 82. Postoperative DREZ follow-up has been 6 months – 6 years. Immediate pain relief occurred in 29 of the 32 patients, but was short-lived, so that after 6 months, only 25% of the patients were relieved. In the ten patients in which the pain did recur, they rated it as less severe than preoperatively. The major risk of this DREZ operation in the thoracic spinal cord is postoperative ipsilateral leg weakness probably due to involvement of the adjacent pyramidal tract. Eight of these patients use a cane to walk, a price that may be too dear for an elderly person. It is important for the neurosurgeon to warn the patient of this risk, and recently we have been reducing the number of DREZ lesions in an effort to reduce the leg weakness.

Chronic head and neck pain

DREZ lesions of the nucleus trigeminal caudalis

Head and neck pains are among the most complex that the neurosurgeon has to deal with. Four cranial nerves (V, VII, IX, X) innervate the head and neck regions and all four singly or in combination may be involved in pain syndromes. The trigeminal nerve innervates the greater portion of the anterior two thirds of the head, with the 7th, 9th and 10th overlapping in the oropharyngeal and aural regions. Postherpetic or post-traumatic facial pain usually only involves the trigeminal branches of the first, second or third divisions, whereas cancer of the head and neck may involve all or part of the various cranial nerves [5, 7, 9, 10].

Sjoquist (1949) published a monograph entitled 'Studies on Pain Conduction in the Trigeminal Nerve, a Contribution to the Surgical Treatment of Facial Pain'. He advocated sectioning the descending portion of the trigeminal tract just below the inferior olive. At the time, this surgical procedure, although brilliantly conceived, was difficult technically and was mainly adopted by neurosurgeons for treatment of pain due to cancer. Sjoquist did operate on a few patients with postherpetic facial pain, but relief from pain was short-lived. Sjoquist explained these failures as due to the possibility that herpetic facial pain was central in origin with the abnormality of the trigeminal nucleus. At the present time there is evidence that postherpetic pain and certain post-surgical pains of the trigeminal nerve may indeed be of a central variety or of a deafferentation type of pain. Neuroanatomists have subdivided the trigeminal nucleus into three divisions and neurophysiologists have shown that the major pain afferents from the face via the trigeminal nerve end in the secondary neurons of the trigeminal nucleus caudalis. This nucleus lies at the cervicomedullary junction between the obex of the fourth ventricle and the dorsal rootlets of C_2. It was Kerr (1961, 1966) who first suggested destroying the caudalis nucleus for facial pain. This was based on his own experimental work in cats. Prior to his suggestion, attempts had been made to destroy the trigeminal tract and nucleus at the cervicomedullary junction by stereotactic surgical techniques.

In the late 1970's we decided to destroy the nuclear complex of the trigeminal caudalis using an open microsurgical procedure combined with intraoperative evoked potential recordings by stimulating the cutaneous branch of the trigeminal nerve (Fig. 11.4). Facial pain of anaesthesia dolorosa or postherpetic trigeminal neuralgia has always been difficult to treat. The details of the caudalis nucleus DREZ operation have already been described (Nashold et al., 1986). Briefly, the trigeminal nucleus caudalis can be lesioned between the obex and the dorsal rootlets of C_2 on the same side as the pain. The region is surgically exposed and a special RF lesion electrode is introduced under microscopic control in the lateral

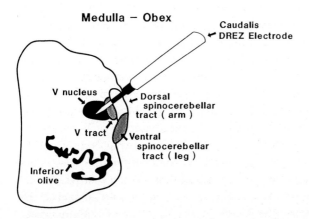

Fig. 11.4. Schematic drawing of target for trigeminal nucleus caudalis lesions.

surface of the brainstem for a depth of 3 mm. A series of 20–30 coagulations are made in a line with the dorsal nerve rootlets ending at, or slightly above, the level of the obex of the fourth ventricle. After the lesion, these patients have complete analgesia in the distribution of the trigeminal nerve both on the face and in the oral cavity. Most patients will also exhibit a mild ipsilateral ataxia in the arm due to partial involvement of the nearby dorsospinocerebellar tract, which lies superficial to the caudalis nucleus. Recently we reported 18 patients with facial pain mainly due to postherpetic neuralgia involving the first division (Bernard et al., 1987). Fifty percent of the patients were relieved after a caudalis DREZ, with a follow-up of 2 years. Postherpetic pain was relieved in 75% of these patients. A favourable surgical outcome could be correlated with a restricted preoperative sensory loss or pain confined to the trigeminal nerve distribution only or when the pain was described by the patient as burning or lancinating. Recently we have been able to relieve the pain in two patients with orbital cancer and in one patient with posterior pharyngeal oesophageal cancer.

Thalamic syndrome with pain

Pain following a stroke is well known and was first described by Dejerine and Roussy in 1906. The vascular lesion usually involves the sensory thalamus and the adjacent midbrain and it is thought that the pain originates from partial injury of the neospinothalamic pathways. It has always been difficult to treat.

The pain may occur immediately after the stroke and usually involves large areas of the body on the paralyzed side. In some patients the pain may be centred more in the head and neck regions. There are varying degrees of sensory loss on the involved side. There seems to be a steady state of pain, but light sensory stimulation or emotional aggravation will increase the intensity of the pain. Active or passive movements of the involved arm or leg can also intensify the discomfort. There is some physiological evidence that the episodes of pain may be due to hyper-irritable neurons in the damaged thalamus or adjacent midbrain (Wilson and Nashold, 1968). The exact incidence of thalamic pain is unknown and medical treatment has been mainly unsuccessful. Numerous surgical treatments have been devised, such as interruption of the limbic pathways (cingulumotomy), which may reduce the suffering but not the pain (Bouckoms, 1984). Hypophysectomy has been reported to reduce the pain (Miles, 1984). The disadvantage of hypophysectomy may be the associated changes in endocrine function, which require additional treatment. The stereotactic introduction of chronic stimulating electrodes into the thalamic or midbrain areas has also been employed on a relatively small scale for pain relief (Richardson, 1985). Forty years ago, Wycis and Spiegel (1962) introduced the stereotactic mesencephalic tractotomy for relief of thalamic pain. Its major disadvantages were ocular dysfunction due to the proximity of the lesions to the midbrain ocular pathways and the crude methods of producing the lesions. With improvements in both lesion and stereotactic techniques we have been able to treat a group of 27 patients with thalamic pain and produce good pain relief (Shieff and Nashold, 1987); thalamic pain was relieved in 21 patients from a stereotactic lesion placed in the ascending neospinal pathways in the mid-brain. Five years later, 24 of these patients were reviewed and 16 (66.7%) still had pain relief. The stereotactic operations were performed under local anaesthesia in an attempt to reduce complications. In our series two patients did develop severe aspiration pneumonia postoperatively and two died later after discharge. Ocular defects due to the midbrain lesions are well known and were noted in 12 of our patients, the defects consisting of conjugate gaze and palsies in the lateral vertical direction. However, none of these ocular defects was considered disabling by the patient.

Pain due to cancer

The neurosurgical treatment of pain due to cancer is still difficult despite the numerous neurosurgical procedures available. Three important factors must be considered in the patient with cancer. One is the timing of the operation with the course of the disease; second is the effectiveness of the operation in terms of the length of time the patient will be relieved; third is selection of the appropriate operation which has the fewest side effects. The type and nature of the cancer as well as its location will influence the timing of the operation. Pain may be an initial symptom before the discovery of the cancer. On the other hand, metastasis of the cancer, especially breast or prostatic cancer, may not occur for several years. Generally it can be said that the decision to perform a neurosurgical operation for pain relief is often made too late. Cancer pain can result in other distressing symptoms requiring treatment. Neurosurgical operations that combine relief of pain and spasticity may be necessary if the spinal cord is involved. Adjunct treatments for cancer such as radiation therapy directed to the brachial or pelvic areas may cause pain. Nowadays most patients with cancer undergo multiple complex medical treatments using experimental drugs and treatment protocols that complicate any decision for surgical treatment.

The pain experienced by a patient with cancer may have an added dimension – the presence of 'suffering'. This is a complex psychological state with emotional changes often associated with autonomic dysfunction (sweating, hyperventilation, increased cardiac rate, anxiety). Treatment which reduces the pain or even relieves it significantly may not alter the suffering component of the disorder. Psychological and psychiatric treatment is important, but in a few persons in whom the suffering is producing a serious disability, a stereotactic cingulumotomy should be performed. Suffering will be relieved and even the need for narcotics diminished (Bouckoms, 1984).

Dorsal root rhizotomy

As we have already commented in the section on the treatment of chronic intractable pain, dorsal rhizotomy is not recommended for chronic pain. This is based on numerous reports in the literature (Loeser, 1974) and our own experience. In 1986, we carried out dorsal root rhizotomy in a group of 25 patients whose pain was due to cancer or chronic coccydynia. The patients were followed for 3 years. In the patients with malignancy involving the sacrum and/or pelvis, 53% had good pain relief following a bilateral sacral dorsal rhizotomy (L_5-S_5), while only 22% with chronic coccygeal pain were relieved (Saris et al., 1987). Selective chemical rhizotomy using either alcohol or phenol injected in the subarachnoid space is also an effective method for the treatment of malignant pain originating below the level of the T_6 dermatome. It is a simple procedure from the patient's point of view, but it does add some additional risk to bladder and bowel function when done bilaterally (see Chapter 8).

Selective posterior rhizidotomy

Sindou et al. (1974, 1976), in 1972, introduced a selective section of the nociceptive fibres ventrolateral to the dorsal roots of the posterior lateral sulcus of the spinal cord. The operation is carried out under microscopic control with a 1–2 mm incision into the spinal cord to divide the ventrolateral nociceptive fibres and adjacent Lissauer's tract (Fig. 11.5). The operation was devised to relieve both pain and spasticity associated with cancer. In 1976, 20 patients with intractable pain due to cancer were reported following rhizidotomy, and complete relief of pain was obtained in 13 (Sindou et al., 1976). An advantage of this operation is the relative sparing of sensation, while its disadvantages include hypotonia and areflexia in the extremity involved. Recently, Sindou and Lapvas (1982) reported 27 patients were reported of whom 13 were suffering from pain associated with lung cancer, and 3 with oesophageal cancer and involvement of the brachial plexus. Good results were noted in this group although the exact duration of the pain relief was not indicated. The long-term results of the rhizidotomy may be limited since the patients operated on were often debilitated with a limited life expectancy.

Commissural myelotomy

The basis for the use of commissural myelotomy is the interruption of the decussating fibres of the spinothalamic tract resulting in a bilateral loss of pain and thermal sensation (Fig. 11.6). It is best used in patients with widespread abdominal or pelvic cancer. Armour (1927) carried out the first dorsal longitudinal incision of the spinal cord in a patient with severe pain of tabetic gastric crises. Later, the

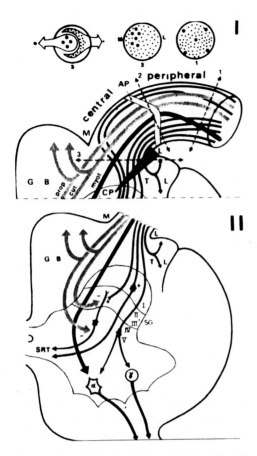

Fig. 11.5. *Top*: Organization of fibres at the posterior rootlet-spinal cord junction in man. Each rootlet comprises a peripheral and a central segment. The junction between the two constitutes the pial ring (*AP*). Peripherally, the fibres have no organization, as shown in the transverse section of the rootlet (*1*). In the neighbourhood of the pial ring, the small fibres are situated on the rootlet surface, predominantly on its lateral side (*2*). Then, in the central segment, they regroup laterally (*3*) to enter the tract of Lissauer (*TL*) and the posterior horn (*CP*). The large fibres are situated centrally for the myotactic fibres and medially (*2, 3*) for the lemniscal (proprioceptive and cutaneous) ones. Selective posterior rhizotomy affects the black triangle. Reproduced with permission from Sindou, 1972; Medical Thesis, Lyon. *Bottom*: Posterior rootlet projections to the spinal cord. The small fibres terminate on the spinoreticulothalamic cells (*SRT*), which they activate, and by polysynaptic arcs on the gamma (γ) and alpha (α) neurons of the anterior horn. The short collaterals of the large fibres (of cutaneous or proprioceptive origin) terminate on the SRT cells, which they inhibit. Reproduced with permission from Sindou et al., 1974 by courtesy of the Editors of the *Journal of Comparative Neurology*.

procedure was used to treat the pain of cancer. Sourek (1969) reported 25 patients with carcinoma receiving good immediate relief; however, the effects tend to wear off in a few months. It appears that good relief can be obtained in about 60% of

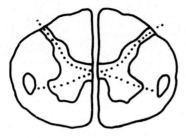

Fig. 11.6. Schematic drawing shows principle of mediolongitudinal myelotomy. Reproduced with permission from Sourek (1969) *J. Neurosurg.*, 31, 524–527.

patients with cancer; however, the disadvantage of the open myelotomy is the development of transient postoperative dysaesthesias and alterations of certain sensory modalities in the segments being treated for the pain. In an effort to simplify the operative procedure, especially in patients ill with cancer, Hitchcock (1970) introduced the percutaneous technique of making a series of midline coagulations in the upper cervical cord (Fig. 11.7). Later, Schvarcz (1976) refined the technique using pre-lesion electrical stimulation to localize the position of the needle. Pain relief was noted in 30 out of 45 patients for up to 6 months and there appeared to be fewer side effects involving the bladder, bowel or sensory deficits. Both stereotactic methods are 'blind', even though X-ray control is employed. The spinal cord lesions involve the central portions of the cervical cord so that the lesions produce widespread sensory changes with varying degrees of asymmetry. The operation using the microscope is probably more precise, whereas the percutaneous technique puts less stress on the patient but requires greater surgical skill than the stereotactic method.

Anterior lateral cordotomy

The spinal lateral cordotomy is one of the most important pain-relieving operations in cancer. With the development of the percutaneous cordotomy technique, many debilitated patients who were unable to stand the surgical stress of an open operation have benefitted (Mullan et al., 1965). The first cordotomy was carried out in 1911 by Martin at the suggestion of Spiller and Martin, who had observed a patient with bilateral loss of pain and thermal sensation due to compression of the anterior lateral part of the cord due to a spinal tuberculoma (Spiller and Martin, 1912). Since that time, lateral spinothalamic cordotomy has been used extensively for the treatment of cancer pain. Extensive literature is available on the effects of both open and closed cordotomy, which have recently been reviewed by Sweet and Wepsic (1974). The percutaneous technique originated by Mullen et al. (1965)

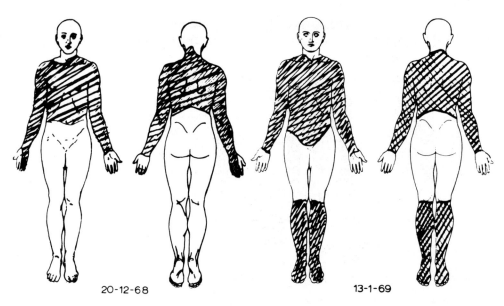

20-12-68   13-1-69

Fig. 11.7. Stereotactic myelotomy of case 1 of Hitchcock with sensory loss (analgesia to pinprick). Reproduced with permission from Hitchcock (1970) *J. Neurol. Neurosurg. Psychiatry*, 33, 224–230.

is the operation of choice at the present time; its advantage is its simplicity in skilled hands. Open unilateral cordotomy results in good pain relief in over 80% of the patients until death (White and Sweet, 1979). The morbidity is greater following cervical than thoracic cordotomy, with an overall mortality rate of 3–13%. Bilateral open cordotomy has about the same mortality as bilateral percutaneous cordotomy (2–11%). Rosomoff et al. (1965) noted 93% pain relief initially following percutaneous cordotomy, and 2 years later about half of the patients continued to be relieved of their pain. The major complications of any cordotomy consist of the development of disagreeable sensations in the analgesia area (4–10%) and muscular weakness in 5%, but these are doubled in patients with bilateral operations. Respiratory insufficiency is a greater risk after cervical cordotomy, and the incidence of sleep-induced apnoea after bilateral percutaneous cordotomy ranges from 3 to 30%. Bladder, bowel and sexual function may also suffer after cordotomy. A unilateral cordotomy usually results in transient disturbances while severe urinary symptoms occur in 5–15% of patients after a bilateral open cordotomy. The ability of a male to maintain an erection and of a woman to experience orgasm remains after bilateral cordotomy, but the male does not experience orgasm. The overall incidence of these complications is not well known. Autonomic dysfunction is also manifest by the loss of the ability to sweat in certain parts of the body associated with postural hypotension. The percutaneous cordotomy is the most effective operation for cancer pain that originates below the clavicles and should be performed as early as possible (Fig. 11.8).

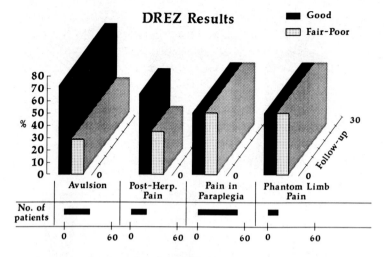

Fig. 11.8. Complications of cordotomy.

Cancer pain of the head and neck

Caudalis trigeminal nucleus DREZ

Pain of the head and neck can be due to involvement of four cranial nerves (V, VII,IX,X). The trigeminal innervates the largest area of the head and oral cavity and is often involved by cancer. If only one or two divisions of the trigeminal are involved, a percutaneous retro-gasserian coagulation may be a simple and useful treatment. However, often the cancer invades the territory of all four of these cranial nerves. At one time, intracranial surgical section of these nerves via the posterior fossa was used as a method of pain relief, but this is a major neurosurgical procedure which is often complicated by the presence of tumour along the route of the surgical operation. Recently we have reported the localized coagulation of the trigeminal nucleus caudalis at the level of the cervicomedullary junction for relief of pain of the head and neck. The trigeminal nucleus caudalis receives the majority of pain afferents from the trigeminal system, and the cancer rarely involves this area of the medullary cervical junction. The neurosurgical operation is designated as the caudalis DREZ. It has been reported extensively in the literature (Bernard et al., 1987). It consists of making a series of small coagulations at the level of the cervicomedullary junction in the trigeminal caudalis nucleus. This results in a loss of pain in all three divisions of the trigeminal nerve as well as in cranial nerves VII,IX and X. More recently, we have had some direct experience in five patients with cancer who have been followed for periods of 14 months. Forty percent of these individuals experienced good pain relief without the use of drugs (analgesics, narcotics). The remainder of the patients (60%) reported less pain but continued to take some drugs and experienced some limitations of physical activity. The pathological causes of the pain in this group of patients were a meningioma in the posterior fossa with compression of the trigeminal nerve at the pontine level, a tumour invading the lacrimal gland, tumours involving the orbital areas and the parasellar region and middle fossa. When the tumour invades the nasopharynx and oesophageal region, not only will the trigeminal nerve be involved but there will also be involvement of cranial nerves VII, IX and X. Three of the patients had received cobalt radiation which had probably complicated the pain. The average age of the patient was approximately 56 years and the pain had been present for about 36 months (longer than in the average cancer patient). The reason for the longer time was that the tumours were the relatively slow-growing type. The patients had previously undergone surgical operations which had been unsuccessful in relieving the pain. The one serious side effect of the caudalis DREZ is the occurrence of ataxia on the side of the operation probably due to involvement of the adjacent spinocerebellar tracts. Fortunately this ataxia resolves without any serious functional disability to the patient.

If the patient has a life expectancy of 6 months or less, drug treatment is more appropriate.

Stereotactic mesencephalic tractotomy for relief of pain from cancer

Even though the trigeminal nerve or its branches are most often involved when cranial cancer spreads, it frequently also involves the cranial nerves. There are several advantages of stereotactic mesencephalic tractotomy. A therapeutic lesion in the dorsolateral midbrain contralateral to the pain results in complete analgesia over the entire half of the body including the head and neck. The early open operation devised by Walker (1942) sectioned the entire spinothalamic input from the lower body and the face. This open operation did not gain wide-spread use because of its technical difficulties and postoperative hazards. There was a mortality rate of 7% and a serious risk of developing post-lesion dysaesthesia, which is often more severe than the patient's original pain. With the development of stereotactic neurosurgical techniques by Spiegel at al. (1947), it became possible to reach these deeper midbrain regions through a burr hole and small selective RF lesions could be made with a small probe, thereby reducing the high morbidity and the post-lesion dysaesthesia (Spiegel et al. 1962). As experience from the stereotactic operation was gained, it was found that by including the ascending spinoreticular pathways lying medial to the spinothalamic tract, not only was good pain relief obtained, but also the patient's anxiety and suffering were reduced. In 1972 we reported good relief of pain in patients with extensive cephalic and oral cancer. After stereotactic midbrain lesions, we found that the pain originating from the

324

oropharyngeal area subsided and that reflex coughing spasms and trismus often associated with the pain were relieved. Over 70% of the patient's cancer pain was relieved for over a year. Frank and associates (1982) reported their European experience of 91 patients, 83.5% of whom were free of pain after a followup of 2–7 months. Their mortality and morbidity were minimal. The one permanent side effect of mesencephalic tractotomy is the occurrence of post-lesion ocular dysfunction with effects such as vergent and conjugate gaze defects. These ocular defects as a rule do not disturb the patient. The greatest advantage of the stereotactic procedure is the use of local anaesthesia along with localization of the target area by physiological electrical stimulation.

PITUITARY ABLATION AND PAIN RELIEF

Pain originating from metastatic bone lesions from breast and prostate cancer can be relieved by destruction of the pituitary gland. Initially the pain relief was thought to be due to changes in pituitary hormone function, while currently the effect may be mediated via the hypothalamus with the release of endorphins resulting in pain relief. Huggins and Hodges in 1941, noted the effects of castration on prostatic cancer and noted changes in metastatic cancer of the male breast. The temporary regression of the tumour was accompanied by alleviation of bone pain in these patients.

Destruction of the pituitary gland can be accomplished by open surgery (transsphenoidal hypophysectomy) or stereotactically via the nasal cavity (Wilson and Saglan, 1973b). A variety of destructive agents have been used to destroy the pituitary gland including radon, yttrium-90 and coagulation from hot or cold, but the simplest approach is the use of an injection of absolute alcohol and was first proposed by Morrica (1974). As with any surgical treatment for cancer pain, the simplest procedure should be employed and this appears to be injection of absolute alcohol. The needle for injection can be introduced under radiographic control through the nasal cavity and the sphenoid sinus into the base of the pituitary gland where 1–2 ml of absolute alcohol are injected. The clinical effect appears to be equal to more complex treatments, especially those using radioactive substances. Both the transnasal and transfrontal craniotomy have been used but are no better as far as pain relief is concerned and add the extra problems associated with major neurosurgery.

The indication for pituitary ablation is the man (prostate) or woman (breast) with severe generalized pain due to bone metastasis. Contraindication to ablation would include intracranial metastasis, extensive involvement of lungs, kidneys, etc. The early experience for breast cancer metastasis suggested that pre-menopausal women with hormone-sensitive tumours were best suited for pituitary ablation, but this has not been the case and older post-menopausal women may have an equal benefit. Prostatic cancer and breast cancer patients are quite similar in their response to pituitary ablation and the above indications hold for both groups of patients.

According to Miles (1984), 80% of the pain can be relieved in breast cancer and about 90% in prostatic cancer. There is no correlation between the hormonal alterations caused by the ablation and pain relief. Pain relief may persist for at least a year in most patients. The mortality rate from alcohol injection is probably about 1%, but serious complications can result from all techniques, and the most serious include changes in visual field function and CSF leaks. The loss of pituitary function including diabetes insipidus can be treated medically without much discomfort to the patient.

CONCLUSIONS

There have been important advances in the treatment of long-term chronic pain, yet our understanding of chronic pain lags behind. This is due in part to the fact that chronic pain may have multiple mechanisms depending on the site in the nervous system where the pathological impact falls. We now realize that chronic pain is more than a symptom; it is a 'disease' process in itself, generated by the complex circumstances of various diseases. Singular treatment modalities are now insufficient to deal with most chronic pain and improvements have occurred where a multidisciplinary treatment approach is used. Long-term pain still extracts a high price from the suffering individual, involving physical, psychological, emotional and economic deterioration. Only concentrated research in the clinic and the laboratory along with 'cross-fertilization' between scientists and treating physicians will improve the lot of 'man in pain'.

REFERENCES

Abbe, R. (1896) Intradural section of spinal nerves for neuralgia. *Bost. Med. Surg. J.*, 135, 329–335.

Armour, D. (1927) Lettsgrian Lecture on the surgery of the spinal cord and its membranes. *Lancet*, 1, 691–697.

Bennett, W.H. (1889) Cited by Abbe, R. Acute spasmodic pain in the left lower extremity. *Med. Chir. Trans.*, 72, 329–348.

Bernard, E.S., Nashold, B.S., Jr., Caputi, F. and Moossy, J.J. (1987) Nucleus caudalis DREZ lesions for facial pain. *Br. J. Neurosurg.*, 1, 81–92.

Bouckoms, A.J. (1984) Psychosurgery. In: *Textbook of Pain*, Editors: P.D. Wall and R. Melzack. Churchill Livingstone, New York, pp. 666–676.

Dejerine, J. and Roussy, G. (1906) Le syndrome thalamique. *Rev. Neurol. (Paris)*, 14, 521–535.

Frank, F., Tognetti, Gaist, G., Frank, G., Galassi, E. and Sturiale, C. (1982) Stereotactic rostral mesencephalotomy in treatment of malignant faciothoracobrachial pain. *J. Neurosurg.*, 56, 807–811.

Friedman, A.H., Nashold, B.S., Jr. and Ovelmen-Levitt, J. (1984) Dorsal root entry zone lesions for the treatment of post herpetic neuralgia. *J. Neurosurg.*, 60, 1258–1262.

Hitchcock, E. (1970) Stereotactic cervical myelotomy. *J. Neurol. Neurosurg. Psychiat.*, 33, 224–230.

Huggins, C.B. and Hodges, C.V. (1941) Studies on Prostatic Cancer 1. The effects of castration of estrogen and of androgen injection on serum phosphatase in metastatic carcinoma of the prostate. *Cancer Res.*, 293–297.

Jannetta, P.J. (1967) Arterial compression of the trigeminal nerves at the pons in patients with trigeminal neuralgia. *J. Neurosurg.*, 26, 159–162.

Kerr, F.W.L. (1961) Structural relation of the trigeminal spinal tract to upper cervical roots and the solitary nucleus in the cat. *Exp. Neurol.*, 4, 134–148.

Kerr, F.W.L. (1966) Spinal V nucleolysis. Intractable facial pain. *Surg. Forum*, 17, 419–421.

Loeser, J.D. (1974) Dorsal rhizotomy. Indications and Results. In: *Advances in Neurology, Vol. 4.*, Raven Press, New York, pp. 615–619.

Loeser, J.D. (1977) The management of tic douloureux. *Pain*, 3, 155–162.

Miles, J. (1984) Pituitary destruction. In: *Textbook of Pain*. Editors: P.D. Wall and R. Melzack. Churchill Livingstone, New York, pp. 656–665.

Moossy, J.J., Nashold, B.S., Jr. and Osborne, D. (1987) Conus medullaris nerve root avulsions. *J. Neurosurg.*, 66, 835–841.

Morrica, G. (1974) Chemical hypophysectomy for cancer pain. In: *Advances in Neurology*. Editor: J.J. Bonica. Raven Press, New York, pp. 707–714.

Mullan, S., Heckmat Panah, J. and Dobben, G. (1965) Percutaneous interruption of spinal pain tracts by means of a strontium needle. *J. Neurosurg.*, 20, 931–939.

Nashold, B.S., Jr. (1984) Current status of the DREZ operation. *Neurosurgery*, 15, 942–944.

Nashold, B.S., Jr. and Bullitt, E. (1981) Dorsal root entry zone lesions to control central pain in paraplegia. *J. Neurosurg.*, 55, 414–419.

Nashold, B.S., Jr. and Vieira, J. (1988) Pain and spinal cysts in paraplegia. In press.

Nashold, B.S., Jr., Lopes, H., Chodakiewitz, J. and Bronec, P. (1986) Trigeminal DREZ for craniofacial pain. In: *Surgery In and Around the Brain Stem*. Editor: M. Samii. Springer-Verlag, Heidelberg, pp. 53–58.

Nashold, B.S., Jr. and Ostdahl, R.H. (1979) Dorsal root entry zone lesions for pain relief. *J. Neurosurg.*, 51, 59–69.

Richardson, D.E. (1985) Deep brain stimulation for pain relief. In: *Neurosurgery, Vol. 3*. Editors: R.H. Wilkins and S.S. Rengachary. McGraw Hill Book Co., pp. 2421–2426.

Rosomoff, H.L., Carroll, F. and Brown, J. (1965) Percutaneous radiofrequency cervical cordotomy: Technique. *J. Neurosurg.*, 23, 639–644.

Saris, S.C., Vieira, J.F.S. and Nashold, B.S., Jr. (1987) Dorsal root entry zone coagulation for intractable sciatica. In press.

Saris, S.C., Iacono, R.P. and Nashold, B.S., Jr. (1985) Dorsal root entry zone lesions for post-amputation pain. *J. Neurosurg.*, 62, 72–76.

Schvarcz, J.R. (1976) Stereotactic extralemniscal myelotomy. *J. Neurol. Neurosurg.*, 39, 53–57.

Shieff, C. and Nashold, B.S., Jr. (1987) Stereotactic mesencephalic tractotomy for relief of thalamic pain. *Br. J. Neurosurg.*, 1, 305–310.

Sindou, M., Quoey, C. and Baleydier, C. (1974) Fiber organization at the posterior spinal cord-rootlet junction in man. *J. Comp. Neurol.,* 153, 15–20.

Sindou, M., Fischer, G. and Mansuy, L. (1976) Posterior spinal rhizotomy and selective posterior rhizidotomy. In: *Progress in Neurological Surgery, Vol. 7*. Editors: P.E. Maspes and W.H. Sweet. S. Karger, Munich, pp. 201–250.

Sindou, M. and Lapvas, C. (1982) Neurosurgical treatment of pain in the Pancoast-Tobias Syndrome. Selective posterior rhizotomy and open anterolateral C2 cordotomy. In: *Advances in Pain Research and Therapy, Vol. 4.* Editors: J.J. Bonica, V. Vittorio and C. Pagni. Raven Press, New York, pp. 199–206.

Sjoquist, H.G. (1949) Surgical section of pain tracts and pathways in the spinal cord and brain stem. *Proc. of the 4th Congress on Neurology,* 1, 119–132.

Sourek, K. (1969) Commissural myelotomy. *J. Neurosurg.,* 34, 524–527.

Spiegel, E.A., Wycis, H.T., Marks, M. and Lee, A.J. (1947) Stereotaxic apparatus for operations on the human brain. *Science,* 106, 349–350.

Spiller, W.G. and Martin, E. (1912) The treatment of persistent pain of organic origin in the lower part of the body by division of the anterolateral column of the spinal cord. *JAMA,* 58, 1489–1490.

Sweet, W.H. and Wepsic, J.G. (1974) Controlled thermocoagulation of trigeminal ganglion and rootlets for differential destruction of pain fibers. *J. Neurosurg.,* 40, 143–156.

Tasker, R.R., Organ, L.W. and Hawrylyshyn, P. (1980) Deafferentation and causalgia. In: *Pain.* Editor: J.J. Bonica. Raven Press, New York, pp. 329–350.

Walker, A.E. (1942) Relief of pain by mesencephalic tractotomy. *Arch. Neurol. Psychiat.,* 48, 865–883.

Wall, P.D. (1980) The role of substantia gelatinosa as a gate control. In: *Pain.* Editor: J.J. Bonica. Raven Press, New York, pp. 205–231.

Wilson, C.B. and Saglan, S. (1973a) Pathophysiology of and indications for hypophysectomy. In: *Neurological Surgery.* Editor: J.R. Youmans. W.B. Saunders Co., Philadelphia, pp. 1901–1907.

Wilson, C.B. and Saglan, S. (1973b) Stereotaxic hypophysectomy. In: *Neurological Surgery.* Editor: J.R. Youmans. W.B. Saunders Co., Philadelphia, pp. 1908–1914.

Wilson, W.P. and Nashold, B.S., Jr. (1968) Epileptic discharges occurring in the mesencephalon and thalamus. *Epilepsia,* 9, 265–273.

Wycis, H.T. and Spiegel, E.A. (1962) Long range results in the treatment of intractable pain by stereotaxic midbrain surgery. *J. Neurosurg.,* 19, 101–107.

M. Swerdlow and J.E. Charlton (eds.) Relief of Intractable Pain
© 1989, Elsevier Science Publishers B.V. (Biomedical Division)

12

Radiotherapy, chemotherapy and hormone therapy in the relief of cancer pain

Thelma Bates

Pain may be a feature of both early and late cancer. It can be caused by the cancer itself, by the cancer treatment or by factors which are totally unrelated.

Three basic principles apply to the control of pain: first to diagnose the cause, which can be multifactorial and highly complex; second, to provide appropriate treatment, and this can include radiotherapy, chemotherapy or hormones; third, to monitor the situation regularly in order to assess the efficacy of the treatment relative to the changing circumstances of the patient. Control of pain is an end in itself, whatever the stage of the disease.

Radiotherapy, chemotherapy and hormones control pain mainly by their anti-tumour effects. They can be used separately or in combination, and sometimes together with surgery, with either radical or palliative intent. Pain relief can be achieved either by local therapy, as with radiotherapy, or by systemic measures using chemotherapy or hormones.

In the patient with early cancer receiving treatment aimed at cure, pain relief is important but is incidental to the treatment of the disease itself. Understandably, radiotherapists and medical oncologists put emphasis on the curative treatment of cancer, but in our present state of knowledge, the majority of cancer patients are not cured (Waterhouse, 1974; Haybrittle, 1983), and a high percentage of our time is occupied with the palliative management of patients with advanced cancer, not least with the control of chronic pain. Here an important skill lies in judging when the benefits of therapy clearly outweigh the disadvantages. This involves not only knowing how to treat, but also when to treat and when to withold active treatment. The oncologist must also understand how to control pain by other means, and not least, how to function as part of a complex multidisciplinary team which includes the hospital, the community and sometimes the hospice services.

LOCAL PAIN RELIEF BY RADIOTHERAPY

Radiotherapy has a particularly important role in the control of severe chronic cancer pain and it can be of value even in the last weeks of life. The aim of radiotherapy in patients with incurable cancer and a limited prognosis is to relieve pain quickly and so improve the quality of life. In such cases treatment is rarely given to prevent a pain which may never arise, although there are a few clear-cut exceptions.

The general principles of palliative radiotherapy at this stage of the disease are dictated by the limited expectation of life and the need to avoid causing the patient additional discomfort. If indicated, radiotherapy should be given with as little delay as possible and if a patient is at home, preferably as an out-patient. Many symptoms, including cancer pain, can be relieved, often completely, in a few treatment sessions and by a low dose of radiotherapy with few or no associated side effects (Bates, 1984). Severe pain due to bone secondaries can even be relieved in a single treatment (Price et al., 1986). Prolonged courses of daily fractions over several weeks are rarely necessary and are not appropriate for patients where the aim is palliation and not cure. In all cases the benefits of treatment have to be carefully balanced against the price the patient has to pay in time and discomfort.

It is never easy to refuse a patient treatment. Very often a radiotherapist has treated the patient over several years and has helped in the past, and both the patient and the relatives may beg for help once again. In addition, his medical colleagues, who themselves have nothing more to offer but wish to give some positive help, may press him to treat a patient. In all cases he must be clear in his own mind what he can hope to achieve by this therapy and, although psychological factors are taken into consideration, he must be motivated by the possible physical benefit to his patient. Occasionally a radiotherapist may be asked to 'pretend to treat' a patient, but such deception is never justified and indeed is unnecessary in the context of a good team approach to palliative cancer care (Bates, 1988).

About 40% of all cancer patients in the UK receive radiotherapy at some stage of their disease (Cohen et al., 1981) and about half the machine workload of a modern radiotherapy department is concerned with palliative treatment. Effective treatment requires a full range of radiotherapy equipment to deal with tumours at different depths and sites and an efficient organization which permits treatment without delay.

Three factors influence the potential value of radiotherapy:

(1) *The radio-sensitivity of the tumour.* Adult bone and soft tissue sarcomas, gliomas and melanomas are radio-resistant; lymphomas and seminomas are radio-sensitive; squamous cell carcinomas and to a lesser extent, adenocarcinomas are moderately radio-sensitive.

(2) *The radio-tolerance of the adjacent normal tissues.* The bowel is particularly

radio-sensitive and large volume abdominal radiotherapy invariably causes nausea and diarrhoea.

(3) *The degree of previous radiotherapy*. Fully irradiated tissues cannot be re-irradiated without the risk of necrosis.

PAIN DUE TO BONE METASTASES

Approximately 15% of the workload of a modern radiotherapy department is concerned with treatment of painful bone metastases and worthwhile pain relief can be achieved in approximately 80% of patients.

Radiotherapy has several roles to play in the management of patients with bone metastases:
— Relief of bone pain with local or hemi-body radiotherapy.
— Prevention of painful pathological fractures or vertebral collapse.
— Promotion of healing in pathological fractures (preferably following surgical fixation).
— Manipulation of the endocrine environment of the tumour (for example, by ovarian irradiation in hormone-sensitive breast carcinoma with bone metastases).

RELIEF OF BONE PAIN

The pathogenesis of bone pain is not well understood, nor is its relief by radiotherapy. No doubt, radiation-induced tumour shrinkage accounts for the relief of pain associated with nerve root or periosteal compression, but this cannot be responsible for the rapid onset of pain relief (often within 24 h) which can follow hemi-body irradiation and endocrine procedures such as pituitary ablation. Even following local irradiation, as many as 30% of patients experience pain relief within the first week irrespective of the degree of radio-sensitivity of the tumour, and this is unlikely to be due to tumour shrinkage. An alternative or additional mechanism may well involve an inhibiting effect on the host cells which secrete chemical mediators of the pain response, such as prostaglandins. Low dose radiotherapy is well known to give excellent pain relief in patients with ankylosing spondylitis.

LOCALISED BONE METASTASES

The literature shows that a variety of radiotherapy techniques for localised bone metastases achieve worthwhile pain relief in about 80% of patients (50% complete, 30% partial relief). Two randomised prospective trials (Schocker et al., 1981; Tong et al., 1982) looked at total dose levels in the range 15–25 Gy given in daily treatments over 5 days and found no dose-response relationship for pain control. Five retrospective studies compared single and multiple treatments (Vargha et al., 1969; Penn, 1976; Allen et al., 1976; Jensen and Rosendahl, 1976; Qasim, 1977) and showed similar pain relief from a single treatment in the range 4–15 Gy as from multiple treatments with a total dose in the range 20–40 Gy.

An important randomised prospective study at the Royal Marsden Hospital (Price et al., 1986) compared a single treatment of 8 Gy with the more conventional ten daily treatments delivering a total dose of 30 Gy. They found no difference in response rate, speed of onset, or duration or degree of pain relief at any site or for any tumour histology, and no difference in early or late radiation morbidity. Patients with severe pain initially were found to be more likely to respond than those with mild or moderate pain. Clearly the single treatment technique is preferable because of the convenience for patients with a short life expectancy. If pain is not relieved or if it returns, retreatment is possible.

GENERALISED BONE METASTASES

When there are generalised pains due to widespread bone metastases, hemi-body irradiation may be indicated. Either the upper or lower half of the body is irradiated in a single treatment of 6–8 Gy, followed if necessary with treatment to the other half of the body 6 weeks later. Treatment to the upper half does, however, require admission to hospital and will probably be associated with nausea and vomiting for up to 3 days. Treatment to the lower half causes more haematological toxicity but is generally better tolerated. Salazar et al. (1986) recorded pain relief in 73% of 168 cases and the median time to onset of pain relief was 48 h.

PATHOLOGICAL FRACTURES

Pathological fractures are usually best treated by surgical fixation whenever possible. Postoperative radiotherapy will further relieve local pain and promote recalcification (Ford and Yarnold, 1983) and a dose sufficient to cause tumour destruction will aid healing at the fracture site. A dose of 25 Gy delivered in five treatments over 15 days is sufficient. This dosage is also appropriate for pathological fractures which cannot be immobilised surgically, such as in the pubic ramus. For a localised fracture of a rib, however, a single treatment of 8–10 Gy is adequate.

PREVENTION OF PATHOLOGICAL FRACTURES OR VERTEBRAL COLLAPSE

Prophylactic irradiation of painless bone metastases is not indicated unless there is a risk of pathological fracture. Large lytic lesions, especially those in the neck or shaft of the femur or in the humerus should be treated promptly. A course of radiotherapy similar to that given for established pathological fractures (25 Gy in five treatments over 15 days) is probably more effective than a single treatment.

In patients with spinal metastases, it is important to be aware of the possibility of vertebral collapse due to metastases as this could precede the development of spinal cord compression. Vertebral collapse, even if painless, is worth irradiating in order to prevent cord, nerve root or cauda equina compression and the resultant pain, paralysis or incontinence.

Radiotherapy is of no benefit for a patient with established *spinal cord compression* due to structural collapse of a vertebra; the only effective treatment at that stage is immediate surgical decompression and spinal fixation and this must be carried out before the onset of paraplegia. However, in non-structural cord compression by radio-sensitive tumours, immediate radiotherapy with concurrent dexamethasone may be as effective as surgery, but again only in early cases and while the patient is still ambulatory (Tomita et al., 1983; Closs and Bates, 1988).

ENDOCRINE MANIPULATION BY RADIOTHERAPY

Patients with bone metastases secondary to hormone-sensitive tumours, such as breast and prostatic cancer, may benefit from endocrine manipulation. Pain may be relieved and previously abnormal radiographs and isotope bone scans can revert to normal. Surgical ablative procedures, such as oophorectomy and hypophysectomy, are more satisfactory than radiotherapy (being quicker and more complete), but when surgery is not possible, irradiation of the ovaries can yield considerable benefit to selected patients as first line endocrine manipulation. Doses of 10–20 Gy in 2–5 treatments will induce an artificial menopause, younger women requiring the higher dose.

A radioactive implant of Yt 90 in the pituitary fossa is an alternative to hypophysectomy as second line endocrine treatment. Both methods have fallen out of favour but either can be associated with very rapid relief of bone and other pain, although the mechanism is not fully understood.

SIDE EFFECTS OF PALLIATIVE RADIOTHERAPY FOR BONE PAIN

Localised bone metastases requiring palliative radiotherapy can occur in any part of the skeleton. Side effects of treatment are unusual at the doses recommended but they depend on the site treated and are predictable. Thus, irradiation of metastases in or near the first lumbar vertebra will inevitably be associated with temporary nausea and possibly vomiting on the day of treatment. A prophylactic anti-emetic such as prochlorperazine can be given 20 min before treatment, and also following treatment according to need. With irradiation at other sites, except for hemi-body radiotherapy, nausea and vomiting are rare.

Large volume irradiation of the pelvis and lower hemi-body can cause diarrhoea. Irradiation of skull metastases within the hair line will cause temporary hair loss. Late damage to important normal tissues such as the spinal cord will not occur at the doses recommended, even for the single treatment technique of 8 Gy.

Some radiotherapists have used a single treatment of 8–10 Gy for bone metastases for many years. It is to be hoped that increasing numbers of patients will be given the convenience of the one treatment technique.

PELVIC PAIN DUE TO ADVANCED OR RECURRENT GYNAECOLOGICAL CANCER

The pain arising from gynaecological malignancy can be most distressing and difficult to manage. The pain takes a variety of forms:
– *Lower abdominal aching pain* arising from involvement of the cervix itself;
– *Suprapubic pain* or a feeling of pressure from direct involvement of the bladder or from distension of the uterus due to pyometra;
– *Low back pain* as a symptom of pelvic disease or a more sinister sign of metastases in the lumbar spine or para-aortic lymph nodes;
– *Pain in the groin, hip or leg* resulting from involvement of the lumbosacral plexus;
– *Dysuria* (and associated distressing frequency of micturition) from bladder neck invasion or urinary tract infection;
– *Loin pain* from urinary tract infection, hydroureter or hydronephrosis.

The pain most commonly seen is that characteristically described as originating in the buttocks and radiating to the hip and lateral aspect of the thigh to the knee (L_2 and L_3 dermatomes). This pain can arise from involvement of the peripheral nerves on the pelvic side wall or from the roots of L_2 and L_3 due to direct invasion from para-aortic lymph node metastases. The lumbosacral trunk may also be involved by parametrial or iliac node invasion, giving rise to pain in the L_5 and S_1 nerve root distribution, while extension of disease into the sacral hollow involving the sacral plexus may give rise to pain in the foot and perineum.

In all cases, a diagnosis of the precise cause of pain has to be made in order to provide the most appropriate treatment. The clinician should always be aware of pain arising from the secondary effects of malignancy, such as obstruction and infection, and must be active in the control of urinary infection and pyometra. The pain of constipation is common in patients taking regular analgesic drugs and advice will be needed on diet and regular aperients. The clinician must also be aware of the possibility that pain may be due to post-radiation bowel damage, which can mimic recurrent disease very closely. This is a curable condition and must be distinguished.

ROLE OF PELVIC RADIOTHERAPY

Patients may present with pain from locally advanced carcinoma of the cervix or body of the uterus. Whenever possible, every effort should be made to eradicate pelvic disease, generally with aggressive radiotherapy but possibly with chemotherapy and sometimes by surgery. However, it must be remembered that radiotherapy and chemotherapy may make matters worse if the tumour is invading a neighbouring structure such as bladder or bowel. In these circumstances, destruction of the tumour can cause a fistula, resulting in symptoms which are even more distressing than the original tumour itself. Similarly, in patients developing uraemia, radiotherapy may well relieve ureteric obstruction and prolong life but it can also allow a patient to develop even more distressing symptoms. Individual value judgements have to be made.

In suitable cases, the volume irradiated in aggressive radiotherapy includes the whole of the pelvis and must cover the common iliac nodes and the nodes on the side walls of the pelvis. A course of external irradiation lasting 4–5 weeks may be followed by intracavitary radiotherapy. Patients generally experience pain relief before the end of their radiotherapy with continuing improvement during the subsequent weeks.

For recurrent pelvic cancer, palliative radiotherapy using a lower dose is an option for pain relief in patients who have not received previous full dose radiotherapy to this site. However, pelvic pain due to nerve involvement is difficult to relieve with radiotherapy although it can be tried if other methods, such as nerve blocks, have failed. A course of treatment given over about 3 weeks is usually necessary. Halle et al. (1987) report effective palliation with a single treatment of 10 Gy to the pelvis, but recommend this only for patients with a life expectancy of less than 1 year.

PAIN DUE TO LUNG CANCER

Lung cancer is the commonest cancer in males. Very few patients present with curable disease and the majority have advanced malignancy suitable only for palliative therapy. The symptomology of lung cancer is variable but pain is a common feature. Radiotherapy to the thorax may be appropriate for three types of pain.

- *Chest wall pain* arising from direct involvement of the chest wall with malignant invasion of ribs or intercostal nerves. This can give rise to very severe pain which may radiate some distance from the site of origin.
- *Pancoast syndrome* is a special example of chest wall invasion. The classical picture first described by Hare in 1838 (Deeley, 1981) is of an apical carcinoma of the lung with invasion and erosion of one or more of the upper ribs, direct extension into the brachial plexus and Horner's syndrome. As a result of the involvement of the brachial plexus, these patients suffer very severe persistent pain radiating into the shoulder and arm, the exact distribution depending on the extent of the disease in the individual.
- *The painful joints of hypertrophic pulmonary osteoarthropathy* secondary to a carcinoma of the bronchus present a distressing syndrome which may be relieved rapidly by palliative radiotherapy to the primary bronchial carcinoma.

The usual palliative dose prescribed for a carcinoma of the lung is 40 Gy in 20 treatments over 4 weeks delivered by parallel opposed fields. The following prescriptions may give equally effective palliation and are more appropriate for patients with a limited prognosis: 20 Gy delivered in five treatments over 5 days; 25 Gy delivered in five treatments over 15 days; or a single treatment of 8 Gy repeated a week later.

Pain is often the first distressing symptom due to lung cancer to be relieved following palliative radiotherapy. This is especially true for mediastinal and chest wall pain, although the pain of Pancoast tumour is much more difficult to relieve.

PAINFUL FUNGATION

Fungating tumours, especially if they are infected, can be very painful. The most painful are those in sites which are either very sensitive such as the vulva, or subject to friction from adjacent tissues or clothing, such as the breast. For previously unirradiated tumours, radiotherapy has a great deal to offer including pain relief, reduction of discharge and tumour control. Control of infection by antibiotics is of course, essential.

Fungating tumours on the surface of the body are accessible and therefore easily treated by radiotherapy with minimal doses to the normal tissues. Techniques will vary depending on the site, size and depth of tumour, the general condition of the patient and the possible length of prognosis. A painful, advanced and fungating breast carcinoma in an untreated patient with a possible prognosis of months or years may warrant full dose radiotherapy. Megavoltage therapy delivered via tangential fields encompassing the whole breast will give a high probability of complete local tumour control and pain relief (Fig. 12.1a and b). A conventional course of radiotherapy would comprise daily treatments delivering 50–60 Gy in 4–5 weeks. The author's technique is to give 35 Gy in six treatments over

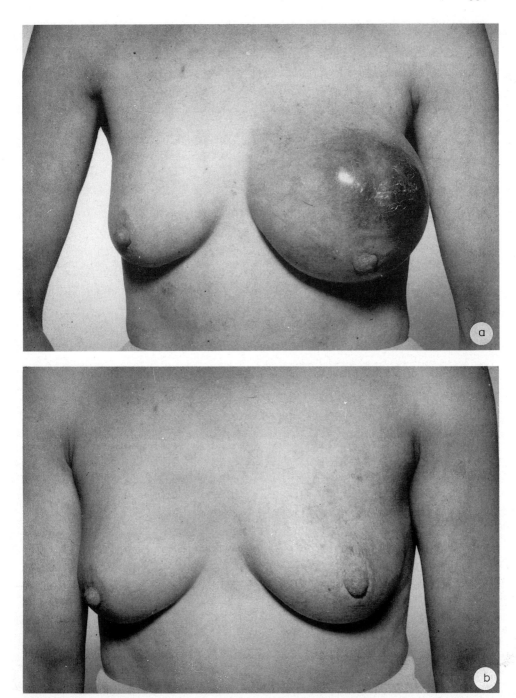

Fig. 12.1. Painful locally advanced carcinoma of the left breast before (a) and after (b) full dose radio-therapy delivered by two opposed tangential fields (Courtesy of Dr. B.A. Stoll.)

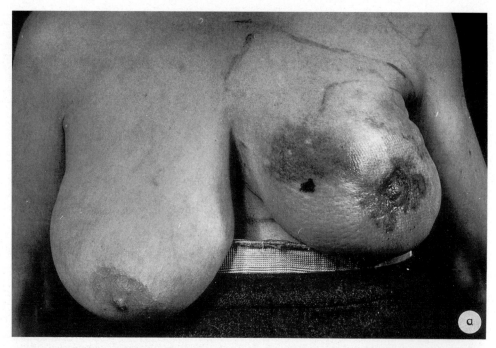

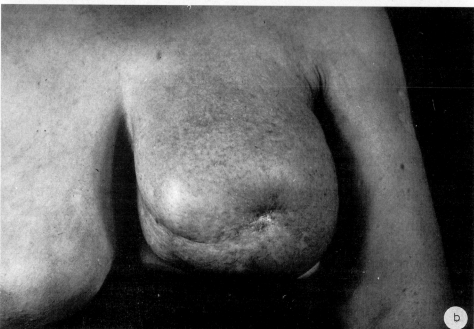

Fig. 12.2. Painful locally advanced carcinoma of the left breast before (a) and after (b) palliative radio-therapy (maximum tissue dose 20 Gy in two treatments over 8 days) by two opposed tangential fields (Courtesy of Dr. B.A. Stoll.)

18 days. This dose gives good tumour control and acceptable early and late normal tissue reactions.

A similar tumour in a patient with a short prognosis requires a modified technique aiming for a realistic level of palliation. For the most frail patients, a single tumour dose of 10 Gy, repeated once if necessary, via tangential fields or a single direct field will reduce or heal the ulcer (Fig. 12.2a and b) (Stoll, 1964) and for the less frail, 30 Gy delivered in six treatments over 18 days gives good pain relief and promotes healing in most patients.

Superficial X-ray or electron therapy may help to heal and reduce pain and discharge in recurrent vulval tumours, but irradiation at this site will inevitably be associated with a temporary painful local reaction.

The effectiveness of radiotherapy for fungating lymph node metastases, e.g., in the supraclavicular fossa from a bronchial carcinoma or in the neck from a head and neck tumour, will depend on the dosage of previous radiotherapy. Irradiated nodes can be treated by the six treatment dose schedule described above but all fields must be treated at each treatment and the maximum dose to the spinal cord must not exceed 3.25 Gy (Dische, 1981).

Painful tenesmus due to a fungating rectal carcinoma is difficult to control but radiotherapy is worth trying if other methods, such as a coeliac block, have failed. A course of megavoltage radiotherapy delivering 30 Gy in six treatments over 18 days (or 40 Gy in 20 treatments over 4 weeks) is the minimum dose likely to be effective for pain relief.

HEADACHE DUE TO BRAIN SECONDARIES

Radiotherapy may be inappropriate in patients with brain secondaries where there is a very short life expectation (e.g. with carcinoma of the bronchus), but may be appropriate where there is a better prognosis (e.g. with carcinoma of the breast), especially if there are distressing symptoms such as paresis, visual disturbances or short-term memory loss. Large opposed fields are usually used with concurrent administration of dexamethasone. A large collaborative study (Borgelt et al., 1980) compared radiotherapy dose-time-fraction schedules and found no difference in response between a dose of 20 Gy in five daily treatments and longer schedules such as 40 Gy in 20 daily treatments. Headache was relieved in 82% of these cases (52% completely relieved). Radiotherapy will cause temporary hair loss and the patient will need a wig, but such treatment may well prolong life as well as relieving pain.

PAINFUL SWALLOWING

This is a complex symptom with several different causes in the cancer patient. As with other types of pain, the precise aetiology needs to be defined in each patient. The appropriate treatment may well include several modalities including analgesic drugs, corticosteroids, dietary advice and occasionally radiotherapy.

Causes which may warrant radiotherapy include intrinsic carcinoma of the oesophagus and external oesophageal pressure by a carcinoma of the thyroid or bronchus or metastatic lymph nodes. External radiotherapy is a useful option for radio-sensitive tumours such as malignant lymphomas or anaplastic thyroid tumours. A single application of intra-oesophageal radiotherapy given under general anaesthetic using an afterloading device (the Selectron) has been found to be particularly useful for oesophageal tumours (Rowland and Pagliero, 1985).

PAIN IN HEAD AND NECK CANCER

Except for carcinoma of the vocal cord and nasopharynx, many early carcinomas of the head and neck are painful from the start and it is beyond the scope of this chapter to deal with the curative management of these tumours. However, as these tumours advance locally and involve bone, nerves and meninges and spread beyond to cervical lymph nodes or become infected, they can be a major cause of severe chronic pain. Many will have had prior radiotherapy and it is unlikely that further radiation therapy will be advisable. The management will then be symptomatic treatment by other means, with or without chemotherapy or commando surgery.

Pain associated with metastatic cervical lymph nodes is generally an indication that a surgical block dissection is unlikely to be successful. If previously unirradiated, such nodes can be usefully treated by radiotherapy using either an opposed pair of megavoltage fields, or a direct 10 MeV electron beam (Jackson, 1970).

PAIN UNLIKELY TO BE RELIEVED BY RADIOTHERAPY

It must be stressed that radiotherapy will not relieve pain of pleural effusions or ascites, nor that caused by radio-resistant tumours. Large field radiotherapy to the abdomen will not relieve the pain of carcinomatosis due to ovarian or bowel tumours, although recent reports suggest that a single 10 Gy dose of radiotherapy using a smaller field directed at an intrapelvic metastasis causing pain has been effective (Adelson et al., 1987).

SIDE EFFECTS OF RADIOTHERAPY

Side effects of radiotherapy are due to the unavoidable irradiation of the normal tissues, and their severity depends on the dose received by these tissues. When palliative doses are given, morbidity should be minimal but with a full radical dose, a temporary, and possibly painful, acute radiation reaction may occur.

The aim of palliative radiotherapy is to relieve pain with the lowest possible dose in the fewest possible treatments. Side effects at the low level of dosage described above are unlikely to be severe and are predictable. Irradiation of tumour on the surface of the body may be associated with temporary skin erythema. This can be kept to a minimum by keeping the skin dry and avoiding the application of ointments, lotions or adhesives containing metal salts such as zinc. Fungating tumours have to be kept clean and free from infection but unnecessary washing should be avoided when possible. When irradiating sites such as the perineum, the benefits of brief bathing far outweigh those conferred by the avoidance of washing.

Mucosal reactions in the mouth and oesophagus are unusual at palliative dosage, but as irradiation predisposes to mucosal infection with *Monilia*, it is wise to accompany irradiation with a prophylactic course of an anti-monilial drug such as Nystatin. Irradiation of the mouth reduces the secretion of saliva and tends to dry the mouth, and good oral hygiene can prevent a great deal of suffering.

Temporary diarrhoea may follow palliative radiotherapy to the pelvis. A kaolin and morphine mixture and codeine phosphate tablets are the most commonly prescribed remedies and, with adequate fluid replacement, should control this side effect.

Nausea is not a common symptom with palliative radiotherapy, but it is inevitable when fields are directed in the region of the first lumbar vertebra or the epigastrium. Prochlorperazine is probably the most useful drug to control radiation-induced nausea and vomiting, and a liberal intake of glucose fluids also helps.

RADIOTHERAPY IN THE RELIEF OF PAIN IN BENIGN CONDITIONS

In the past, radiotherapy has been used in the management of a variety of painful non-malignant conditions. These include tenosynovitis, subacute parotitis, Peyronie's disease of the penis, chronic paronychia, small plantar warts, postherpetic neuralgia and ankylosing spondylitis. However, radiotherapy is rarely recommended in these conditions today primarily because of the late carcinogenic risk following even low doses of ionising radiation (Doll, 1981). Patients with ankylosing spondylitis treated with only a single course of X-rays showed a subsequent statistically significant increase in their incidence of leukaemia and cancers of the tissues in the path of the beam (Smith and Doll, 1982).

Rheumatoid arthritis can become resistant to all conventional therapy, and in some cases low dose external radiotherapy to painful joints or intra-articular radi-

342

oisotopes (Bridgman et al., 1973) can give pain relief. Unfortunately, this relief is very temporary and it is unwise to re-treat. Such local radiotherapy is no longer recommended. More recently, total lymph node irradiation in this disease has been reported to cause relief of joint tenderness and swelling and improvement of function (Kotzkin et al., 1981). Treatment is, however, associated with a sustained fall in the absolute lymphocyte count and deaths have been reported in some of these patients who are so often ill and frail (Calin, 1985). In addition, the long-term value of such treatment is not confirmed.

PAIN RELIEF BY SYSTEMIC CHEMOTHERAPY AND HORMONES

Systemic therapy also has an important role in pain control and may involve hormone-modulating or cytotoxic drugs. Hormone therapy is generally less toxic than cytotoxic therapy and duration of response tends to be longer. However, only about 30% of all cancers of the breast, endometrium and prostate show response to such treatment and the time to the onset of symptomatic improvement is slow (about 4–6 weeks).

Cytotoxic chemotherapy is a relatively new but rapidly developing form of treatment. It offers the possibility of cure in a few individual tumours such as lymphomas, some leukaemias, choriocarcinomas, testicular tumours and some childhood tumours, which are beyond the scope of this chapter. In most other tumours, the role of cytotoxic drugs is purely palliative and as with radiotherapy, symptomatic benefit has to be balanced against toxicity. No cytotoxic drug has yet been discovered which is cancer-specific, and unpleasant side effects are common. They include a variable degree of nausea and vomiting, possible hair loss and marrow depression and may be toxic to the skin, heart, lungs, kidneys, nerve tissue or bladder. It is therefore important that their prescription and preparation are under the control of a cancer team experienced in their use.

Many cancer patients receive cytotoxic drugs in the context of a clinical trial, and it is essential in such trials that the assessment of a patient's response should include also a measure of the side effects and their effect on the quality of the patient's life (Priestman and Baum, 1976). There is a current tendency to over-treat with chemotherapy outside clinical trials merely as a demonstration of 'we never stop trying'. This is inappropriate treatment and it must not be overlooked that many of these drugs are expensive. A survey in the USA suggests that 17% of cancer patients are currently receiving cytotoxic chemotherapy (de Vita, 1983) and in most of these patients, it is given in the knowledge that cure is not possible.

Tumours vary in their response to cytotoxic drugs and hormones. Response is conventionally defined as 'complete response' (CR) when there is complete disappearance of all observable disease for a period of 1–3 months (depending on the trial criteria) and a 'partial response' (PR) when there is a measurable decrease of 50% or more in the tumour size. Pain relief often precedes such objective tumour response, but despite its importance to the patient, it is rarely used as one of the criteria of response. It is frequently not mentioned and is only very rarely quantified. The following are examples of the role of systemic therapy in pain relief.

Breast carcinoma

In pre- and peri-menopausal patients with painful deposits from hormone-sensitive metastatic breast carcinoma, ovarian ablation by surgery or radiotherapy will be first line treatment. In post-menopausal patients, hormone therapy with tamoxifen is likely to be used for soft tissue disease and an androgen (intramuscular decadurabolin) or aminoglutethamide with cortisone for bone metastases. Objective response to such treatment will be no more than 30–40% in unselected cases (Stoll, 1969). Although response rates for bone metastases are said to be lower than those for soft tissue disease, relief of bone pain in the absence of objective response is common with androgens (Stoll, 1969), medroxyprogesterone acetate (Pannuti et al., 1979) and aminoglutethamide (Smith and Macaulay, 1985).

Cytotoxic chemotherapy, being more toxic, is reserved for suitable patients who fail to respond to hormone therapy or who have very rapidly progressing disease. Combination chemotherapy with cyclophosphamide, fluorouracil, methotrexate and adriamycin will produce objective remission rates of 50–80%, with a median duration of 8–10 months. A single agent such as mitoxantrone gives a slightly lower response rate but is considerably less toxic (Smith 1983). Selection of systemic therapy is well covered by Henderson and Canellos (1980).

Prostatic carcinoma

Pain from bone metastases throughout the skeleton is characteristic of advanced prostatic carcinoma. They respond poorly to cytotoxic therapy but about a third of cases will show objective response to hormone therapy and this may last for several years. Well differentiated tumours respond better than poorly differentiated types. First line treatment is usually orchidectomy followed by oestrogens or for patients who are unfit for surgery, the anti-androgen cyproterone acetate (Drug and Therapeutic Bulletin, 1986). Other hormonal methods include progestins, aminoglutethimide and an oestrogen-mustine complex (estramustine). Reports of pain relief from such treatment vary from 35% (Stoll, 1981) to 70% (Pannuti et al., 1979).

Endometrial carcinoma

Medroxyprogesterone acetate (MPA) is the hormone of choice for this tumour in the advanced stages with a response rate of about 30% (Ehrlich and Young, 1981). Well differentiated tumours again are more likely to respond than poorly differentiated types. Alternate 2 week cycles of MPA and tamoxifen may give better palliative results and are under investigation.

Ovarian carcinoma

Most patients with ovarian carcinoma present with advanced disease and pain is a common result of ascites or intestinal obstruction. Neither radiotherapy nor hormone therapy are of significant value in this situation but cytotoxic chemotherapy has an important role in selected cases (Tattersall, 1985). Single agents such as Chlorambucil can result in worthwhile remission with few distressing side effects in about 30% of cases. The median survival of those responding is 17–22 months, although long-term responses lasting several years are not uncommon.

More aggressive chemotherapy with intravenous Cis Platin or Paraplatin gives a higher response rate of 50–60%, which again may be long lasting. These drugs are more toxic but they are the drugs of choice for the younger and fitter patient. Cis Platin causes severe nausea and vomiting and is nephrotoxic, necessitating pre- and post-treatment intravenous hydration. Paraplatin causes less nausea and vomiting and less nephrotoxicity but leads to more marrow depression. Treosulphan either orally or intravenously is a useful second line treatment, especially for patients with ascites. Of the hormones, only progestins have shown any activity in the palliation of ovarian cancer.

Lung cancer

Only small-cell carcinoma of the lung shows a worthwhile response to chemotherapy. Combination chemotherapy is more effective than single drug therapy. A combination of cyclophosphamide, methotrexate, vincristine, adriamycin and VP16 has resulted in complete response in 70% of patients with limited disease and in 25% of patients with extensive disease (Arnold and Williams, 1979). The patients who respond achieve good relief of pain.

Multiple myeloma

This disease often causes severe generalised bone pain. It is a chemo-sensitive tumour and good pain relief can be obtained by the skilful combination of systemic chemotherapy (usually melphalan and prednisolone) with local or very occasionally hemibody radiotherapy. A response rate of 60% with a median duration of 53 months is reported by Scarffe (1982).

CONCLUSION

One of the most important advances in oncology in recent years has been the rapid growth of knowledge in palliative cancer management, not least the control of severe pain. Quality of life is given a great deal more emphasis than it was twenty years ago. However, the current generation of clinicians has unfortunately had very inadequate teaching in pain control, and the subject is only just beginning to be emphasised adequately in undergraduate and postgraduate teaching. Palliative radiotherapy, chemotherapy and hormone therapy all have an important role in the control of chronic cancer pain and they are best practised by oncologists who understand the fundamental differences between the goals of radical and palliative treatment. Particularly in the management of pain, oncologists should work as part of the multidisciplinary team which takes responsibility for patients both in the hospital and in the community.

REFERENCES

Adelson, M.D., Taylor, Wharton, J. Delclos, M.D., Copeland, L. and Gershenson, D. (1987) Palliative radiotherapy for ovarian cancer. *Int. J. Radiat. Oncol. Biol. Phys.*, 13, 17–21.

Allen, K.L., Johnson, T.W. and Hibbs, C.G. (1976) Effective bone palliation as related to various treatment regimens. *Cancer*, 37, 984–987.

Arnold, A.M. and Williams, C.J. (1979) Small-cell lung cancer: a curable disease? *Br. J. Dis. Chest*, 73, 327–348.

Bates, T.D. (1984) Radiotherapy in terminal care. In: *The Management of Terminal Malignant Disease. 2nd Edition.* Editor: C.M. Saunders, Edward Arnold, London.

Bates, T.D. (1988) The provision of good palliative care. In' *Contemporary Palliation of Difficult Symptoms. Clinics in Oncology.* Editor: T.D. Bates. Bailliere Tindall, London.

Bates, T.D. (1987) The management of bone metastases: radiotherapy. *Palliative Med., 1,* 117–120.

Borgelt, B., Gelber R., Kramer, S., Brady, L.W., Chang, C.H., Davis, L.W., Perez, C.A. and Hendrickson, F.R. (1980) The palliation of brain metastases: final results of the first two studies by the Radiation Therapy Oncology Group. *Int. J. Radiat. Oncol. Biol. Phys.*, 6, 1–9.

Bridgman, J.F., Bruckner, F., Eisen, V., Tucker, A., Bleehen, N.M. (1973) Irradiation of the synovium in the treatment of rheumatoid arthritis. *Quart. J. Med.*, 42, 347–367.

Calin, A. (1985) X-radiation in the management of rheumatoid disease. *Br. J. Hosp. Med.*, 33, 261–265.

Closs, S. and Bates, T.D. (1988) The management of spinal cord compression. In: *Contemporary Palliation of Difficult Symptoms. Clinics in Oncology.* Editor: T.D. Bates, Bailliere Tindall, London.

Cohen, S.S., Conolly, C.C., Matthews, G.C. and Skeet, R. (1983) Information needs for radiotherapy services. *Br. J. Radiol. Bull.*, B51–B54.

Deeley, T.J. (1981) Superior pulmonary sulcus syndrome. In: *Proceedings International Seminar on Management of Pancoast's Syndrome.* Stresa.

De Vita, V.T. (1983) Progress in cancer management. *Cancer*, 51, 2401–3409.

Dische, S. (1981) Radiation myelopathy in patients treated for carcinoma of the bronchus using a six fraction regime of radiotherapy. *Br. J. Radiol.*, 54, 29–35.

Doll, R. (1981) Radiation hazards: 25 years of collaborative research. Sylvanus Thompson Memorial Lecture. *Br. J. Radiol.*, 54, 179–186.

Drug and Therapeutic Bulletin (1986) Management of metastatic prostatic carcinoma. *Drug Ther. Bull.*, 24, 85–88.

Ehrlich, C.E. and Young, P.C.M. (1981) Endometrial cancer: rationale for hormone therapy. In: *Hormone Management of Endocrine-Related Cancer.* Editor: B.A. Stoll. Lloyd-Luke, London.

Ford, H.T. and Yarnold, J.R. (1983) Radiation therapy – pain relief and recalcification. In: *Bone Metastasis: Monitoring and Treatment.* Editors: B.A. Stoll and S. Parbhoo. Raven Press, New York.

Halle, J.S., Rosenman, J.G., Varia, M.A., Fowler, W.C., Walton, M.D. and Currie, J.L. (1986) 1000 cGy single dose palliation for advanced carcinoma of the cervix or endometrium. *J. Radiat. Oncol. Biol. Phys.*, 12, 1947–1950.

Haybrittle, J.L. (1983) What is cure in cancer? In: *Cancer Treatment, Endpoint Evaluation.* Editor: B.A. Stoll. John Wiley, Chichester.

Henderson, I.C. and Canellos, G.P. (1980) Cancer of the breast. The past decade. *N. Engl. J. Med.*, 302, 79–90.

Jackson, S.M. (1970) The clinical application of electron beam therapy with energies up to 10 MeV. *Br. J. Radiol.*, 43, 431.

Jensen, N.H. and Rosendahl, K. (1976) Single dose irradiation of bone metastases. *Acta Radiol. Ther. Phys. Biol.*, 15, 337–339.

Kotzin, B.L., Strober, S., Engelman, E.G., Calin, A., Hoppe, R.T., Kansas, G.S., Terrell, C.P. and Kaplan, H.S. (1981) Treatment of intractable rheumatoid arthritis with total lymphoid irradiation. *N. Engl. J. Med.*, 305, No. 17, 969–976.

Pannuti, F., Martoni, A., Rossi, A.P. and Piana, E. (1979) The role of endocrine therapy for relief of pain due to advanced cancer. In: *Advances in Pain Research and Therapy, Vol. 2.* Editors: J.J. Bonica and V. Ventafridda. Raven Press, New York.

Penn, C.R.H. (1976) Single dose and fractionated palliative irradiation for osseous metastases. *Clin. Radiol.*, 27, 405–408.

Priestman, T.J. and Baum, M. (1976) Evaluation of quality of life in patients receiving treatment for advanced breast cancer. *Lancet*, 1, 899–901.

Price, P., Hoskin, P.J., Easton, D., Austin, D., Palmer, S.G. and Yarnold, J.R. (1986) Prospective randomised controlled trial of single and multifraction radiotherapy schedules in the treatment of painful bony metastases. *Radiother. Oncol.*, 6, 247–255.

Qasim, M.M. (1977) Single dose palliative irradiation for bony metastases. *Strahlentherapie*, 153, 531–532.

Rowland, C.G. and Pagliero, K.M. (1985) Intracavitary irradiation in palliation of carcinoma of the oesophagus and cardia. *Lancet*, 981–983.

Salazar, O.M., Rubin, P., Hendrickson, F.R., Komaki, R., Poulter, C., Newall, J., Asbell, S., Mohiuddin, M. and Van Ess, J. (1986) Single-dose half-body irradiation for the palliation of multiple bony metastases from solid tumours. *Int. J. Radiat. Oncol. Biol. Phys.*, 7, 773–781.

Scarffe, H. (1982) Multiple myeloma. In: *Treatment of Cancer.* Editor: K.E. Halnan. Chapman & Hall, London.

Schocker, J.D., Brady, L.W., Risch, V.R., Venuto, J. and Mowry, M. (1981) Radiation therapy for bone metastasis; The Hahnemann Experience. In: *Bone Metastasis.* Editors: L. Weiss and H.A. Gilbert. Hall, Boston.

Smith, I.E. and Macaulay, V. (1985) Comparison of different endocrine therapies in management of bone metastases from breast carcinoma. In: *Bone Metastases from Breast Carcinoma*. Editor: T.D. Bates. Royal Society of Medicine Supplement No. 9.

Smith, I.E. (1983) Mitoxantrone (novantrone): a review of experimental and early clinical studies. *Cancer Treat. Rev.*, 10, 103–115.

Smith, P.G. and Doll, R. (1982) Mortality among patients with ankylosing spondylitis after a single course of X-rays. *Br. Med. J. (Clin. Res.)*, 284, 249–460.

Stoll, B.A. (1964) Rapid palliative irradiation of inoperable breast carcinoma. *Clin. Radiol.*, 15, 175–178.

Stoll, B.A. (1969) *Hormonal Management in Breast Cancer*. Pitman Medical, London, pp. 38–67.

Stoll, B.A. (1981) Breast and prostatic cancer: methods and results of endocrine therapy. In: *Hormonal Management of Endocrine-Related Cancer*. Editor: B.A. Stoll. Lloyd-Luke, London.

Tattersall, M.H.N. (1985) Chemotherapy in ovarian cancer. In: *Ovarian Cancer*. Editor: C.N. Hudson. Oxford University Press, Oxford.

Tomita, T., Galicich, J.H. and Sundaresan, N. (1983) Radiation therapy for spinal epidural metastases with complete block. *Acta Radiol. Oncol.*, 22, 135–143.

Tong, D., Gillick, L. and Hendrickson, F.R. (1982) The palliation of symptomatic osseous metastases. *Cancer*, 50, 893–899.

Vargha, Z.O., Glicksman, A.S. and Boland, J. (1969) Single-dose radiation therapy in the palliation of metastatic disease. *Radiology*, 93, 1181–1184.

Waterhouse, J. (1974) *Cancer Handbook of Epidemiology and Prognosis*. Churchill Livingstone. Edinburgh and London.

M. Swerdlow and J.E. Charlton (eds.) *Relief of Intractable Pain*
© 1989, Elsevier Science Publishers B.V. (Biomedical Division)

Appendix I

(I AND II) PREPARATION OF NEUROLYTIC SOLUTIONS

(I) Phenol (hydroxybenzene)

At 20°C, one part phenol dissolves in twelve parts of water. Accordingly, phenol may be prepared in aqueous solution only in lower concentrations. If a stronger preparation is required a water/glycerine mixture is used as the solvent.

Product:	aqueous phenol 5%	phenol injection 8%	phenol injection 10%
Formula:	phenol crystals 5 g water for injections to 100 ml	phenol crystals 8 g glycerine 50% v/v in water for injections to 100 ml	phenol crystals 10 g glycerine 50% v/v in water for injections to 100 ml

Method of preparation
Pass through sintered glass filter, pack in ampoules and sterilize by autoclaving at 115° C for 30 min.

Packaging
2 ml or 5 ml ampoules. Protect from light. Store in cool place.

Precautions
Avoid prolonged contact with rubber or plastics.

Stability
One year from date of sterilization.

Product: *phenol injection 5% in glycerine*

Formula: phenol crystals 5 g glycerine
(previously dried at 120°C
and cooled) to 100 g

Method of preparation
Dissolve the phenol in glycerine with the aid of gentle heat. Whilst still warm pass through a No. 3 sintered glass filter.

Packaging
Pack in 2 ml or 5 ml ampoules. Protect from light. Store in a cool place.

Sterlization
Dry heat 150°C for 1 h.

Stability
1 year from date of manufacture.

(II) Chlorocresol (parachlormetacresol)

Chlorocresol (parachlormetacresol) is 4-chloro-3-methylphenol. At 20°C it is soluble (1 part in 260 parts of water):

Product: chlorocresol 1 in 40   chlorocresol 1 in 50
in glycerine   in glycerine

Formula: chlorocresol 1 g   chlorocresol 1 g
glycerine (dried at 120°C   glycerine (dried at 120°C
for 1 h) to 40 g   for 1 h) to 50 g

Method of preparation
Dissolve the chlorocresol in the glycerine, using gentle heat. Whilst the solution is still warm pass through a No. 3 sintered glass filter. Pack in 2 ml or 5 ml ampoules.

Sterilization
150°C for 1 h in hot-air oven.

Precautions
Prolonged contact with rubber and plastics must be avoided. Protect from light. Store in a cool place.

Stability
1 year from date of preparation.

(III) INJECTION ABSOLUTE ALCOHOL

Method of preparation
In order to avoid absorption of moisture the infiltration procedure is best carried out under positive pressure, using solvent inert membrane filters. The preparation is then packed in 2 ml or 5 ml ampoules.

Sterilization
Autoclave at 155°C for 30 min.

Special precautions
Absolute alcohol absorbs moisture from the atmosphere; once the ampoule is opened the contents should be used at once.

Stability
2 years from date of sterilization.

(IV) AMMONIUM SULPHATE INJECTION

Product:	ammonium sulphate *injection* – 10%	ammonium sulphate *injection* – 20%
Formula:	ammonium sulphate 10 g water for injections to 100 ml	ammonium sulphate 20 g water for injections to 100 ml

Method of preparation
Dissolve the ammonium sulphate in water for injections; pass through a sintered glass filter. Pack in ampoules.

Sterilization
Autoclave at 115°C for 30 min.

Stability
In view of the fact that there is no official assay process, an expiry date of 1 year from date of sterilization is suggested.

Appendix II

DRUG INTERACTIONS

A large number of adverse drug reactions have been described, but not all are clinically important. Many of the most significant involve drugs used in the management of pain or that are likely to be prescribed in a pain clinic population.

Warfarin – phenytoin, carbamazepine, aspirin

Warfarin is the most commonly used anticoagulant throughout the world. It is extensively protein-bound and is metabolized in the liver; thus, enzyme-inducing drugs such as phenytoin and carbamazepine may produce therapeutic failure. Warfarin has a narrow therapeutic index and small variations in the effect of warfarin may lead to excessive anticoagulation and bleeding. Aspirin interacts with warfarin by reducing plasma prothrombin levels and inhibiting platelet function, which may potentiate anticoagulation. Other NSAIDs do not have this effect, but the effects upon the gastrointestinal tract should be borne in mind.

Beta-adrenergic blockers – NSAIDs

NSAIDs can attenuate the hypotensive effects of many antihypertensives. This effect has been seen most often with indomethacin, but other NSAIDs have been implicated. The mechanism is unknown.

Phenytoin – cimetidine, carbamazepine

This drug is extensively protein-bound, and exhibits 'zero-order' pharmacokinetics. Thus, small increases in dose may produce large increases in plasma concentration with consequent toxicity. Cimetidine will inhibit the metabolism of phenytoin, whereas carbamazepine is a potent enzyme inducer and may increase phenytoin clearance causing therapeutic failure.

Angiotensin-converting enzyme (ACE) inhibitors – NSAIDs

ACE inhibitors are becoming used more frequently in the management of hypertension and heart failure. NSAIDs reduce the hypotensive effects through an unknown mechanism.

Lithium – thiazide diuretics

Lithium may exhibit serious dose-dependent toxicity including renal damage. Diuretics, particularly the thiazides, can cause an increase in the reabsorption of lithium leading to elevated plasma levels. A reduced dose of lithium should be used.

Diuretics – NSAIDs

Diuretics interfere with the efficacy of diuretics, particularly the loop diuretics. This may lead to loss of control in congestive failure.

Oral contraceptives – phenytoin, carbamazepine

These are amongst the most commonly prescribed drugs and they are cleared by hepatic metabolism. Enzyme inducing agents such as phenytoin and carbamazepine may cause increased clearance and lead to failure of contraception. Sodium valproate does not have this effect.

Methotrexate – aspirin, NSAIDs

Methotrexate is used extensively in cancer chemotherapy. Concurrent administration of aspirin and methotrexate may lead to serious methotrexate toxicity. This is thought be due to effects upon protein binding and upon its renal excretion. NSAIDs may have the same effect.

Subject index

A-fibres, 3
  myelinated, 5, 6
  stimulation responses, 4
  synapses, 7
Abdominal pain, 260, 265, 318, 334
Acetaminophen *see* Paracetamol
Acetylsalicylic acid, 126
Acupressure, 173
Acupuncture
  Chinese, 169, 170, 173
  clinical implications, 175
  ear, 170
  history, 169
  hypersensitivity, 171
  laser, 174
  low-frequency stimulation, 172
  mechanism of action, 171
  methods, 172
  sympathetic dystrophies, 275
  trigger points and pain, 175–182
  use, 173
Addictions, opioids, 109
Adenosine monophosphate, 151, 152
Adverse reactions (side effects)
  baclofen, 147
  carbamazepine, 130
  clonazepam, 133
  cordotomy, 321
  fluphenazine, 144

  intrathecal block, 241–245
  non-steroidal anti-inflammatory drugs,
  122–125
  opioid analgesics, 97
  opioids, 107, 108
    epidural, 114
    subarachnoid, 112
  pentazocine, 117
  phenothiazines, 51, 53, 54, 144
  phenytoin, 132
  radiotherapy, 333, 334, 340, 341
  shortwave diathermy, 184
  sodium valproate, 133
  tricyclic antidepressants, 139, 141, 142
  ultrasound, 186
  vascular decompression, 309
Age and headache, 27
Aggression
  pain, 36–38
  and trauma, 36
Alcohol *see* Ethyl alcohol
Alcohol neuritis, 244
Aldose reductase inhibitors, 152
Algodystrophy, drug treatment, 150
Algologist, 79
  investigations, 89
  pain history, 82
Amitriptyline
  analgesic effects, 50

programme, 51
in migraine, 149
postherpetic neuralgia, 53
Ammonium sulphate
nerve block, 197, 240
solution preparation, 351
Anaesthesia dolorosa, 211, 291, 309
Analgesia, vibration-induced, 8 *see also*
individual analgesics
Analgesic ladder, 97
Analgesics, adjuvants, 97 *see also* individual
compounds and techniques
Angiotensin-converting enzymes, drug
interactions, 354
Animal experiments, 2
Animal models, 14
Anticholinesterases, 151
Anticonvulsants, 17, 129, 130
Antidepressants *see also* Tricyclic antidepressants
chronic pain, 134
5-HT reuptake, 16
pain in depression, 50
Antihistamines, 52
dosage, 146
Anxiety
muscle tension and pain, 31
and pain, 34
reduction, 32, 52, 55
Arthritis and tricyclic antidepressants, 137
Ascending pathways, 10–13
Aspirin, 125, 126
Assessment, 38, 39
patient, chronic pain, 79–90
psychological pain, 39
Atypical facial pain, 84, 309

Back ache *see* Low back pain
Baclofen, 147
side-effects, 147
Barbotage, 241
Beck Depression Scale, 50
Behavioural model, pain clinic, 70
Behavioural modification, 43
Bengues Balsam, 187
Benzodiazepine, 145
Beta-blockers
algodystrophies, 152
drug interactions, 353
in migraine, 149

Biofeedback, 75
uses, 41, 42
Bladder paresis, nerve block, 241, 242
Bone metastases
pain relief, 331, 332
radiotherapy, 331
Bone pain, 84
relief, 331–334
Brachial plexus root avulsion, 310
dorsal root entry zone operation, 311, 312
Breast cancer pain
cytotoxic chemotherapy, 343
hormone therapy, 343
radiotherapy, 336–339
Brompton Cocktail, 103
Buprenorphine
dose, 99
epidural, 113
half-life, 118
use, 118
Butorphanol
dose, 99
half-life, 118
use, 118
Butyrophenones, 145

C-fibres, 3, 4
cell bodies, 5, 6
primary afferent, 6
stimulation responses, 4
synapses, 7
Caffeine, uses, 127, 128
Calcitonin analgesia, 151
Calcitonin gene-related peptide, 4
Calcium channel blockers, migraine, 149
Cancer pain relief, 97, 98 *see also* individual
organs, systems
antidepressants, 138, 139
chemotherapy, 342–345
coeliac plexus block, 268
epidural morphine, 113
head and neck, 199–205, 322–324
nerve blocks, 198–205
neurosurgery, 317–324
radiotherapy, 329–342
stereotactic technique, 323
subarachnoid block, 223 *et seq.*
visceral, 264, 265
Cancer, terminal, and hypnosis, 49

Capsaicin in algodystrophies, 152
Carbamazepine, 130, 131
  in trigeminal neuralgia, 129–131, 206
  side-effects, 130
Cardiac pacemakers in TENS, 285
Cardiovascular toxicity, tricyclic antidepressants,
  141, 142
Care deprivation, 39
Causalgia, 18, 84, 186, 261
Central nervous system examination, 88
Central pain, 17, 316
Chemotherapy, cytotoxic
  complete and partial response, 342
  pain, 342–345
Chlorocresol, 224, 238
  preparation, 350
Chronic pain
  CNS examination, 88
  description, 83, 84
  duration, 85
  frequency, 27
  investigations, 89, 90
  opioids, 95, 96
  oral medication, 95
  patient assessment, 79–90
    overview, 81, 82
  periodicity, 85
  physical examination, 87
  position, 84, 85
  psychiatric illness, 29, 30
  tension, 31
  types, 83
Claudication, intermittent, 82, 177, 262, 274
Clonazepam dose and use, 132, 133
  side-effects, 133
Clonidine, 150
  algodystrophies, 152, 153
Cluster headache, 131, 143, 149
Cocaine, subarachnoid, 223
Coccydynia
  nerve blocks, 212
  neurosurgery, 318
Codeine, 52
  dose, 116
  half-life, 116
Coeliac plexus block, 268–270 see also
  Splanchnic nerve block entry levels, 269, 271
Cognitive therapy, 47, 48, 57
  outcome, 49

pain clinic, 75
  trials, 47
Cold therapy, 186, 187
  application, 187
  effects, 187
Commission on Accreditation of Rehabilitation
  Facilities (CARF), 67
Commissural myelotomy
  cancer, 318, 319
  midline coagulations, 320, 321
  scheme, 320
  uses, 318
Computerized tomography, 89, 189, 312
Coping strategies, 47
Cordotomy
  antero-lateral, 320–322
  cancer pain, 320
  complications, 321, 322
  morbidity, 321
  sexual function, 321
  side-effects, 321
Corticosteroids, 128, 129
  algodystrophy, 150, 151
  mechanism of action, 128
Counter-irritants, 187, 188
Cryoanalgesia, nerve block, 217
Cupping, 175
Cyproheptadine, 149, 150

Dantrolene in pain, 147
Deafferentation pain
  causes, 274, 309, 310
  definition, 1, 83, 309, 310
  electrical stimulation, 291
Deep brain stimulation, 290–293
  conditions treated, 290–291
  electrodes, 291
  hazards, 291, 293
  outcome assessment, 293
Definition, pain, 24, 25
Degerine-Roussy syndrome, 291 see also
  Thalamic syndrome
Denervation states, tricyclic antidepressants, 137,
  138
Denial and persistent pain, 35
Dental fillings, anaesthesia and pain, 45
Dependence, opioids, 109
Depression
  chronic pain, 30, 38

treatment, 24
   outcome, 48, 55
Dermatome innervation chart, 200
Descending inhibition, 14–17
   scheme, 15
Description, pain type, 83, 84
Detrusor instability
   causes, 215
   nerve block, 216
   psychological factors, 215, 216
Dextromoramide, 106
Dextropropoxyphene
   dose, 116
Diabetic neuropathy, 18, 87, 130, 138, 152
Diagnosis, 31, 33
   epidural opioids, 113
   local anaesthetic block, 195, 276
   procedure, 39
Diamorphine (heroin), 103
   dose, 99
   metabolism, 103
   solubility, 103
Dihydrocodeine
   dosage, 116
   use, 116
Dipipanone, 105
Dorsal column stimulation, 286 *et seq.*
Dorsal rhizotomy
   indications, 306, 318
   targets, 307
Dorsal root entry, 5, 6
   gate mechanisms, 8
   surgery, 306, 307
   synaptic arrangements, 7
Dorsal root entry zone (DREZ), 306
   operation, 310–322
      complications, 322
      lesion sites, 310, 311
      results, 311
      risks, 314, 323
Drug combinations, 128, 144
Drug interactions, 353, 354
Drug treatment, 93–153

Electrical stimulation
   history, 281
   implanted, 282–284
   and pain relief, 281–300
Electrodes

combinations, 299, 300
   spinal cord, 286, 288
Emotional disturbances and pain, 27
Emotional effects of continued pain, 36–38
Emotional maladjustment and pain, 37
Encephalins, receptor binding, 9
Encouragement, benefits, 48
Endometrial cancer pain, cytotoxic
   chemotheraphy, 344
β-Endorphin, opioid receptor binding, 9, 16
Epidural block, 245–247
   agents, 245, 246
   alcohol, 247
   assessment, 247
   complications, 251, 252
   continuous, 251
   history, 245, 247
   local anaesthetics, 248–251
   non-neurolytic, 247–250
   results, 249
   steroid, 248
   technique, 246, 247
Epidural electrode placement, 286, 287
Epidural scarring, 289
Epilepsy, psychological referral, 28
Ergotamine in migraine, 148
Ethyl alcohol
   nerve block, 196, 197
   solution preparation, 351
   sympathectomy, 277
Exercise
   and pain, 46, 47
   therapeutic, 189
Experimental pain, 1
Extradural block *see* Epidural block
Eysenck personality inventory, 37

Facet joint, 82, 87, 217
Facial pain
   antidepressants, 135
   atypical, neurosurgery, 309
'Failed back' syndrome, 290
Familial diseases, 86
Family interviews, 57
Family patterns and pain, 55
Fear and pain, 23
Fibrositis, 33, 183
Fluphenazine, 144
Fractures, pathological, 332, 333

Gangrene, sympathectomy, 273, 274
Gasserian ganglion block, 206, 207
  Härtel's route, 207, 208
Gate control theory, 6–8, 31, 281
  acupuncture, 171
  dorsal horn, 8
  scheme, 8
Glossopharyngeal nerve block, 202, 203
  bilateral, 204
  X-ray, 204
Glossopharyngeal neuralgia, 131, 202
  pain and neurosurgery, 307
Glycerol nerve block, 209
  problems, 229
Gold therapy, 129
Group treatment, 55
Guanethidine, 19, 261, 264, 275
  adrenergic block, 276
Gynaecological cancer, pain and radiotherapy,
  334, 335

Half-lives, opioids, 107
Headache, 25, 27
  brain secondaries, 339
  tricyclic antidepressives, 134
Head and neck pain
  cancer, 199–205, 322, 323
  neurosurgery, 314–316, 322, 323
Heat
  therapy effects, 187
  uses, 186
Heroin see Diamorphine
Herpes zoster, pain types, 213 see also
  Postherpetic
Hip pain, nerve block, 214, 215
History, chronic pain, 81, 82
  family, 86, 87
  personal, 86
Hormone therapy, pain, 342–345
Hydromorphone, 107
  dose, 99
5-Hydroxytryptamine (5-HT, serotonin), 16 see
  also Serotonergic
  analogue use, 142
Hypnosis, 34
  anaesthesia, 40
  nature, 40
  terminal cancer, 49

Hypnotherapy, pain management, 40, 41
Hypochondriacal hysteria, chronic pain, 29, 30
Hypochondriasis and outcome of spouse
  treatment, 44
Hysteria
  conditions, 33
  and misdiagnosis, 33
  pain evidence, 32
  support, 56
Hysterical conversion, 31

Implanted stimulation systems, 295–300
  apparatus, 296, 297
  assessment, 295
  cell longevity, 297
  devices, 282, 283
  electrical combinations, 299
  indications, 254, 295
  peripheral devices, 295
  personal computer, 300
  programmable, 298, 299
  pulse generators, 296
  radiofrequency-coupled, 296–299
Incidence of pain, 25–30
Indigestion, minor analgesics, 52
Indomethacin, 125, 126
Intercostal neuralgia, nerve block, 214
Intermittent claudication, 177
  pain features, 84
  sympathectomy changes, 272, 273
Intracisternal neurolysis, 234
Intraspinal narcotics, 250, 251
Intrathecal block, 228–245 see also Subarachnoid
  agents, 228–231, 240, 241
  assessment, 234
  chlorocresol, 231
  complications, 241–245
  failure, 237–240
  hyperbaric solution, 230
  hypertonic saline, 240, 241
  phenol, technique, 228–231
    dose, 230
    results, 230–233
    sensation, 230
  position, 228, 229
  side-effects, 241–245
Intravenous lignocaine test, 90
Intravenous regional sympathetic block, 150
Irritability, chronic pain, 36

Ketanserin, 151, 264

Laboratory investigations, chronic pain, 89
Laminectomy, 289
Lancinating pain, 131
Learning and pain, 45, 46
Levorphanol
  dose, 99
  half-life, 107
Lithium
  drug interactions, 354
  use, 143
Local anaesthetics
  epidural block, 250, 251
  infusions, 152
  sympathetic nerve block, 276
Low back pain, 285, 286
  epidural injection, 245–247
  frequency, 27
  operant conditioning, 43
  surgery and personality assessment, 35
  tricyclic antidepressants, 135, 136
Lower end pain
  neurolytic blocks, 235–237
  patient position, 235–236
Lumbar puncture, 228, 229
Lumbar sympathetic block, 270–275
  anatomy, 272
  approach, 271, 272
  assessment, 275
  complications, 274
  dye spread, 272, 273
  flow response, 272, 273
  single needle, 271
  vascular disease, 270, 271
Lumbosacral avulsion injury, dorsal root entry
  zone operation, 311, 312
Lumbosacral spinal fibrosis
  electrode placement, 287–289
  spinal cord stimulation, 286, 288
Lumbo-sciatic syndrome, 248
Lung cancer pain
  chemotherapy, 344
  radiotherapy, 335, 336

McGill Pain Questionnaire, 3
  use, 83
Mandibular nerve block, 201–203

Manipulation, pain patients, 43
Marital relationship and pain, 34, 35
Massage and exercise, 188
Maxillary nerve
  anatomy, 201
  peripheral block, 199–201
    hazard, 206
Mean effective analgesic concentration, 94, 95
Measurement of pain, 2, 3
Mechanisms of pain, 31–38
Medical model, pain clinic, 70
Meningismus, 245
Meperidine, 105
  dose, 99
Meptazinol
  half-life, 118
  uses, 119, 120
Methadone
  bioavailability, 103
  clearance, 104
  dose, 99
  pharmacokinetics, 104
Methotrexate, drug interactions, 354
Methylprednisolone, extradural block, 249
Methysergide, 149
Migraine, 87
  biofeedback, 41
  drug therapy, 148–150
  and personality, 28
Minimum effective analgesic concentration, 95
Minnesota Multiphasic Personality Inventory
  (MMPI)
  chronic pain patients, 29
  low back pain surgery, 35
  operant conditioning, 44
Mobilization, definition and uses, 188, 189
Monoaminoxidase inhibitors, 142
Morphine
  alternatives, 105–107
  dose, 98, 99
    and plasma levels, 99
  first pass effect, 100
  infusion, continuous, 102
  metabolism, 99, 100
  oral, 100, 101
    dose, 99–101
  pharmacology, 98–100
  pinprick sensation, 10
  receptor binding, 9, 96

routes, 102
slow-release, 101, 102
  dose, 102
synaptic effects, 8, 9
Mortality, nonsteroidal anti-inflammatory drugs, 122
Moxibustion, 174
Multidisciplinary treatment, 45, 293
Multiple myelona pain therapy, 344
Muscle paresis, nerve block, 241, 242
Muscle relaxants, 146–148
Myodil, 224, 240
Myofibrositis, 177

Nalbuphine
  dose, 99
  half-life, 118
  uses, 118
Naloxone, 120
  opioid binding sites, 9
  opioid side-effects, 120
Naproxen, 125
Needle effect, 178
Needle puncture, 177
Nefopam, 120, 121
Nerve blocks, 75 *see also* Intrathecal, extradural
  and subarachnoid
  agents, 196–198, 209
    preparation, 349–351
  aids, 196–198
  contention, 195
  inflammatory response, 197, 198
  peripheral *see also* Peripheral nerve blocks
Nerve entrapment, nerve block, 211, 212
Nerve stimulation, 281 *et seq.*
Neurogenic pain, 1
  allodynia, 17
  anatomical changes, 17
  clinical forms, 18
  definition, 17
  description, 18
  diagnosis, 19
  treatment, 19
Neuroleptic use, 143–145
Neuromata, 18, 183
Neurosurgical relief of pain, 305–325 *see also*
  Dorsal rhizotomy and individual techniques
  conditions treated, 308–324
  dorsal root targets, 307

non-cancerous, 306
trigeminal neuralgia, 307, 308
Nocigenic pain, 1, 19
Non-steroidal anti-inflammatory drugs (NSAID)
  acetic acid derivatives, 125
  clinical use, 124
  dosage, 124
  drug interactions, 353, 354
  fenamates, 127
  gastric effects, 122, 123
    management, 123
  half-life, 122
  indole derivatives, 126
  metabolism, 121, 122
  mode of action, 121
  propionic acid derivatives, 124, 125
  pyrazoles, 126
  renal problems, 123, 124
    management, 124
  salicylates, 126
  side-effects, 122–126
  types, 125

Occipital neuralgia, nerve blocks, 215
Occupational therapy, 72
Operant conditioning, 42–47, 75
  benefits, 49
  comparative study, 44
  limitations, 46
  low back pain, 43, 45
  and patient experience, 45
  treatment programme, 44
Opioid analgesics *see also* Adverse reactions,
  individual drugs
  chronic use, 97
  dosage, 98, 99
  epidural, 112–115
    delivery, 115
    dosage and tolerance, 115
    side-effects, 115
  side-effects, 97
  spinal, 109–112
  strategy of use, 94, 95
  subarachnoid, 110, 111
    chronic use, 111
    side-effects, 112
Opioid peptides, 95–97
  classification, 96
  clinical uses, 96

kappa agonists, 96, 97
Opioid receptors, 8 *et seq.*
Oral contraceptives, drug interactions, 354
Osteoarthritis, 185
Oxycodone
    dose, 99
    use, 106
Oxymorphone, 107
    dose, 99

Pain clinic (pain relief clinic), 67–77
    director, 71
    economics, U.S.A., 67
    expansion, 69, 70
    function, 72–74
    medical options, 75
    multidisciplinary, 69, 70
        structure, 70–74
    numbers, 67
    nurses, 72
    outcome studies, 74–77
    patient features, 28
    personnel, 71
    psychiatrist, 35
    psychological options, 75, 76
    referral, 73
    setting up, 68–70
    small practice, 68, 69
    specialists, 72
    treatment options, 74
    University of Minnesota survey, 76
Pain
    definition, 24
    descriptions, 83, 84
    diary, 86
    games, 46
    modifying factors, 33, 34
    pathways
        ascending, 10–13
        CNS entry, 5, 6
        descending, inhibitory control, 14–17
        scheme, 11
        tissue damage, 13
    syndrome and phenothiazines, 50
    threshold, 2
    tolerance level, 2
    types, 83
Palaeospinothalamic fibres, 10–12
Pancoast Syndrome, 336

Pantopaque, 240
Paracetamol, dose-response, 127
Paraplegia, neurosurgery, 312
Pelvic pain, 265, 318, 334
Penicillamine, 129
Pentazocine
    dose, 99
    half-life, 117, 118
    side-effects, 117, 118
    uses, 117, 118
Perception, pain, 2
Percussion, 183
Periaqueductal grey
    electrical stimulation, 290
        conditions treated, 290, 291
    electrodes, 291, 292
    nociceptive pain, 290
    pain pathway, 15
Peripheral nerve blocks, 195–218
    brachial plexus, 205
    cancer pain, 198–205
    complications, 210, 211
    duration, 201
    glossopharyngeal, 202, 203
    head and neck, 199–205
    intercostal, 205
    local anaesthesia, 207
    mandibular, 200, 201
    maxillary, 199–201
    ophthalmic, 199
    paravertebral root, 218
    superior laryngeal, 204, 205
    T-cells, 195
    trigeminal, 199
        relief duration, 210
    trigeminal neuralgia, 205–211
Peripheral nerve stimulation, 283
    clinical trials, 283, 284
Peripheral vascular disease, neurolytic
    sympathectomy, 262, 263
Personality disorder, 38
    phychological treatment, 48, 49, 57
Pethidine (Meperidine)
    dose, 99
    pharmacokinetics, 105
Phantom limb pain, 145
    nerve stimulation for, 291
    neurophysiology of, 312
    mechanism, 312

neurosurgery, 313
ultrasound, 186
Pharmacodynamics, 93, 94
Pharmacokinetics, 93, 94
Phenazocine, 106
Phenol
  in Conray 420, spectrophotometry, 277
  in glycerine, 207
  nerve block, 197
    sensations, 230
  solution preparation, 349, 350
  spinal nerve roots, 224
  sympathectomy, 269, 270, 272, 273, 277
Phenothiazines
  analgesic effects, 50, 51, 143–145
  side-effects, 51, 53, 54, 144
  treatment regime, 51, 52
    analgesics, 52
    drug interactions, 51
    problems, 54
D-Phenylalanine, 151
Phenytoin
  dose and concentrations, 131, 132
  drug interactions, 353, 354
  half-life, 132
  side-effects, 132
  trigeminal neuralgia, 132
Physical examination, 87, 88
Physiotherapy, 75
Pituitary ablation
  indications, 324
  pain relief, 325
  radiotherapy, 333
  surgery, 324
Pizotifen, 148, 149
Placebo techniques
  and pain, 34
  pain intensity, 41
Postamputation pain, nerve block, 217
Postcentral gyrus lesions, 12
Posterior rhizotomy
  scheme, 318, 319
  selective, 318
Postherpetic neuralgia, 36, 130
  amitriptyline, 53
  anticonvulsants, 129, 131
  nerve blocks, 213, 214
  neurophysiology, 18, 213, 306
  neurosurgery, 313, 314

trigeminal nucleus, 316
therapies, 147, 187, 213, 250, 291
tricyclic antidepressants, 138
Postoperative encouragement and analgesia, 34
Prostatic carcinoma pain treatment, 343
Pruritus, 111
Psychiatric illness, pain frequency, 25, 26
Psychiatric treatment, 34
Psychodynamics, 34, 35
Psychological factors
  chronic pain, 29, 30
  pain origin and treatment, 57
Psychological illness see also individual
  conditions and pain, 48
Psychological treatment, 39–58
  assessment, 55
  benefits, 48, 49, 56
  groups, 80
Psychotropic drugs, 49–53

Radiofrequency lesioning
  intercostal pain, 217
  results, 217
Radio-opaque dye, 269, 270, 272, 273
Radiotherapy for cancer pain, 329–342
  bone pain, 331–334
  breast cancer, 336–339
  doses, 332
  endocrine manipulation, 333
  factors affecting success, 330, 331
  gynaecological malignancy, 334, 335
  headache, 340
  lung cancer, 335, 336
  non-cancer pain, 341, 342
  pelvic, 335
  principles, 330
  side-effects, 333, 334, 340, 341
Raphe-spinal axons, 16
Rat polyarthritis, 14
Raynaud's disease, 150, 263, 264, 275
Receptors see also A-fibres, C-fibres, nociceptors
  opioid, 8–10, 95, 96
    binding affinity, 9
    localization, 9, 10, 13
    spinal cord, 10
    subtypes, 9, 96
Rectus sheath, intercostal nerves, 211, 212
Referral, chronic pain assessment, 80, 82
Referred pain mechanisms, 5

Reflexology, 175
Relaxation techniques
    back pain, 43
    pain, 42
Reserpine, 276
Respiratory depression, 108, 112
    subarachnoid morphine, 112
Rest pain, 273
Reticular formation, pain pathway, 10, 11
Rheumatoid arthritis, 37, 86, 128, 137, 185
    radiotherapy, 341
Rhizotomy, 306, 313, 318
Risk factors, periaqueductal grey, 291, 293
Ryodoraku, 174

Saline nerve block, 240, 241
Sciatica, 82, 283, 294
    neurosurgery, 313
Serotonergic fibres, descending inhibition, 15
Shortwave diathermy
    application methods, 183
    contraindications, 184
    current, 183
    side-effects, 184
Sicknesss diary and GP consultations, 27, 28
Side-effects *see* Adverse reactions and individual
    compounds and techniques
Silver nitrate, 240
Sodium valproate
    side-effects, 133
Soft tissue pain, 32, 33
Somatostatin, 153
Spasticity, 146
Spinal artery thrombosis, 245
Spinal column, 229
Spinal cord compression, 333
Spinal cord stimulation, 286–289
    electrodes, 286–289
    indications, 286, 289, 294
Spinothalamic tractotomy, 305
Splanchnic nerve block, 268–270
    anatomy, 268
    dye spread, 269, 270
    hypotension, 269
    radiographs, 269, 270
    safety, 268
Stellate ganglion block, 265
    approach, 265, 266
    complications, 267

technique, 265–267
Stereotactic technique
    cancer pain, 323, 324
    mesencephalic tractotomy, 323, 324
Stimulation analgesia *see also* individual
    techniques
    mechanisms, 282, 283
Subarachnoid alcohol injection, 224–226,
    231–235
    acute pain, 231
    dose, 231, 232
    management, post-injection, 232
    opioid withdrawal, 233
    position, thoracic pain, 232
Subarachnoid neurolytic injection, 224–228
    alcohol, 224–226, 231–235
    assessment, 233, 234, 237–240
        alcohol, 239, 240
        chlorocresol, 238–240
        phenol, 238
    bladder effects, 242, 243
    chlorocresol, 224
    clinical uses, 226, 227
    complications, 233, 241–245
        duration, 242, 243
    degeneration, 225
    duration and agent, 239
    patient preparation, 227
    phenol, 224–226
    position, 224, 225, 228
    regeneration, 224
Submaximum effort tourniquet test, 2
Substance P, 4, 14
    nociceptors, 9
Swallowing, painful, 339, 340
Sympathectomy, pharmacological, 275, 276
Sympathetic dystrophies, nerve block, 263, 264
Sympathetic nerve block, 260
    adrenergic, 276
    agents, 276, 278
    blood flow, 262, 263
    clinical objectives, 261, 262
    peripheral vascular disease, 262, 263
    sympathetic dystrophies, 263, 264
    techniques, 266–276 *see also* individual blocks
    uses, 262–266
    visceral cancer pain, 264, 265
Sympathetic nervous system
    and central pain, 264

nociception, 260
noradrenaline depletion, 275
pain, features, 260–262
pain, relief, 259, 278

Tension headache, 31, 42, 136
Thalamic nuclei
  electrodes, 292
  intralaminar, 13
  stimulation, 291
Thalamic syndrome, 11, 19, 144, 306 *see also*
  Dejerine-Roussy
  neurosurgery, 316, 317
    pain relief, 120, 291, 317
Thalamus, 10–12
Therapeutic window, 136–139
Thermography
  diagnosis, 89, 189
  infrared, 190
  technique, 189, 190
Thresholds, 2, 3
Thromboangitis obliterans, 263
Tic douloureux, 205
Tolerance, opioids, 108, 114
Transcendental meditation, 42
Transcutaneous Electrical Nerve Stimulation
  (TENS, TNS), 7, 175, 284, 285
  contraindications, 285
  electrode placement, 284
  frequencies, 282
  nervous system effects, 283
  origin, 284
  phenothiazine side-effects, 54
  precautions, 285
  sympathetic dystrophy, 276
Transsacral nerve block, 216, 217
Treatment contract, 43
Tricyclic antidepressants
  analgesic effects, 134
  anticholinergic, 140
    side-effects, 141, 142
  choice, 140, 141
  clinical uses, 135–141
  dosage and timing, 139
  half-life, 139
  5-HT reuptake, 134
  5-HT uptake, 139
  mechanism of action, 19, 134, 135
  pharmacological properties, 140

safety, 141
side-effects, 139, 141, 142
Trigeminal neuralgia, 17, 18, 84
  alcohol block, 206
    approaches, 206, 207
    X-rays, 207–209
  anticonvulsants, 129–132
  carbamazepine, 130
  diagnosis, 205
  nerve block, 206–211
  neurosurgery, 307–308
  pain features, 206, 308
  percutaneous treatment, 309
  radiofrequency lesioning, 217
  vascular decompression, 308, 309
Trigeminal nucleus caudalis
  cancer pain, head and neck, 322, 323
  coagulations, 315, 316
  DREZ lesions, 314–316
  scheme, 315
Trigger points, 84
  acupuncture points, 176, 177
  localization, 176
  and pain patterns, 175–182
  steroids, 182
  treatment, 177
L-Tryptophan, 17, 142
Tumour, fungating
  breast, 336–339
  lymph node, 339
  radiotherapy, 336–339

Ultrasound
  frequency, 185
  side-effects, 186
  therapeutic uses, 184–186

Vane Hypothesis, 120
Vascular decompression, 308
  assessment, 309
  side-effects, 309
Vasoactive intestinal polypeptide, 4
Vertebral collapse prevention, 332, 333
Vibrators and pain control, 7, 182, 183
Visual analogue scale (VAS), 3
  use, 83

Warfarin, drug interactions, 353
Wounding

    and pain, 33, 34
    soldiers, 34

X-ray and nerve blocks, 196

Yttrium, endocrine treatment, 324, 333